Challenging ECGs

Challenging ECGs

Henry J. L. Marriott, MD, FACP, FACC
Clinical Professor of Medicine (Cardiology)
Emory University School of Medicine
Atlanta, Georgia
Clinical Professor of Pediatrics (Cardiology)
University of Florida College of Medicine
Gainesville, Florida
Clinical Professor of Medicine
University of South Florida College of Medicine
Tampa, Florida

Hanley & Belfus, Inc. / Philadelphia

Publisher: HANLEY & BELFUS, INC.
               Medical Publishers
               210 S. 13th Street
               Philadelphia, PA 19107
               (215) 546-7293; 800-962-1892
               FAX (215) 790-9330
               Website: http://www.hanleyandbelfus.com

CHALLENGING ECGs   ISBN 1-56053-547-4

Library of Congress Control Number: 2002102758

Last digit is the print number: 9 8 7 6 5 4 3 2 1

Contents

Preface

This collection of choice challenges is designed to keep you on your diagnostic toes!

At first I thought it would be most challenging and enjoyable for the reader if, rather than presenting the tracings under such general headings as Arrhythmias, Blocks, and Infarctions, they were in no particular order and were therefore true "unknowns." But as the project matured, I found I could not live with the total lack of order. Accordingly, I have assembled the records under eight headings, which means that you know ahead of time the ballpark of at least one of the diagnoses—but you have no prescient idea what additional bandits may lurk within the waves and intervals and relationships confronting you!

Each tracing should be approached as an *exercise in thoroughness.* Leave no diagnostic stone unturned. Just because you quickly spot the atrial flutter and LBBB, don't overlook the subtle Wenckebach sequences that affect the flutter impulses as they negotiate the junction, or the evidence of a probable, associated early inferior infarction.

Two special exhortations: (1) Be on the look-out for *important diagnoses that are often overlooked,* like pulmonary embolism and the very early inferior wall infarction. (2) Don't overlook *important clues that often go unrecognized,* such as inverted U waves, and "Wellens' warning" of critical LAD stenosis.

I am hopeful that these pages may provide a painless introduction to some concepts that are often thought difficult, like parasystole and concealed conduction. Several examples here will serve as a clarion warning not to rely upon the interpretive skills of the willing but wanting computer—consider the patient who was not seen by a cardiologist for several hours and died because the computer interpreted his acute infarction as "old."

I am grateful to the technical staffs of ECG departments at various hospitals who save samples of "intriguing" tracings for me; their contributions account for the majority of the records herein. But a significant minority come from Dr. Bill Nelson, whose store of "fascinomas" is seemingly endless and whose generosity in sharing them is boundless. Unfortunately, I cannot acknowledge each of his contributions individually because they have become immersed in the sea of tracings that swirl about me; but my debt to him is perennially enormous and most gratefully and happily acknowledged.

I am most grateful to Jacqueline Mahon whose skillful editorial touch has greatly improved the entire text.

HJLM

Glossary

Acronyms

AIVR	Accelerated idioventricular rhythm
APB	Atrial premature beat
AV	Atrioventricular
AVB	Atrioventricular block
BB	Bundle-branch
BBB	Bundle-branch block
F	Fusion beat
LA	Left atrial
LAD	Left axis deviation
LAHB	Left anterior hemiblock (or fascicular block)
LBBB	Left bundle-branch block
LPHB	Left posterior hemiblock (or fascicular block)
LV	Left ventricle, left ventricular
LVH	Left ventricular hypertrophy
MI	Myocardial infarction
NSR	Normal sinus rhythm
RA	Right atrial
RBBB	Right bundle-branch block
RV	Right ventricle, right ventricular
RVH	Right ventricular hypertrophy
SA	Sino-atrial (or sinus)
VPB	Ventricular premature beat
VT	Ventricular tachycardia
WPW	Wolff-Parkinson-White syndrome

Terms

Allorhythmia
: The repeated recurrence of an arrhythmic sequence. Example: A sinus beat (SB) followed by an APB, which is followed by a junctional escape (JE) beat, which in turn is followed by a VPB, and this sequence repeats itself—SB, APB, JE, VPB, SB, APB, JE, VPB, SB, etc., etc.

Concealed conduction
: Conduction that can be recognized only from its effect on the subsequent beat, cycle, or interval. Example: When the sinus beat immediately following an interpolated VPB has a prolonged PR interval, it is because the retrograde ventricular ectopic impulse reached the AV junction and made it refractory, so that the next descending impulse was delayed. The fact that retrograde conduction invaded the junction is recognized only from its effect on the subsequent beat—lengthening its PR interval.

In atrial fibrillation, unpredictable concealed conduction of the fibrillatory impulses into the AV node is the cause of the marked variation in the ventricular cycles.

Concordance
: Indicates that all of the precordial QRS complexes, from V1 to V6, have the same polarity: *positive concordance* if they are all upright from V1 to V6; *negative concordance* if they are all inverted.

Coupling
: The dependent relationship of a premature beat (extrasystole) on the preceding beat of the dominant (usually sinus) rhythm. An extrasystole is a *coupled beat;* a series of extrasystoles show *fixed coupling.* A parasystolic beat is independent of the preceding beat, and therefore the beats of a parasystolic rhythm change their relationship to their preceding beats—this is often, but incorrectly (because they are independent beats and therefore not "coupled") described as "variable coupling." It is a convenient inexactitude!

Intrinsicoid
: When a recording electrode is placed on a strip of muscle and that muscle is stimulated at one end, as long as the impulse travels towards the electrode, a positive deflection is recorded. At the moment that the impulse reaches the electrode and passes under it, a sharp downward deflection is recorded, the *intrinsic deflection.* Clinically, as we do not place electrodes right on the heart muscle but situate them on the chest wall several centimeters from the muscle, the corresponding deflection is called intrinsicoid and signals the arrival of the activating impulse under the electrode.

Orthodromic tachycardia
: The most common tachycardia of the WPW syndrome. The circulating wave travels down the AV junction and up an accessory pathway. If it goes the other way, down an accessory pathway and up the junction, it is *antidromic.*

P-terminal force
: This is the terminal, negative part of the P wave in lead V1 (sometimes abbreviated to PTF-V1) expressed as the multiple of its depth in millimeters and width in seconds (mm/s). The normal PTF-V1 does not exceed 0.04 s wide and 1 mm deep, i.e., 0.04 mm/s.

QRS-T angle
: The angle between QRS and T wave in the frontal plane. Normally, the two forces should be in the same general direction and never more than 45–50 degrees apart.

Section I

Extrasystoles and Parasystole

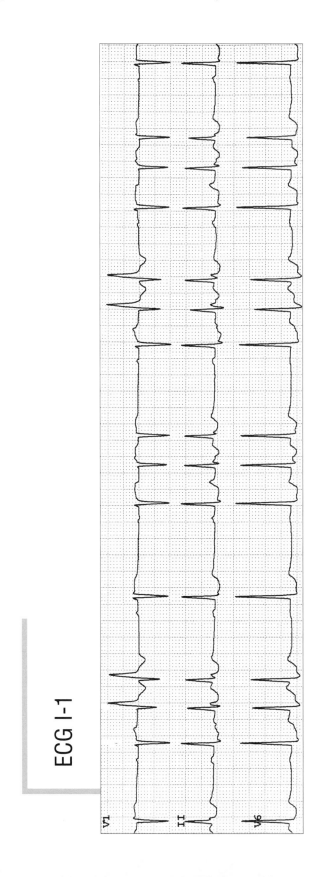

ECG I-1

Diagnoses   ECG I-1

1. Sinus rhythm (? bradycardia—rate not determinable) with . . .

2. . . . paired atrial premature beats (APBs) . . .

3. . . . with and without RBBB aberration

4. Probable myocardial ischemia (horizontal ST depression)

5. Possible left ventricular hypertrophy (voltage in V6)

Clinical Data

84-year-old woman

Comments

Two questions arise:

- Why are some premature complexes aberrant while others are not?
     Answer: In the first and third pair, the coupling interval of the first APB is shorter (43; see ECG below) than that in the second and fourth pairs (47, 48).

- If the short cycle of the first atrial premature in each pair is short enough at times to evoke aberration, why isn't the even shorter cycle of the second APB *always* associated with aberration?
     Answer: The reason presumably resides in the shortened preceding cycle, which shortens the ensuing refractory period of the RBB (as well as of the rest of the ventricular conduction system), so that aberration is side-stepped.

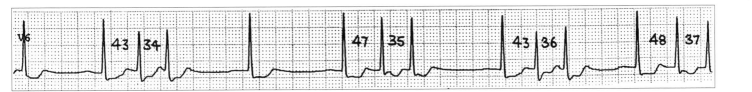

ECG I-2

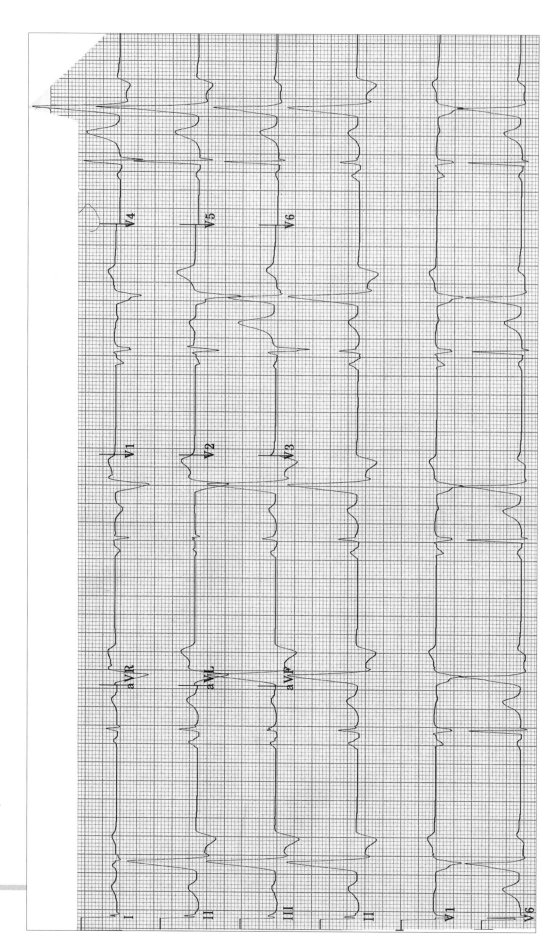

Diagnoses   **ECG I-2**

1. Sinus rhythm (? bradycardia) with . . .

2. . . . right ventricular bigeminy with . . .

3. . . . probable retrograde conduction to atria

4. Left atrial enlargement

Clinical Data

63-year-old man

Comments

A straightforward tracing, but with several notable features:

• The typical morphology of RV ectopy in lead V1—slurring on downstroke of QS complex requiring 0.09 s to reach nadir

• The P-terminal force in V1 = 0.14 (0.07 s wide $\times$ 2 mm deep)—2.5 times the upper limit of normal—indicating LA enlargement

• The rate of the visible P waves is only 29/mm, obviously an unlikely sinus rate. If the rate were double (58), the alternate P waves would be visible at the end of the T waves. Therefore, the most likely option is that there is retrograde conduction to the atria from each VPB. The S-like waves ending the ectopic complexes in the inferior leads are probably "pseudo-S" waves representing the tail-end of inverted (retrograde) P waves.

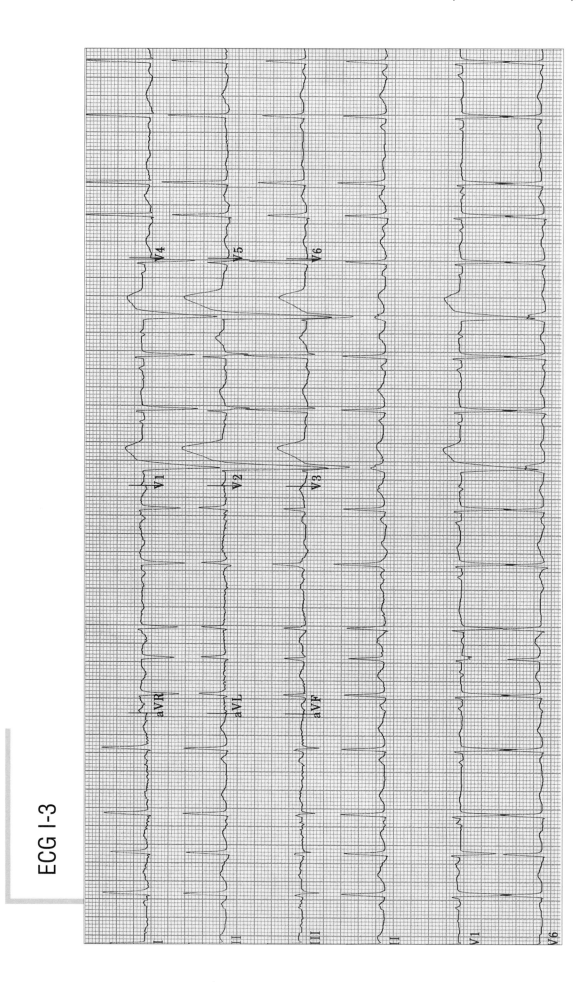

ECG I-3

Diagnoses   ECG I-3

1. Sinus tachycardia (rate is just over 100/min when there are consecutive sinus beats)

2. Atrial premature beats, singly and in pairs, normally conducted and also conducted with minor (probably RBB delay; see Comment) aberration and with LBBB aberration

3. Borderline low T waves in 1, aVL, and V6

Clinical Data

79-year-old woman

Comment

In lead V1, the earliest indication of RBB delay is usually shrinkage of the S wave. The configurations of the 2nd and 6th beats therefore presumably indicate different degrees of minor delay in the RBB.

ECG I-4

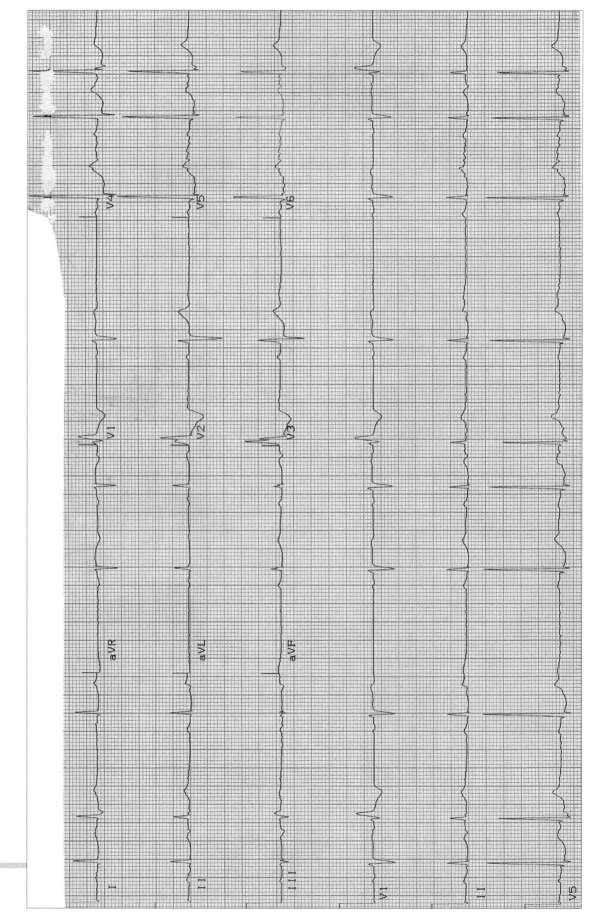

Diagnoses   ECG I-4

1. Sinus rhythm (rate = 72/min) with . . .

2. . . . atrial premature beats, two nonconducted and three conducted with RBBB aberration

3. Abnormal ST depression V3–V6 (? subendocardial ischemia)

Clinical Data

85-year-old man

Comments

Note:

- How impossible it is to recognize the aberration in lead 2, but how obvious it is in V1

- The "overdrive suppression" of the sinus by the APBs (the sinus P-P interval is 88, whereas the post-ectopic P′-P interval is about 106—significant, but not enough to call it a sick sinus).

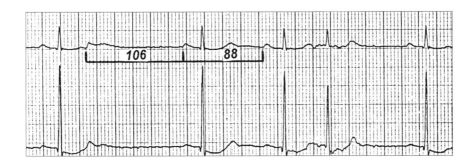

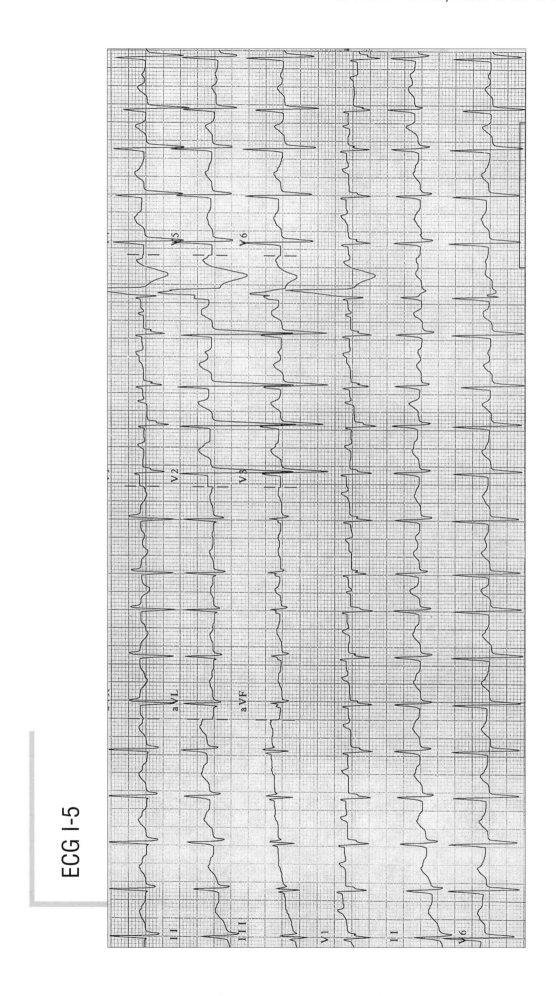

ECG I-5

Diagnoses   **ECG I-5**

1. Sinus tachycardia (rate = 118/min)

2. Atrial premature beats, one conducted with RBBB aberration

3. First-degree AV block (PR = 0.23 s)

4. Minimal RBB delay in sinus beats

Clinical Data

Unknown

Comments

• Slurring on the upstroke of the S wave in V1 is another early sign of RBB delay—the Mexican school calls it "first-degree" RBBB; here this impression is confirmed by the prominent S wave in leads V1, and V5–6.

• The only point of interest in the APBs is that the third one is aberrantly conducted, while the first APB, which ends a cycle of identical length, is not. The answer is in the *preceding* cycle: the cycle preceding the cycle of the third APB is about 0.59 s, whereas that preceding the cycle of the first APB is only 0.52 s. The longer cycle lengthens the refractory period of the conducting fascicles so that the next descending impulse is affected by that longer refractoriness.

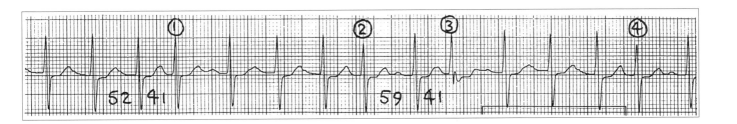

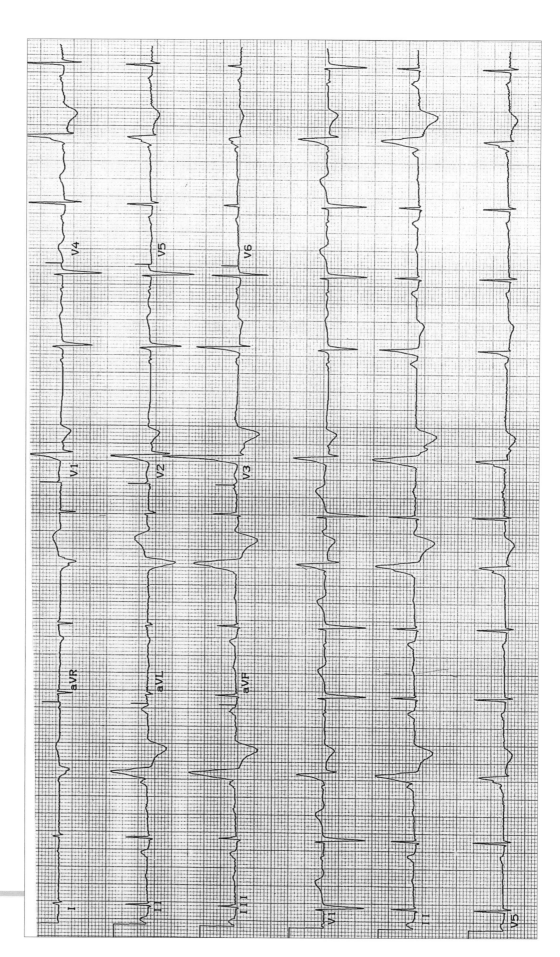

ECG I-6

Diagnoses   **ECG I-6**

1. Ventricular parasystole (rate = 48/min)

2. One fusion beat

3. Nonspecific T wave abnormalities

Clinical Data

Unknown

Comments

The two steps in diagnosing parasystole are:

• *Recognizing independence* of an ectopic rhythm. Here the obvious variation in coupling intervals alerts you to an independent rhythm; furthermore, one of the ectopic beats (the one that produces fusion) is not preceded by a sinus beat, which proves independence.

• *Demonstrating "protection,"* i.e., that the ectopic pacemaker is not discharged by other impulses and so maintains a more or less regular rhythm. The interectopic intervals here are indicated on the strip below; F = fusion beat.

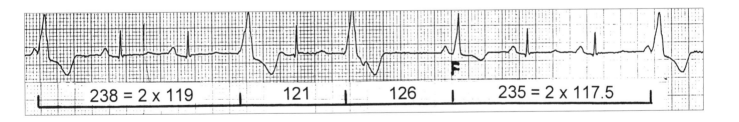

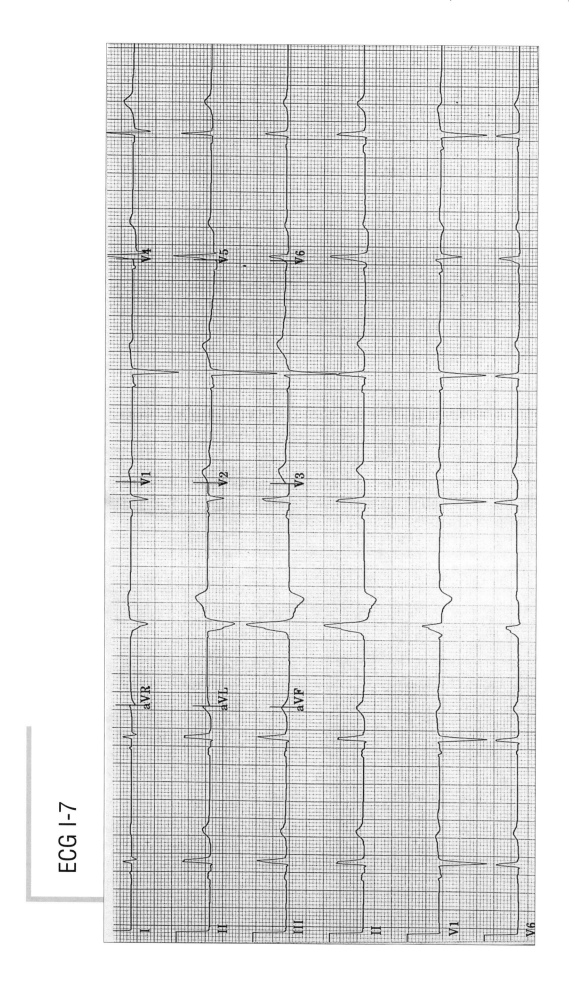

ECG I-7

Diagnoses   ECG I-7

1. Sinus bradycardia (rate = 44/min)

2. Ventricular escape (3rd and 6th beats)—the 6th beat is a fusion beat between the escaping ventricular rhythm and the sinus.

3. Borderline ST-T pattern—horizontality may be secondary to the bradycardia.

Clinical Data

60-year-old man

Comments

The ectopic ventricular beats illustrate the difficulty in defining "escape" beats, which are usually described as *late, ectopic beats* ending cycles *longer* than the dominant cycle. In this case, the late, ectopic beats end cycles that are slightly shorter than the long sinus cycles and are therefore a little bit premature in the context of marked bradycardia. But clearly we shouldn't call them "premature beats," because that term is commonly equated with extrasystoles. Thus, the least unsatisfactory term for them is **escape beats.**

ECG I-8

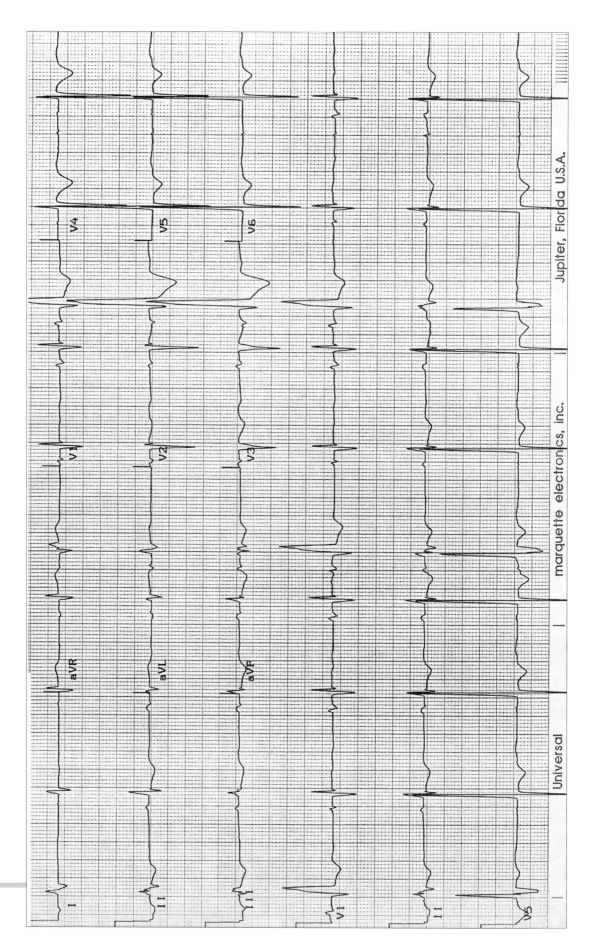

Universal   marquette electronics, inc.   Jupiter, Florida U.S.A.

Diagnoses   **ECG I-8**

1. Borderline sinus bradycardia (rate about 58/min)

2. Frequent atrial premature beats with RBBB aberration

3. Old anteroseptal infarction

4. Probable right ventricular hypertrophy (prominent R in V1 and huge voltage of R in aberrant beats)

5. Probable diffuse ischemia (T-wave abnormalities throughout)

Clinical Data

87-year-old woman

Comments

None

ECG I-9

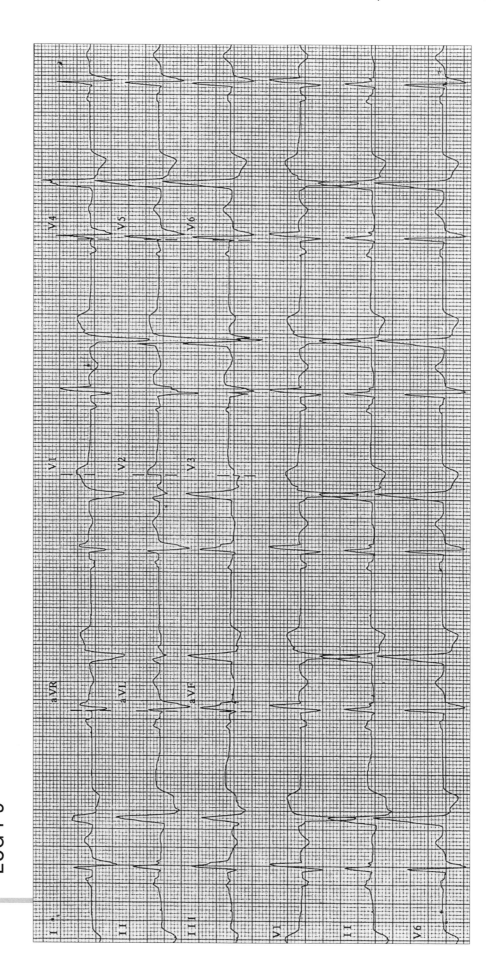

Diagnoses   **ECG I-9**

1. Sinus rhythm with right ventricular bigeminy

2. Left atrial enlargement

3. Right bundle-branch block

4. Anteroseptal infarction of uncertain date, probably recent

Clinical Data

95-year-old man

Comments

Note:

• The "P-terminal force" in V1 = about 12 mm/s (i.e., three times the upper limit of normal), which is typical of left atrial enlargement.

• The slurring on the downstrokes of the VPBs in lead V1, producing a delayed nadir at 0.09 s, is typical of RV ectopy and unlike the slick downstroke and earlier nadir of LBBB.

ECG I-10

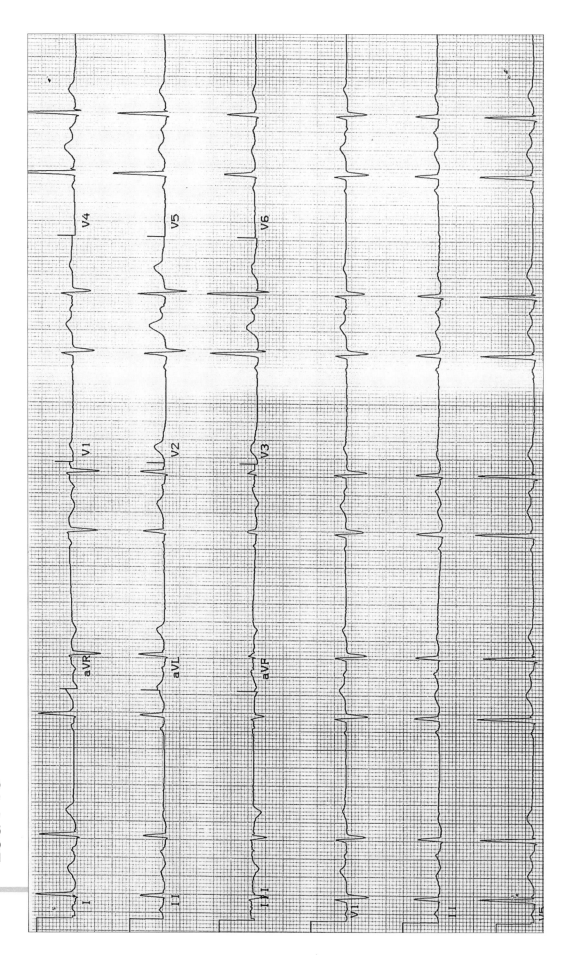

Diagnoses   **ECG I-10**

1. Sinus rhythm, with . . .

2. . . . atrial premature beats (APBs) in bigeminal rhythm (atrial bigeminy)

3. Probable old inferior infarction

Clinical Data

71-year-old man complaining of irregular heart beat

Comments

• At first glance, the correct diagnosis (atrial bigeminy) seems obvious. But then, if you measure the ventricular cycles, the short cycles are so precisely and consistently half the long cycles (consecutive cycles measure 66, 132, 68, 136, 65, 131, 65, 131, 66) that SA exit block seems to become more likely. In favor of atrial bigeminy, however, are the slightly different early P waves; and if you measure the P-P intervals instead of the R-R intervals, the shorter P-Ps (63–64) are *less than half* the longer P-Ps (134–139), and this clinches the diagnosis of APBs rather than SA block.

• The ST-T configuration in lead 3, with the inverted T wave in aVF and a too-low T wave in lead 2, makes an old inferior infarction likely.

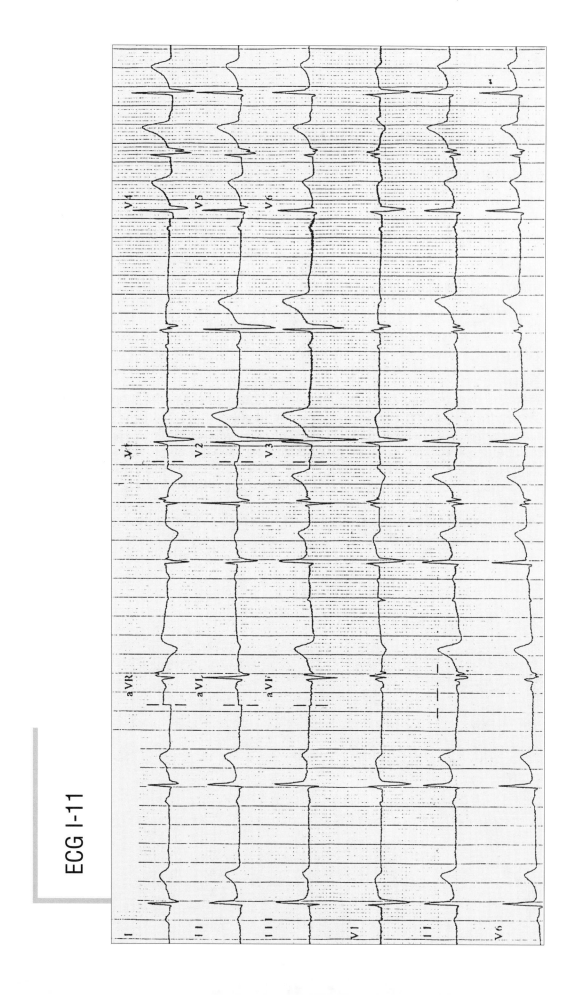

ECG I-11

Diagnoses   **ECG I-11**

1. Sinus bradycardia (rate = 48/min)

2. Probable normal "early repolarization"

3. Ventricular parasystole (rate = 32/min)

4. Fusion beat

Clinical Data

38-year-old man with no symptoms except awareness of cardiac irregularity

Comments

• The obvious variation in the "coupling" intervals of the four ectopic beats tells you that they represent an *independent* rhythm; then the constant interectopic intervals (184, 184, 186; see ECG below) confirm that it is a *"protected"* pacemaker (i.e., cannot be depolarized by other impulses). Independence + protection = parasystole.

• The third parasystolic beat produces ventricular fusion (*F*)—adequate PR for AV conduction + changed QRS, most evident in V1.

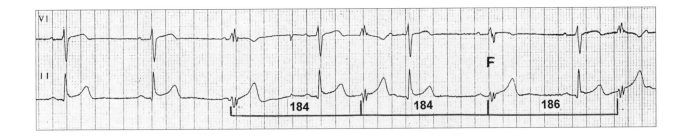

ECG I-12

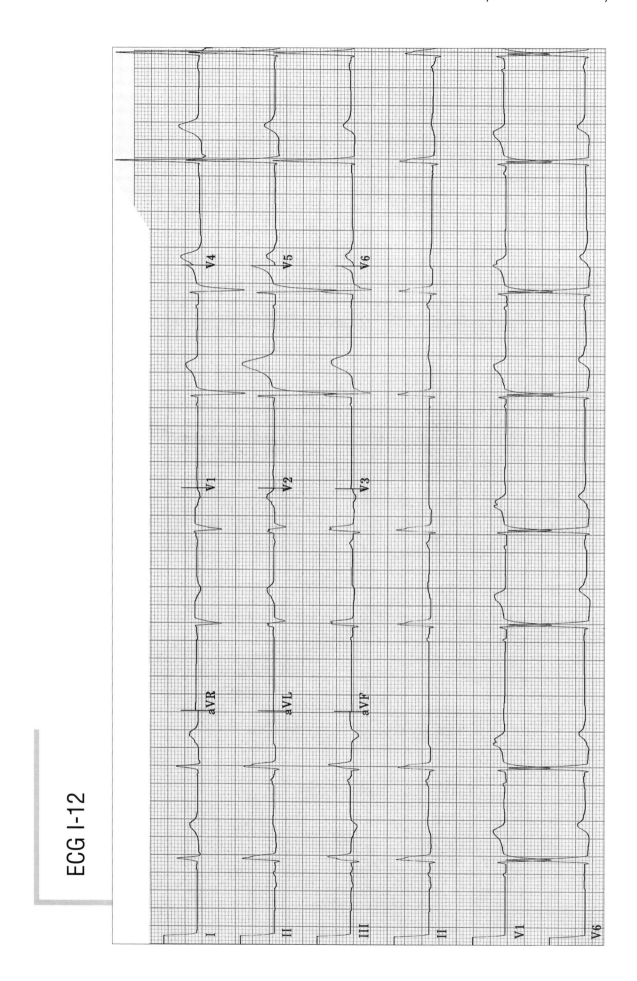

Diagnoses   ECG I-12

1. Borderline sinus bradycardia (rate about 58/min) with shifting atrial pacemaker and . . .

2. . . . a nonconducted atrial premature every third beat

3. Probable left ventricular hypertrophy

4. ST-T pattern (ST horizontality with ST-T angulation) strongly suggesting ischemic disease

5. Inferior infarction of uncertain date

Clinical Data

88-year-old man with history of hypertension, atrial fibrillation, and angina

Comments

• An unusual mechanism of "bigeminy"—every third beat a nonconducted APB

• An excellent demonstration of the value of simultaneous leads: the only lead in which you can see the APBs clearly is V1 where they notch the T waves; but the only lead in which the shift of the pacemaker is obvious is lead 2.

• Of the three longer ventricular cycles resulting from the nonconducted APBs, the second and third end with shorter PR intervals than the first and are probably junctional escapes.

ECG I-13

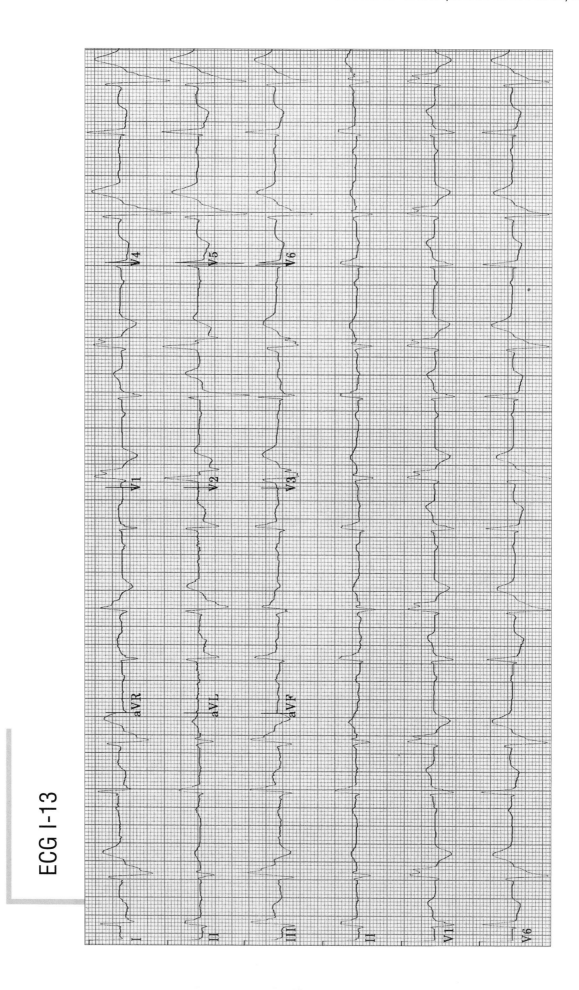

Diagnoses

ECG I-13

1. Sinus rhythm with left ventricular bigeminy

2. Acute, evolving inferior infarction

3. Borderline first-degree AV block (PR = 0.20–0.22 s)

Clinical Data

77-year-old man

Comments

Note:

• The classic morphologic features of left ventricular ectopy in the VPBs: taller left "rabbit-ear" in V1 with rS complex in V6

• That the features of acute infarction are also evident in the VPBs: Q waves, elevated ST, and inverted T waves in leads 3 and aVF, with reciprocal ST depression in leads 1, aVL, and some of the V leads

ECG I-14

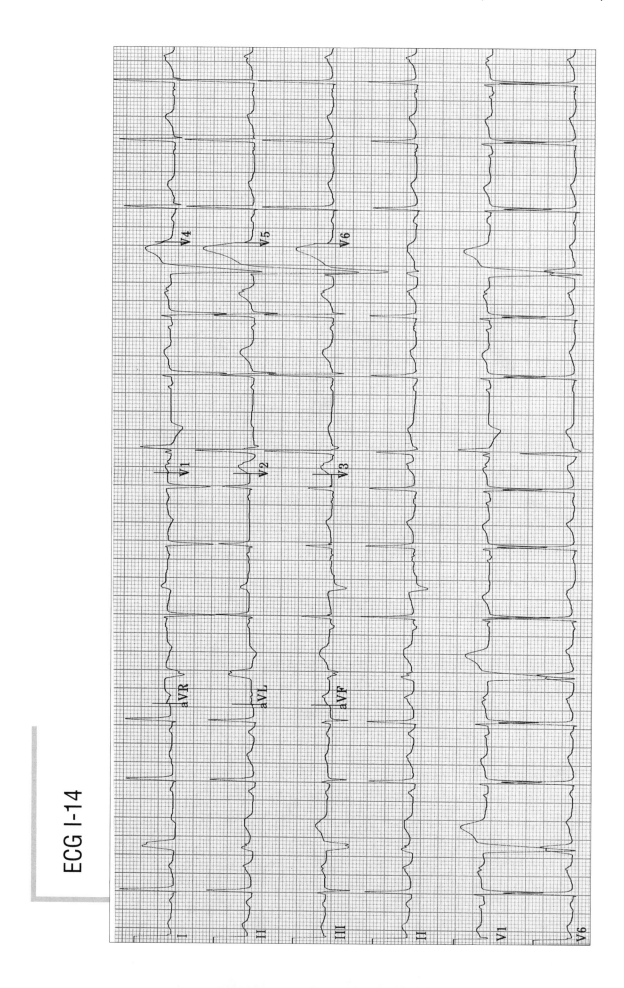

Diagnoses   **ECG I-14**

1. Sinus rhythm (rate = 96/min), with . . .

2. . . . four atrial premature beats, with RBBB aberration in one and LBBB aberration in three

3. After 2nd APB, pacemaker shifts to junctional; after 4th APB it shifts to ectopic atrial (change in P wave, especially in V1)

4. Borderline T-wave pattern and QRS voltage—probable early left ventricular hypertrophy

5. Artifact distorting T wave of 6th beat

Clinical Data

79-year-old woman

Comment

Regarding diagnosis no. 4: The T wave is flat in aVL, with a QRS amplitude of 7 mm, and suspiciously low in lead 1, and the precordial T-wave balance indicates a rather anterior vector (TV1 is at least as tall as TV6), all of which could be early evidence of LVH—with which diagnosis the QRS voltage is certainly compatible.

ECG I-15

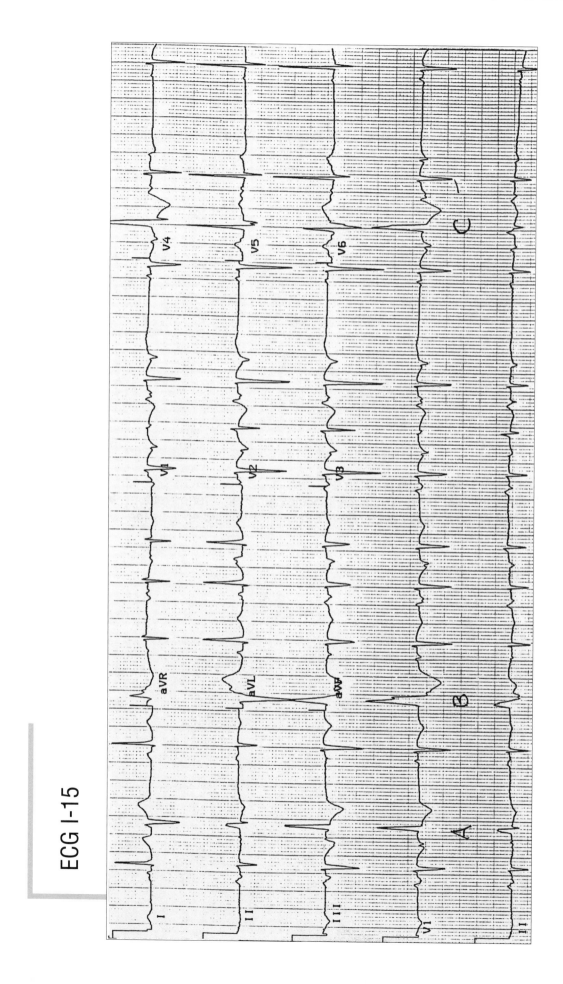

Diagnoses   ## ECG I-15

1. Sinus rhythm with . . .

2. . . . frequent atrial premature beats, two nonconducted

3. Three ventricular premature beats, one typical (*B*) and . . .

4. . . . two (*A* and *C*) producing fusion beats with simultaneous APBs

5. Left axis deviation (−45 degrees)

6. Abnormal T-wave inversion in leads 2, 3, and aVF with simultaneous inversion in V1−3 suggest the possibility of acute cor pulmonale.

Clinical Data

89-year-old woman

Comment

Because the ventricular coupling intervals of beats A, B, and C vary, parasystole is a possibility—but precise measurement of intervals A-B and B-C is not confirmatory.

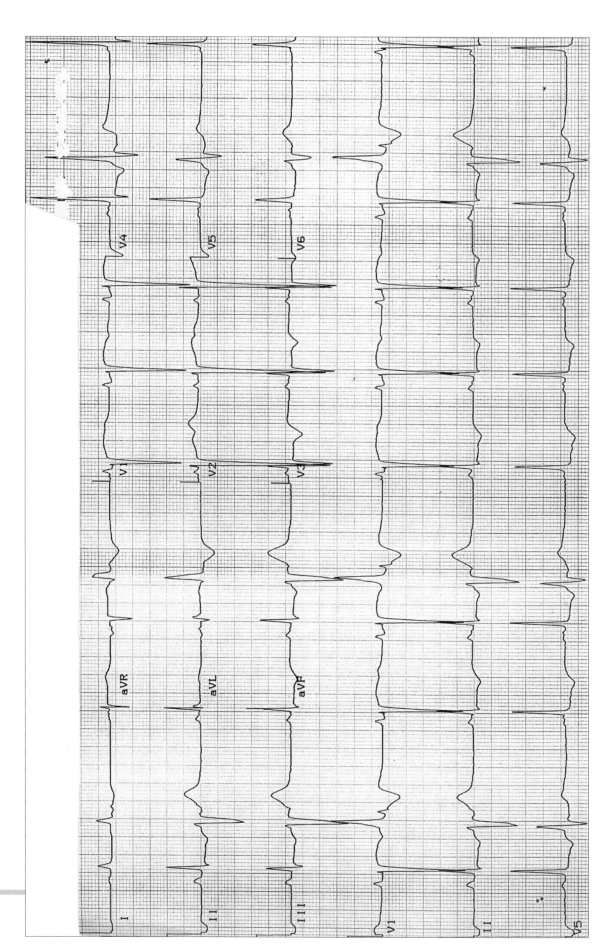

ECG I-16

Diagnoses   **ECG I-16**

1. Abnormal P waves (? bi-atrial enlargement)

2. Three left ventricular premature beats with . . .

3. . . . retrograde conduction to atria, each followed by . . .

4. . . . junctional escape beats

5. Left ventricular enlargement/hypertrophy

Clinical Data

69-year-old woman with hypertension

Comments

• The notched P-wave pattern in leads 2 and V3–6 suggests left atrial enlargement, while the prominent positive P in V1 suggests right atrial enlargement.

• The P waves immediately following the VPBs are retrograde because: they are early; they follow at a constant RP interval; and careful scrutiny reveals a definitely different contour from the sinus P waves.

• After the VPBs, the returning beats are escapes (see ECG I-7) because: their PR intervals have shortened and are varied, and they all end identical (longer-than-sinus) ventricular cycles.

ECG I-17

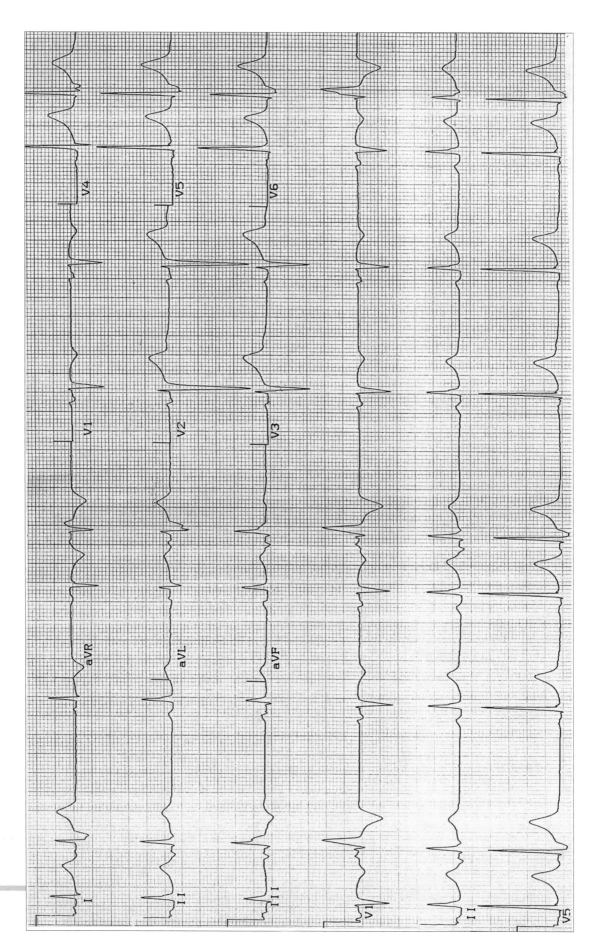

Diagnoses   **ECG I-17**

1. Sinus bradycardia (rate about 50/min)

2. Supraventricular (probably junctional: retrograde-shaped P′ waves with P′R of 0.11 s) premature beats, with . . .

3. . . . RBBB aberration

Clinical Data

50-year-old man, complaining of dizzy spells

Comment

Probably incipient sick sinus in view of the significant "overdrive suppression" of the sinus by the premature (retrograde) activation of the atria: P-P interval = 1.17 s, P′-P interval = 1.45 s (see below)

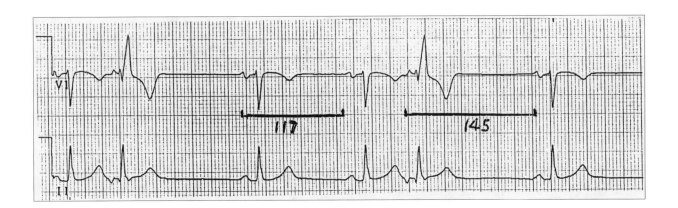

ECG I-18

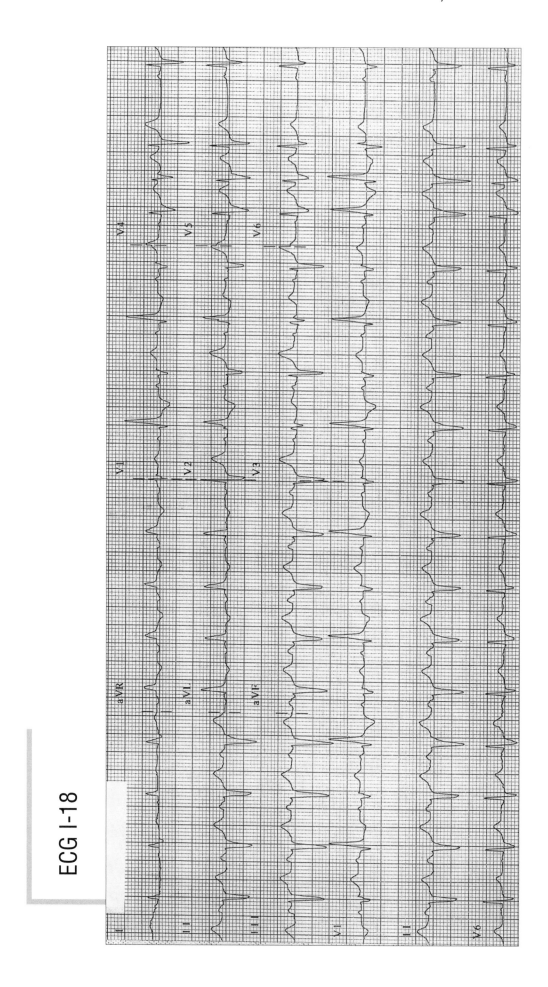

Diagnoses

ECG I-18

1. Sinus tachycardia (rate = 103/min)

2. Left anterior hemiblock

3. Intermittent—mostly alternating—RBBB

4. Two supraventricular (probably atrial) premature beats (see ECG below; *1* and *2*)

Clinical Data

59-year-old man

Comment

The two APBs again demonstrate the role of the *preceding* cycle in determining the fate of intraventricular conduction. Since refractory periods are proportional to rate (i.e., to the preceding cycle): The first APB follows a longer cycle (60) and is aberrantly conducted, whereas the second follows a shorter cycle (37), which shortens refractoriness, and the RBB conducts better.

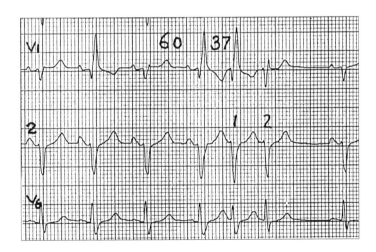

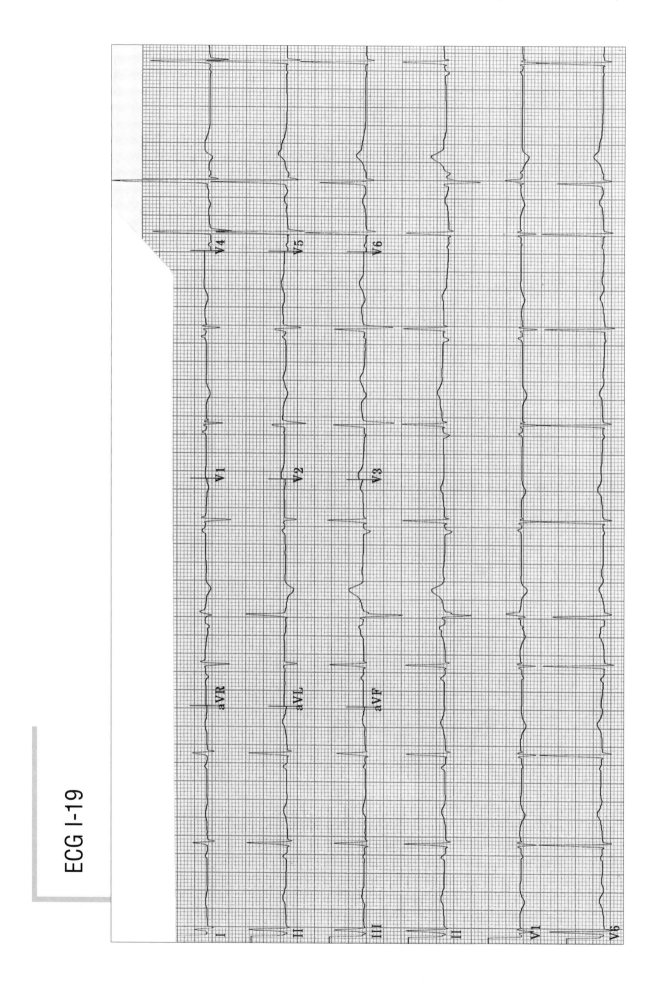

ECG I-19

Diagnoses   ECG I-19

1. Sinus rhythm with shifting pacemaker (rate about 63/min)

2. One atrial and one junctional premature beat, both with . . .

3. . . . bifascicular aberration (incomplete RBBB + LAHB)

4. Nonspecific ST-T abnormalities

Clinical Data

50-year-old man

Comments

• Note that the APB, by suppressing the sinus, induces a shift in the pacemaker from sinus to junctional—a fairly common occurrence.

• The 9th beat has a P wave that differs from both the sinus and the retrograde P wave and therefore represents either an ectopic atrial focus or, more likely, **atrial fusion** (between sinus and retrograde impulses).

ECG I-20

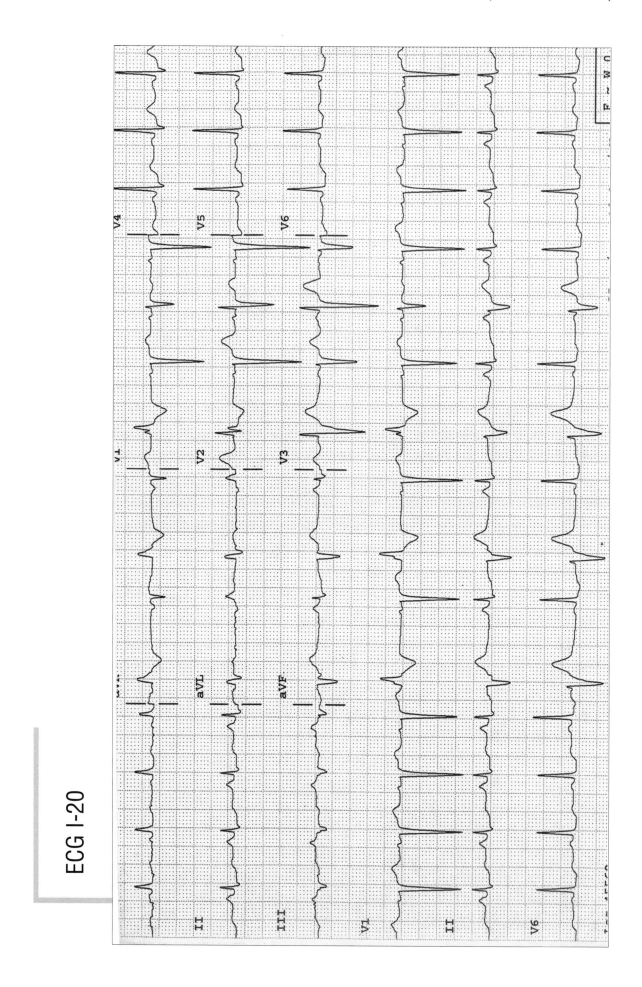

Diagnoses   **ECG I-20**

1. Sinus rhythm (rate = 98/min)

2. Widespread and rather horizontal ST depression, probably due to ischemia

3. Ventricular parasystole—the fourth parasystolic beat produces ventricular fusion

Clinical Data

72-year-old woman

Comments

Parasystole is diagnosed in two stages:

  • First, you note that the "coupling" interval of the ectopic beats varies (here it gets progressively longer with successive beats), which tells you that the ectopics are not extrasystoles.

  • Then you measure the interval between the parasystolic beats (interectopic interval) and find it to be constant. This establishes the interval as an *independent* rhythm not interrupted by the intervening sinus impulses—in other words, it's a natural, fixed-rate pacemaker.

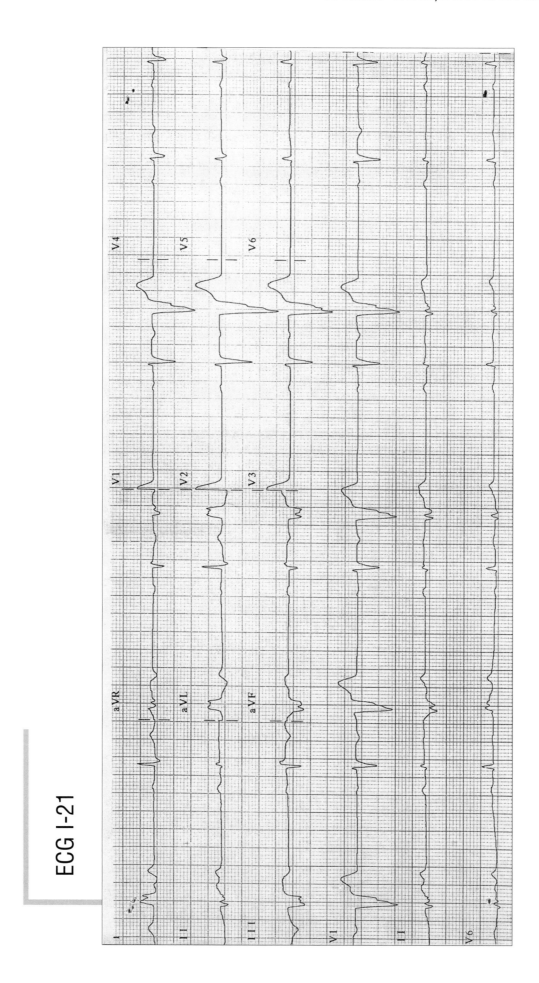

ECG I-21

Diagnoses   ECG I-21

1. Sinus bradycardia (rate = 54/min) with . . .

2. . . . first-degree AV block (PR = 0.28 s)

3. Inferior infarction of uncertain age, probably recent

4. Junctional bigeminy with LBBB aberration

Clinical Data

Unknown

Comments

The coupled (premature) beats have the classic features of LBBB in V1 (i.e., slick downstroke to early nadir—only 0.04 s—with slurring on upstroke), and not of ventricular ectopy, which usually begins with a wide R wave or a slurred downstroke producing a delayed (> 0.06 s) nadir (see RV ectopics in ECGs I.2 and I.9). Of course nothing is 100%, and VPBs cannot be absolutely ruled out, but such typical morphology makes LBBB the much more likely diagnosis.

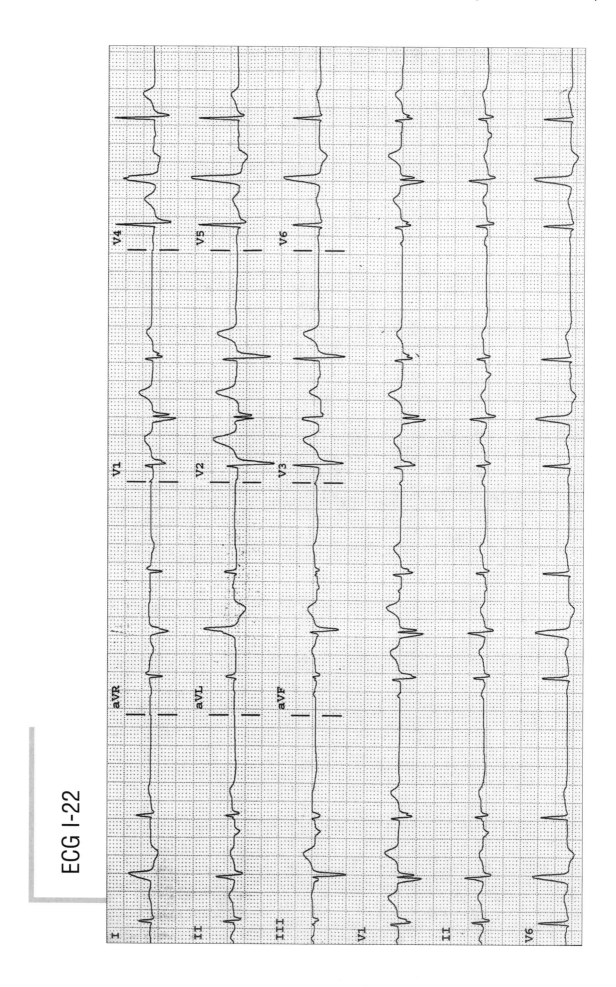

ECG I-22

Diagnoses   **ECG I-22**

1. Sinus bradycardia with . . .

2. . . . ventricular bigeminy (see first two Comments) and . . .

3. . . . reciprocal beating with . . .

4. . . . one probable atrial fusion beat

5. Possible T-wave abnormality (see last Comment)

Clinical Data

85-year-old man with palpitations

Comments

• Because the coupled, ectopic beat in V1 has a slick downstroke and early nadir, and because its morphology in other leads is compatible with LBBB, it is certainly possible that it is junctional with an LBBB aberration (see ECG below, *c*) rather than a ventricular one (*b*).

• The modified retrograde P wave in *a* is most likely due to atrial fusion.

• The T wave in V1 taller than the T wave in V6—implying a too anterior T vector—is always a suspicious finding that requires further assessment.

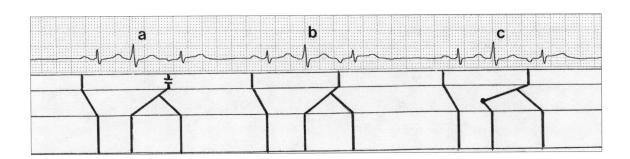

ECG I-23

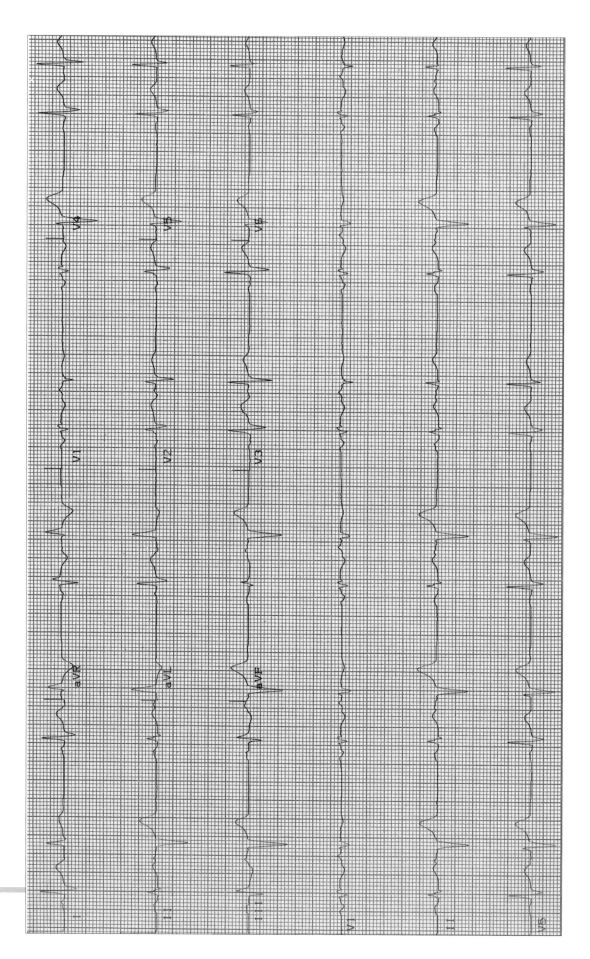

Diagnoses   ECG I-23

1. Atrial premature beats in bigeminal rhythm, with . . .

2. . . . left anterior hemiblock aberration of most of the prematures

3. Incomplete RBBB pattern in the sinus beats

4. Possible old inferior infarction

5. Intra-atrial block/left atrial abnormality (see Comment)

Clinical Data

72-year-old man complaining of irregular pulse

Comment

Abnormally wide P waves, measuring 0.14 s, and abnormal P-terminal force in V1

ECG I-24

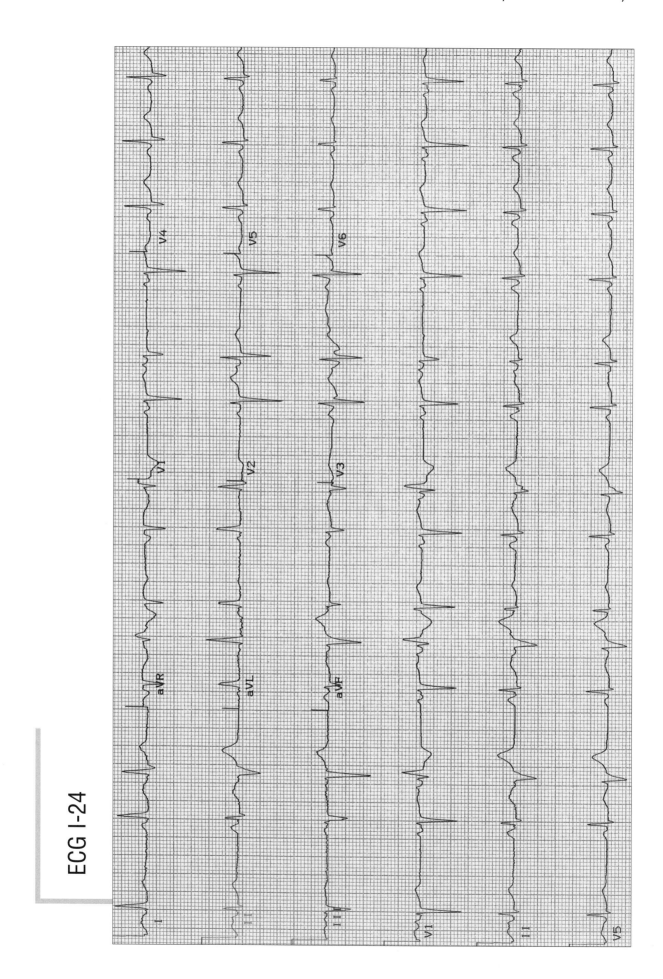

Diagnoses   ECG I-24

1. Sinus rhythm interrupted by a run (four couplets) of atrial bigeminy with . . .

2. . . . RBBB and left anterior hemiblock aberration of varying degrees (see Comments)

3. Borderline low T waves in 1, aVL, and V6

Clinical Data

74-year-old woman

Comments

• The first two aberrant beats show (probably) complete RBBB and (probably) complete LAHB. The third shows still the same RBBB but now less left axis and therefore presumably less anterior fascicular delay. The fourth shows the earliest sign of RBB delay (i.e., shrinkage of the S wave in V1) and lower R waves in V6 than the sinus beats, presumably because of some anterior fascicular delay.

• Why isn't the 6th beat in the strip (the beat after the 2nd aberrant APB) also significantly aberrant, since it ends a cycle even shorter than the cycle of any of the aberrant beats?

Answer: The 6th beat is *preceded* by a shorter cycle than any of the aberrant beats, and that preceding shorter cycle has decreased the ensuing refractory period of both the RBB and the anterior fascicle. Compare the influence of preceding cycles in ECGs I-5, I-8, and I-18.

ECG I-25

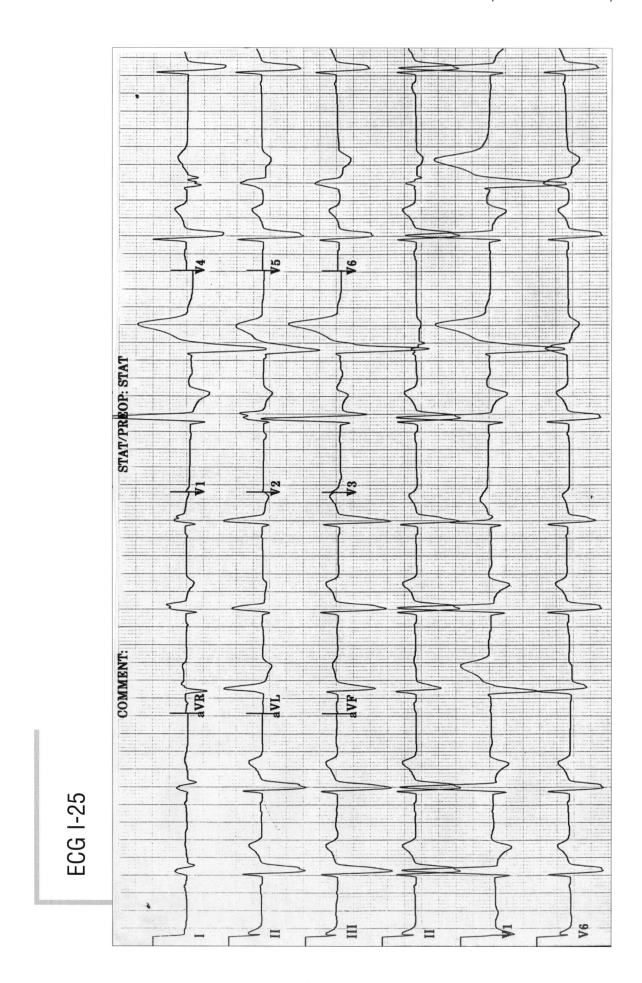

COMMENT:

STAT/PREOP: STAT

Diagnoses   ECG I-25

1. Borderline sinus bradycardia with arrhythmia (average sinus rate = 58/min) and intra-atrial block (P waves > 0.12 s wide)

2. Right bundle-branch block with left anterior hemiblock (axis about −80°)

3. Right ventricular parasystole (rate = 32/min), including fusion beats (see ECG below, *F*)

4. Right ventricular hypertrophy (R in V1 = 27 mm)

5. Possible old anteroseptal infarct (but hemiblock alone can produce q waves in anteroseptal leads)

Clinical Data

90-year-old man with Parkinson's disease and hemiparesis

Comments

None, but see below.

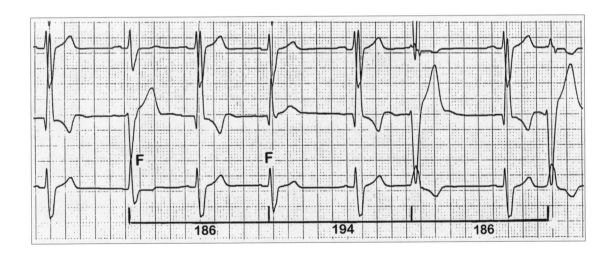

ECG I-26

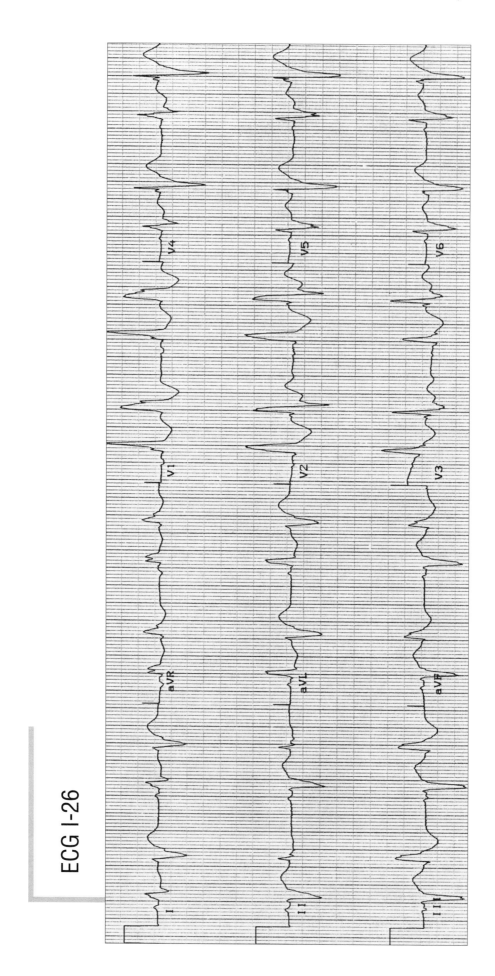

Diagnoses   **ECG I-26**

1. Sinus rhythm (rate = probably 94/min, possibly 47/min)

2. Bifascicular block (RBBB + LAHB)

3. Left ventricular bigeminy

Clinical Data

Unknown

Comments

• In V6, a good example of **mutual mimicry:** the rS shape, usually a good clue to LV ectopy, can also be produced by bifascicular block.

• Note three other characteristic contours: the qR complexes in V1 with early peak in ectopy and delayed peak in RBBB; and the right axis deviation of LV ectopy.

ECG I-27

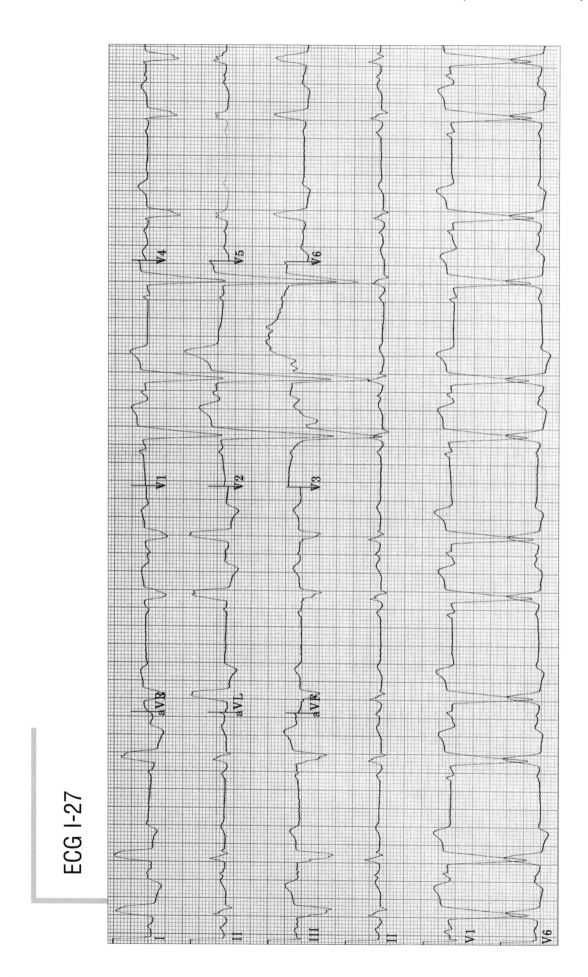

Diagnoses   **ECG I-27**

1. Sinus rhythm with atrial bigeminy

2. Left bundle-branch block

Clinical Data

69-year-old woman

Comments

This ECG was misinterpreted by the computer as 3:2 sinus Wenckebachs. Carefully inspect the P waves in each pair of beats: they clearly differ from each other (best seen in lead 2), establishing an ectopic origin for the second of each pair. Note that the coupling interval of the APBs varies by as much as 0.12 s.

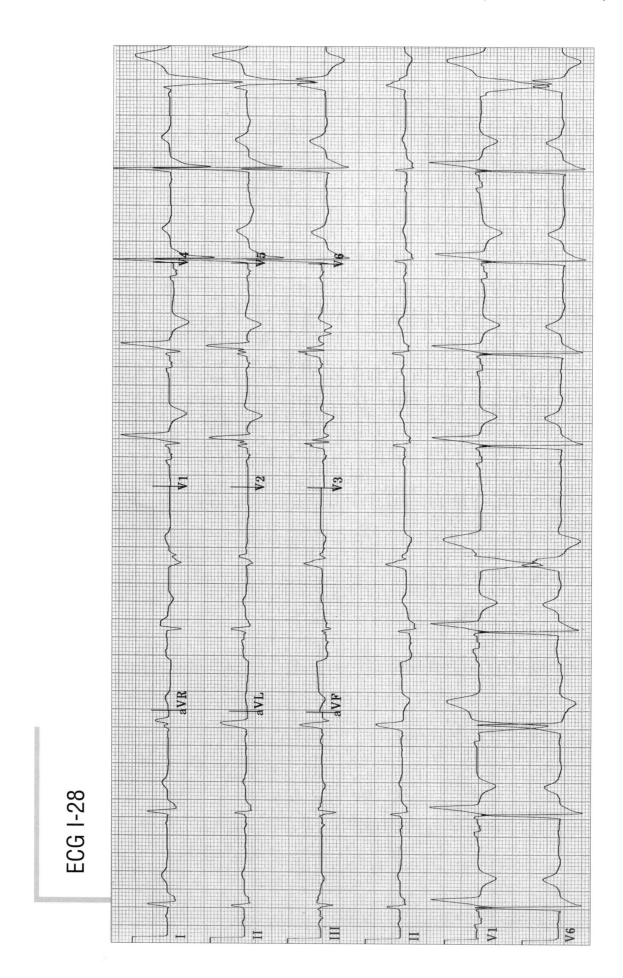

ECG I-28

Diagnoses

ECG I-28

1. Sinus bradycardia (rate = 59/min)

2. Right bundle-branch block

3. Probable left ventricular enlargement (R-wave voltage V5–6)

4. Ventricular parasystole

5. Fusion beat (see ECG below, *a*)

6. Inverted U waves (especially V5–6)

Clinical Data

70-year-old man years post-CABG and transplanted kidney for renal failure

Comments

• Whether 59/min should be called bradycardia is moot—there is a practical movement afoot to redefine normal sinus rates as 50–90 rather than 60–100.

• Parasystole is suspected from the evident variation in the coupling intervals of the ectopic beats, which indicates an independent rather than extrasystolic (fixed coupling) mechanism. Parasystole is then confirmed by measuring the interectopic intervals and finding that there is a common denominator (a-b = 178; b-c = 3 × 177).

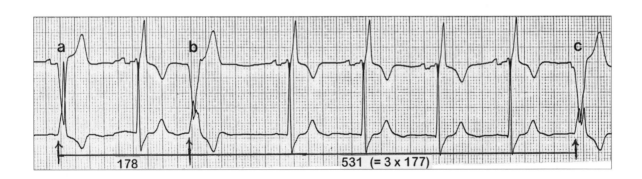

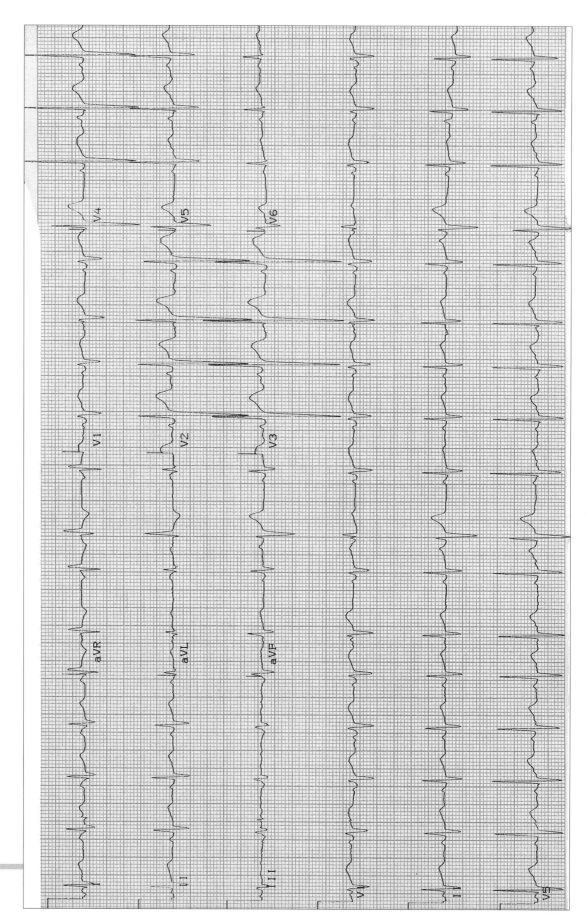

ECG I-29

Diagnoses

1. Sinus tachycardia (rate = 100/min) with . . .

2. . . . frequent atrial premature beats, with and without . . .

3. . . . incomplete RBBB and left anterior hemiblock aberration

4. Short PR interval (0.11 s)

5. "Indeterminate" axis

Clinical Data

53-year-old man

Comment

No axis is truly indeterminate, but it's the lazy or sensible (choose your descriptor) person's way out when all the limb leads have equiphasic complexes: the initial and terminal forces are in opposite directions; the "mean" axis is therefore meaningless; two axes—initial and terminal—must be determined; and "indeterminate" is the resulting cop-out.

ECG I-30

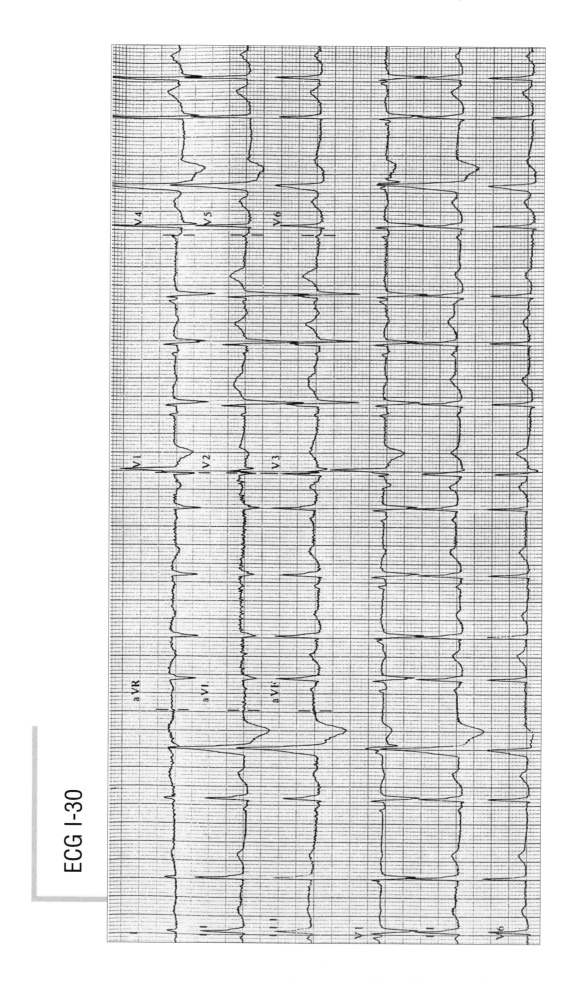

Diagnoses

1. Two ventricular premature beats (see ECG below, *V*)

2. Four junctional premature beats (*J*)

3. One atrial premature beat (*A*) with RBBB aberration

4. A junctional beat of uncertain description (*?*)

Clinical Data

90-year-old woman

Comment

An exercise in multilevel ectopy, otherwise a normal—especially at this age!—tracing

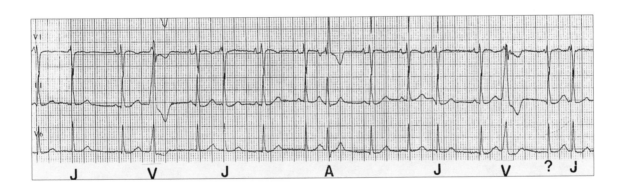

ECG I-31

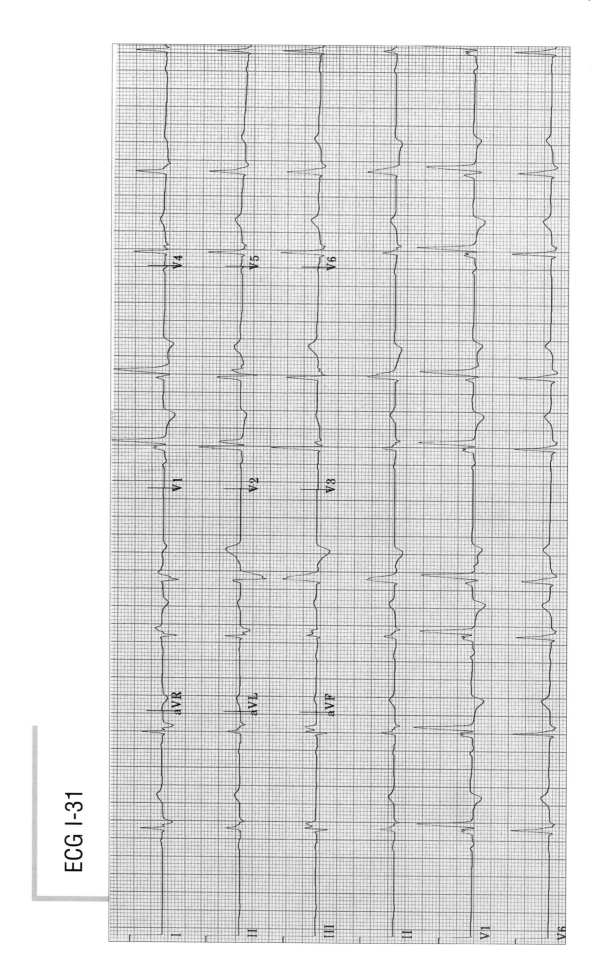

Diagnoses

1. Sinus bradycardia (rate = 56/min)

2. Right bundle-branch block

3. Junctional parasystole with posterior hemiblock aberration

4. Borderline P wave width (about 0.12 s)

5. Borderline first degree AV block (PR = about 0.22 s)

Clinical Data

76-year-old woman

Comments

• Parasystole is diagnosed because the "coupling interval" (see ECG below; *63, 78, 89*) of the ectopic beats is changing—which excludes extrasystoles—while the interectopic intervals (*228, 229*) remain constant.

• The posterior hemiblock aberration is apparent in the first parasystolic beat showing marked right axis deviation (leads aVL and aVF).

• Note the slight but definite notching of the initial R wave of the sinus beats in V1, absent in the parasystolic beats. Significance?

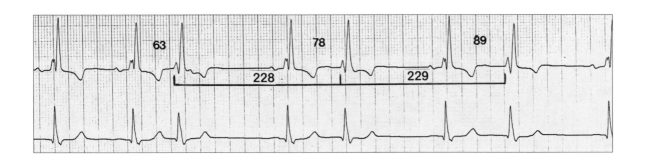

ECG I-32

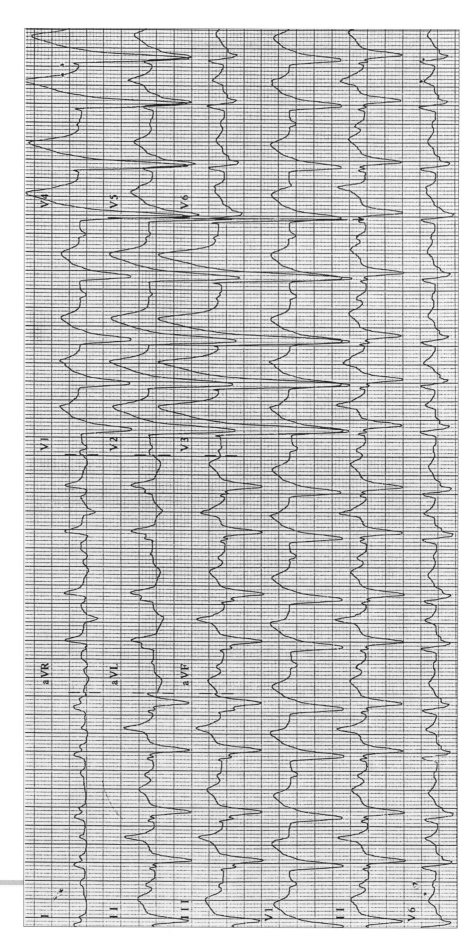

Diagnoses   **ECG I-32**

1. Sinus rhythm with frequent atrial premature beats, mostly in bigeminy, but including one pair (beats 11 and 12)

2. Left atrial enlargement (PTF-V1 = 0.18 mm/s)

3. Left bundle-branch block with unusually wide QRS (0.20 s) and . . .

4. . . . marked left axis deviation (about −75 degrees)

Clinical Data

70-year-old man

Comments

Points of special note:

- The unusually wide QRS complexes, more often seen with ectopy than with BBB

- The very tall P′ waves in lead 2, at first glance looking like peaked T waves

Section II

Wide-QRS Rhythms

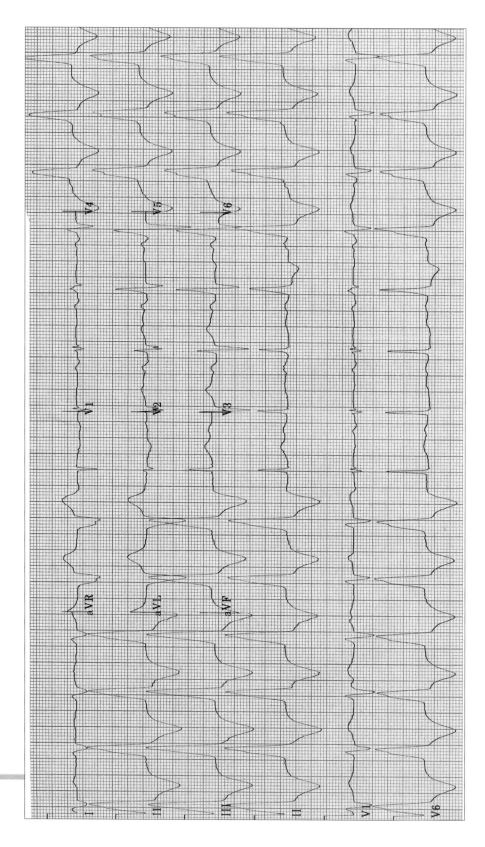

ECG II-1

Diagnoses   **ECG II-1**

1. Accelerated idioventricular rhythm (rate = 85/min) with . . .

2. . . . one—maybe more—ventricular fusion beats

3. ST-T abnormalities

Clinical Data

74-year-old man

Comments

• The tracing begins with the accelerated idioventricular rhythm (AIVR) dissociated from the slightly slower sinus rhythm; but when the P wave lands far enough beyond the QRS, the sinus captures the ventricles and remains in control for three beats. The fourth beat is a ventricular fusion beat as the slightly faster AIVR resumes control.

• The conducted sinus beats in leads 2 and V6 manifest an abnormal ST-T pattern (but this may be due to minimal fusion with the almost isorhythmic ectopic beats).

ECG II-2

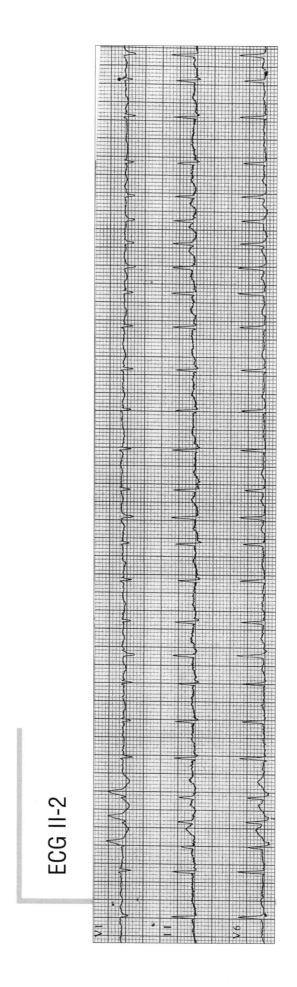

Diagnoses   **ECG II-2**

1. Atrial fibrillation with rapid (about 160/min) ventricular response

2. A 3-beat run of RBBB aberration

3. Rather low voltage

4. Nonspecific ST-T abnormalities

Clinical Data

Unknown

Comment

Note that the aberration is, as usual, precipitated by a longer-shorter cycle sequence and shows characteristic RBBB morphology (rsR′ in V1, qRs in V6).

ECG II-3

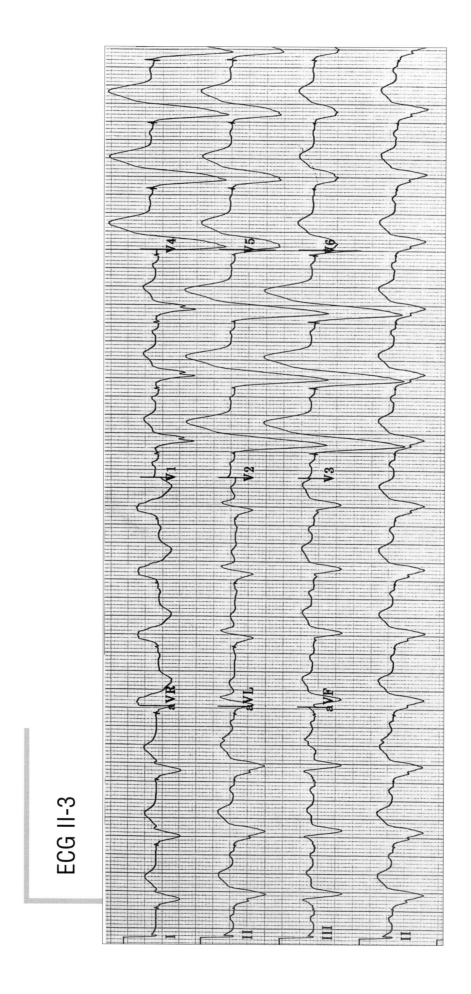

Diagnoses   **ECG II-3**

1. Sinus rhythm with . . .

2. . . . right ventricular pacemaker in atrial-tracking mode (rate = 84/min)

Clinical Data

66-year-old man

Comments

• Another simple one, but still too much for the computer, which failed to perceive the pacemaker stimuli and diagnosed "normal sinus rhythm" with "nonspecific intraventricular block."

• A particularly good example of two of the best clues to ventricular ectopy: axis in upper right quadrant ("no-man's land") and negative concordance in the chest leads—both of which are commonly seen with right ventricular pacemakers.

ECG II-4

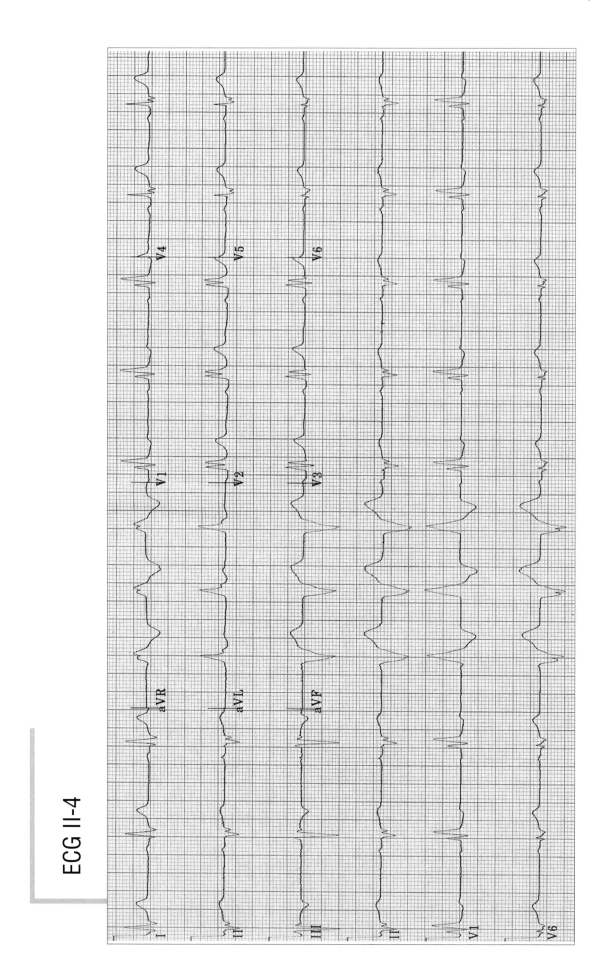

Diagnoses   **ECG II-4**

1. Borderline sinus bradycardia (rate = 58/min) interrupted by . . .

2. . . . a 3-beat run of accelerated idioventricular rhythm from the left ventricle

3. Right bundle-branch block

4. Left axis deviation (about −40 degrees), possibly left anterior hemiblock

5. Primary T-wave changes

6. Possible old inferior infarct

Clinical Data

Unknown

Comment

None

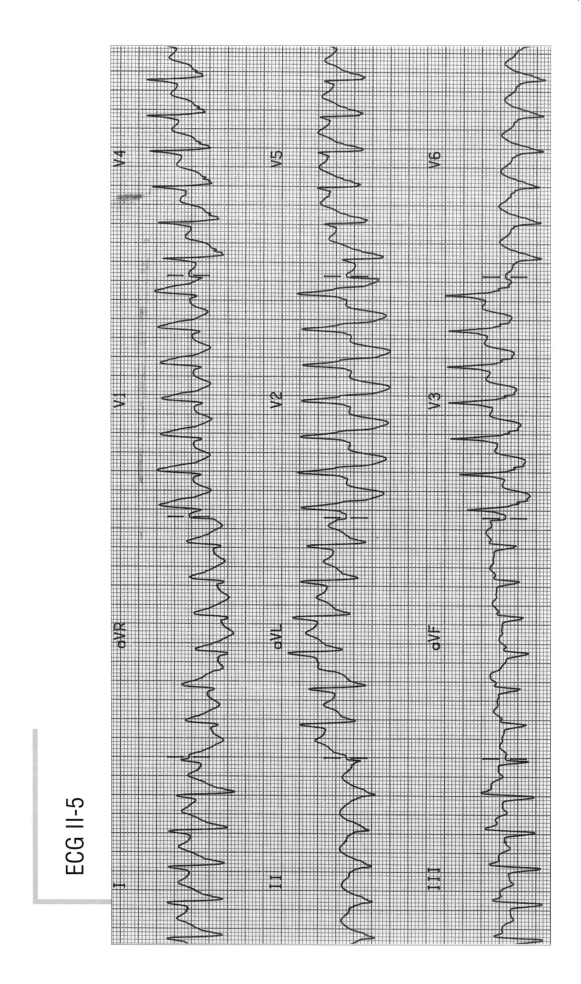

ECG II-5

Diagnoses   **ECG II-5**

1. Ventricular tachycardia (rate = 160/min)

2. Acute inferior infarction

Clinical Data

84-year-old man with severe chest pain, BP 85/40

Comments

Note:

• The characteristic features of VT (axis in no-man's land, steep upstroke with slurred downstroke in V1, and QS complex in V6)

• How clearly—despite the ectopic rhythm—the indicative changes of acute infarction show up in lead 3 (Q wave, ST elevation, T wave beginning to invert), with reciprocal ST depression in leads 1 and aVL.

ECG II-6

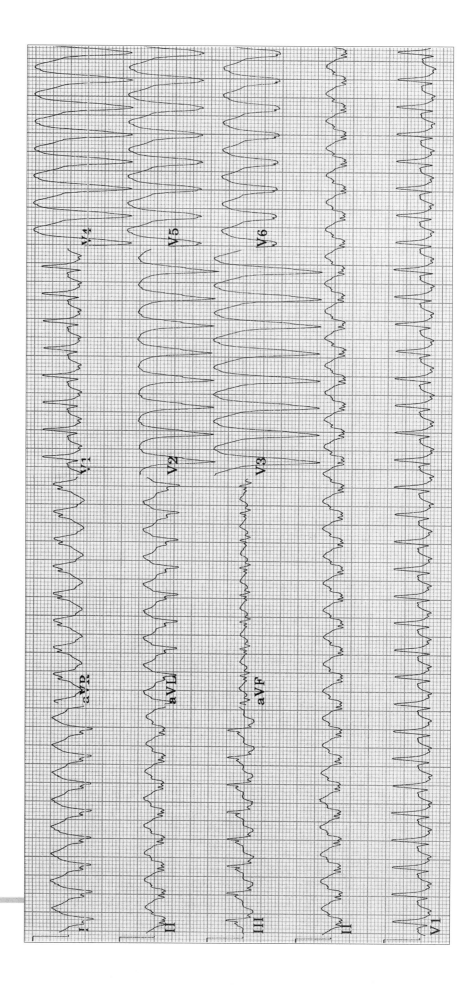

Diagnosis   **ECG II-6**

Ventricular tachycardia (rate = 204/min) with probable 1:1 retrograde conduction to atria

Clinical Data

57-year-old man whose tracings during sinus rhythm showed old anteroseptal infarction and left anterior hemiblock

Comments

• The important clues to VT are the QS complexes in both lead 1 and V6.

• When confronted with a wide-QRS tachycardia, one is always concerned that it might be a preexcited (WPW) tachycardia; in this case, accessory pathway conduction is excluded by the wholly negative complexes in V4–6.

• In lead V1 there is a tiny positive wave just following the QRS that precisely corresponds with a negative wavelet in lead 2—possibly retrograde P waves.

ECG II-7

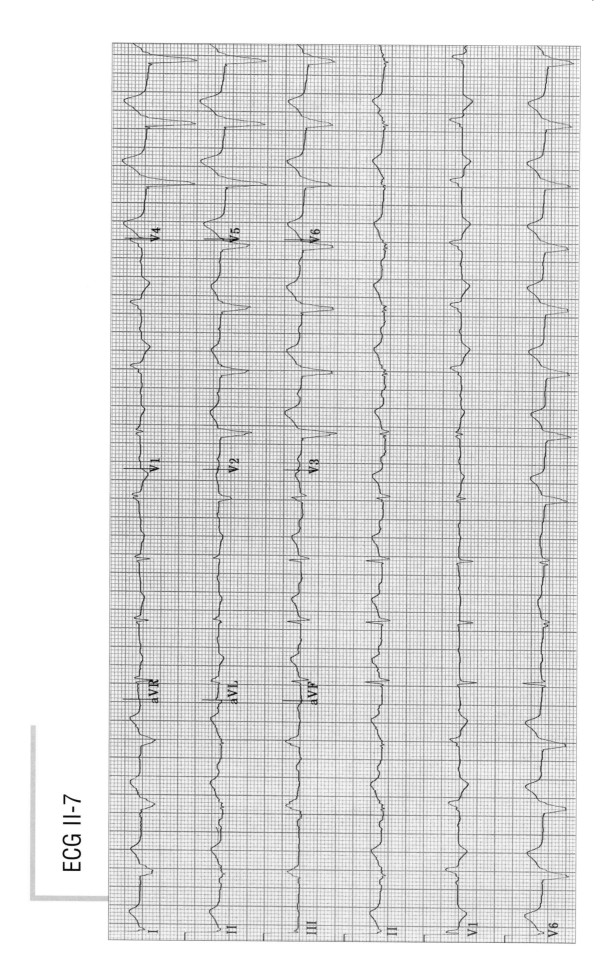

Diagnoses

ECG II-7

1. Accelerated idioventricular rhythm (rate = 88/min) dissociated from . . .

2. . . . sinus rhythm (rate = 86/min) with . . .

3. . . . one ventricular capture beat (see ECG below, *C*) followed by . . .

4. . . . four fusion (partial capture) beats (*F*)

Clinical Data

89-year-old man with acute anterolateral infarction

Comment

QS complexes in leads 1 and V6 are characteristic of ventricular ectopy.

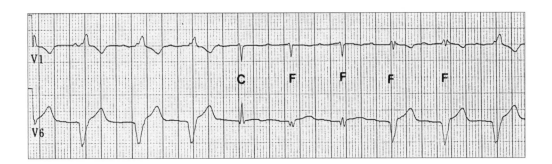

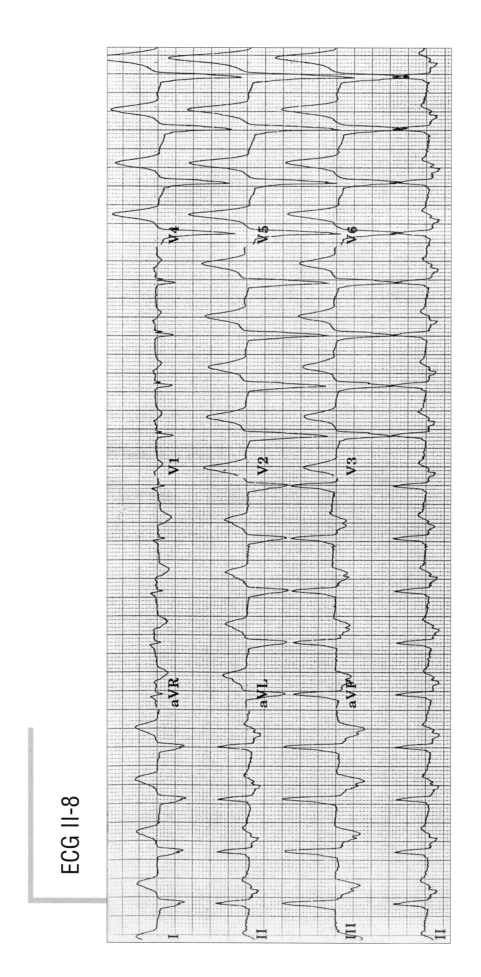

ECG II-8

Diagnoses

1. Ventricular tachycardia (rate = 110/min) with . . .

2. . . . 1:1 retrograde conduction to atria

Clinical Data

62-year-old woman, clinically stable

Comments

• The right axis combined with negative concordance in the V leads provides strong evidence favoring VT; while the QRS pattern, so unlike either BBB, makes any SVT most unlikely.

• Negative QRSs from V4–6 exclude a preexcited (WPW) tachycardia.

ECG II-9

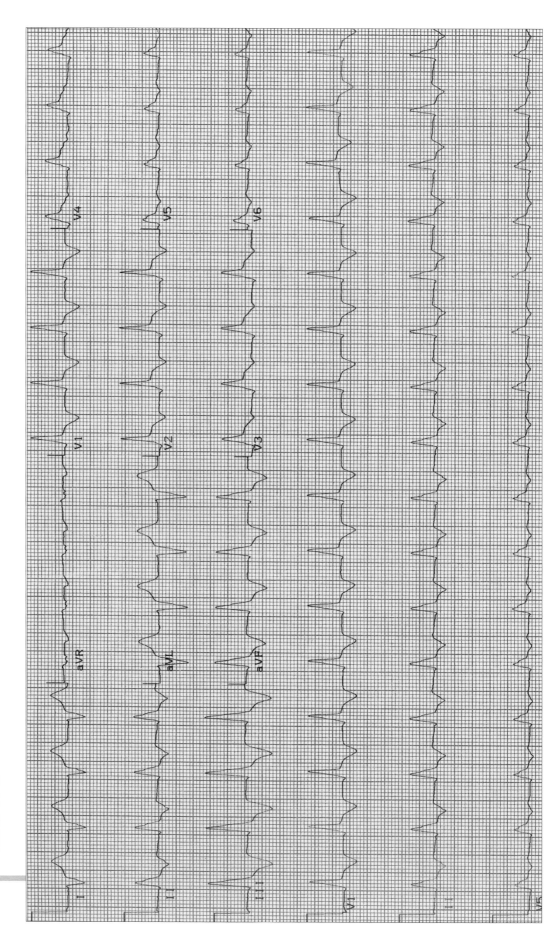

Diagnoses

ECG II-9

1. Accelerated idioventricular rhythm (rate = 99/min)

2. Acute extensive anterior (anterolateral) infarction

Clinical Data

58-year-old woman with retrosternal pain

Comments

• There is no recognizable evidence of atrial activity; retrograde activation (P′ wave lost in QRS-T) cannot be ruled out.

• Points favoring ventricular ectopy are: right axis deviation in a wide-QRS rhythm, and positive concordance in the V leads.

• It's notable that the current of injury is evident—not masked by the ectopic rhythm.

ECG II-10

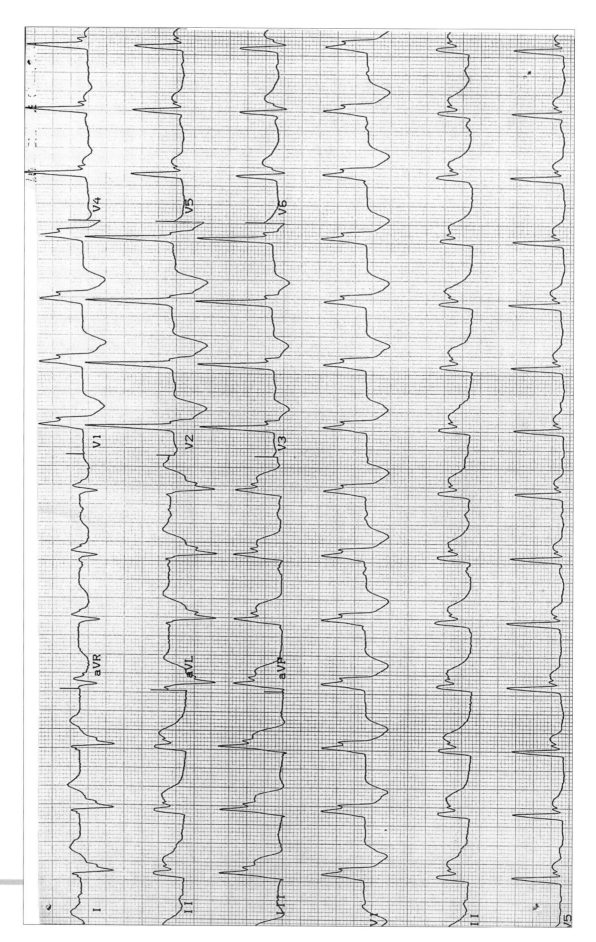

Diagnoses

1. Accelerated idioventricular rhythm (rate = 88/min) dissociated from . . .

2. . . . sinus tachycardia (rate = 102/min)

3. Acute inferolateral infarction

4. Some indefinable degree of AV block

Clinical Data

Unknown

Comments

• Note the typical left ectopic morphology of the QRS in V1 (taller left "rabbit-ear"), and the fact that the acute injury shows clearly despite the ectopic rhythm.

• Although an idioventricular rhythm is much more likely, you cannot absolutely exclude a junctional rhythm with bifascicular aberration (RBBB + posterior hemiblock).

• Regarding the infarction, the tall early peak in V1 and high early voltage in V2 should lead you to also suspect involvement of the posterior wall.

• The presence of AV block is proven by the PRs of at least 0.24 s in the 7th and last beats without any evidence of AV conduction—not even a whisper of fusion. The block itself may be quite minor, but it is an undoubted contributor to the complete AV dissociation.

ECG II-11

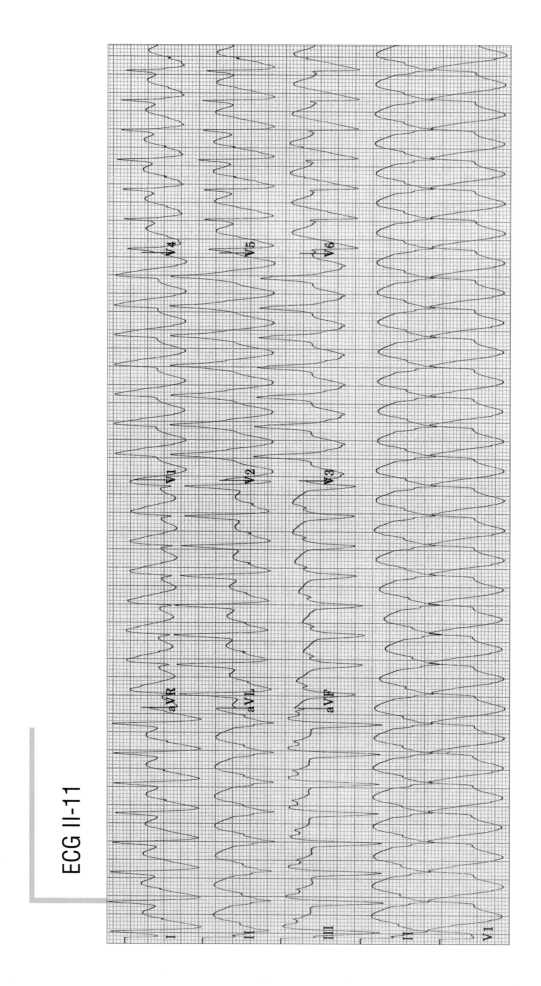

Diagnosis

(Left) ventricular tachycardia (rate = 182/min)

Clinical Data

51-year-old, diabetic, overweight, and hypercholesterolemic man 6 years after myocardial infarction

Comments

ECG features favoring ventricular ectopy rather than aberration include:

- QRS is "wide-wide" (i.e., > 0.14 s) rather than just wide (computer reads this QRS interval as 0.186 s)

- Steeper R-wave upstroke than downstroke in V1 (taller left "rabbit-ear" equivalent)

- rS in V6

- QRS axis in upper right quadrant (about −120 degrees), often referred to as "no-man's land."

Note: What look like retrograde P waves in leads 3 and aVF are actually occurring *during* the QRS (judging by simultaneous leads) and are therefore part of the ventricular complex rather than atrial waves.

ECG II-12

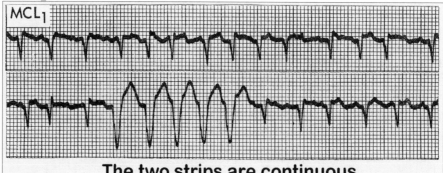

The two strips are continuous.

Diagnoses   **ECG II-12**

1. Atrial flutter-fibrillation with rapid and irregular ventricular response (rate = 180/min)

2. A 5-beat run of *either* LBBB aberration *or* ventricular tachycardia

Comments

• First glance suggests atrial fibrillation, but careful scrutiny reveals regular atrial activity at 320/min (see ECG below, *dots*).

• The flurry of wide beats is probably due to aberration rather than VT—but therapeutically it doesn't matter.

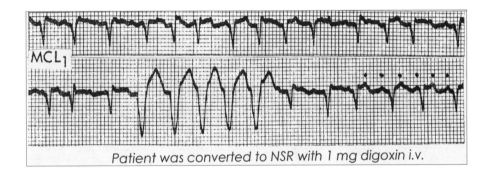

Patient was converted to NSR with 1 mg digoxin i.v.

Treatment

In this context (wide beats in presence of rapid response to atrial flutter or fibrillation), lidocaine is *CONTRAINDICATED*. (Unfortunately, it is often used, partly thanks to ACLS guidelines.) In fact, using lidocaine is a fourfold blunder!

(1) It breaks the "golden rule": RESTORE A NORMAL *VENTRICULAR* RATE. (Lidocaine is aimed at the ugly beats, not at the ventricular rate.)
(2) Lidocaine may do just the opposite: increase the already dangerous ventricular rate by slowing the atrial rate and favoring AV conduction.
(3) It amounts to treating what you're guessing at (VT), rather than what you're sure of (rapid ventricular response to atrial tachyarrhythmia).
(4) It delays correct therapy (digitalis, propranolol, diltiazem, or cardioversion).

ECG II-13

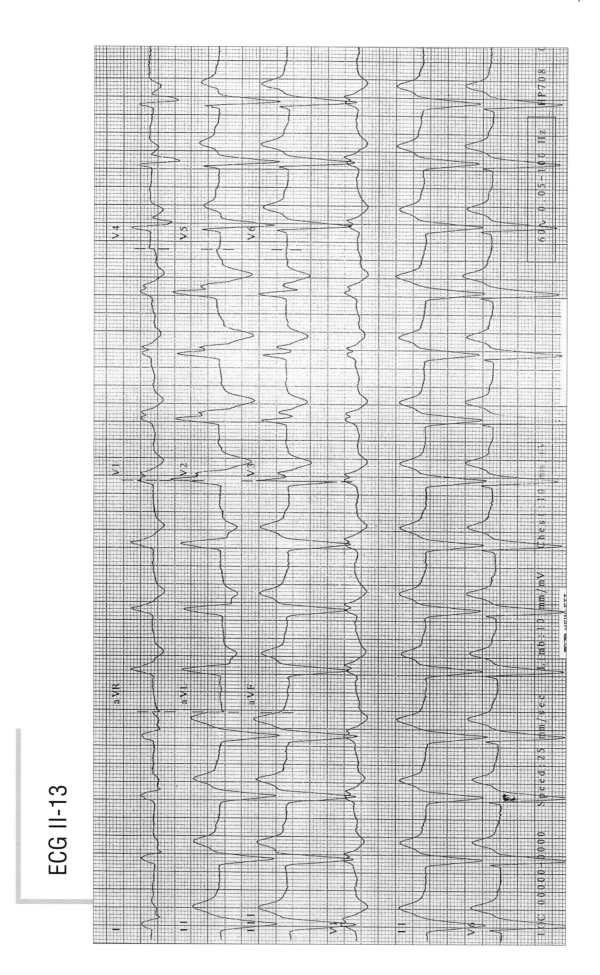

Diagnoses   **ECG II-13**

1. Accelerated idioventricular rhythm (rate = 85/min)

2. Underlying atrial rhythm is uncertain, but is probably atrial fibrillation

3. Misplaced electrodes

Clinical Data

Unknown

Comments

Obviously this is not as firm a diagnosis as some, but the **clues** that favor ventricular ectopy include:

- The QS complexes in 2, 3, aVF

- The rS complex in V6 with . . .

- . . . S wave of more than 15 mm depth

- QRS duration of 0.15 s.

The negative QRS (rS) complexes in V4–6 also serve to exclude accessory pathway conduction.

Did you spot the technician's error that concealed the best clue of all? The lead labeled V2 is obviously V1 with typical taller left "rabbit-ear"; lead V3 is really V2; and the lead labeled V1 is V3.

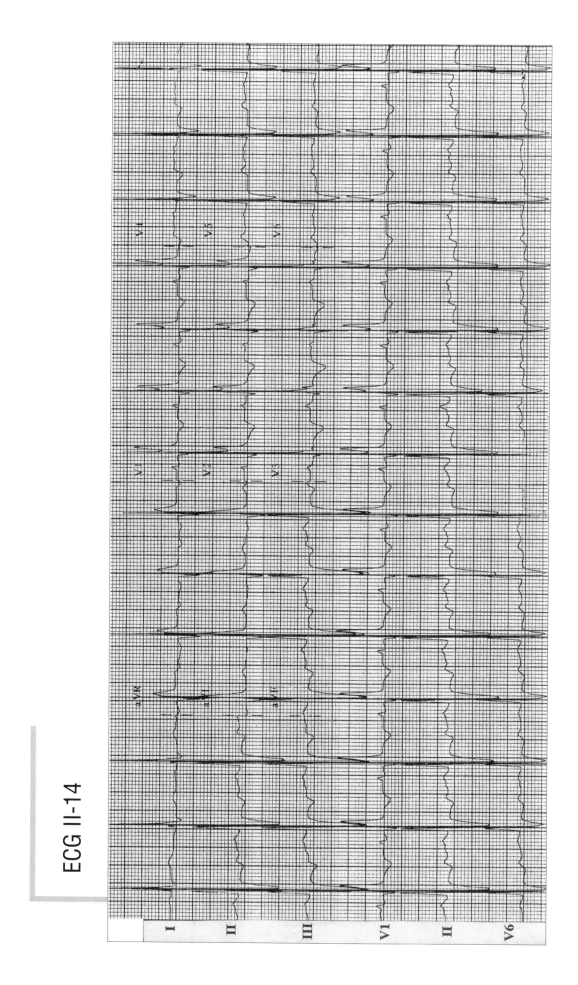

ECG II-14

Diagnoses

ECG II-14

1. Sinus rhythm with RBBB and left axis deviation

2. Right atrial hypertrophy

3. Ineffective electronic pacemaker in atrial-tracking mode

4. Old anteroseptal infarction

5. Primary T-wave changes—? ischemia

Clinical Data

Unknown

Comments

• The PR interval (0.18 s) is shorter than the programmed AV delay (apparently about 0.19 s); therefore, since AV conduction is intact, the pacemaker is frustrated (there is, at most, an element of fusion). You may wonder what the indication for implantation was—in view of the normal PR and BBB, perhaps at some point there was additional evidence of type II AV block.

• The left axis shift is not due to anterior hemiblock because it mainly involves the second half of the QRS, i.e., during activation of the *right* ventricle (by either natural or paced impulses—or both, which is fusion).

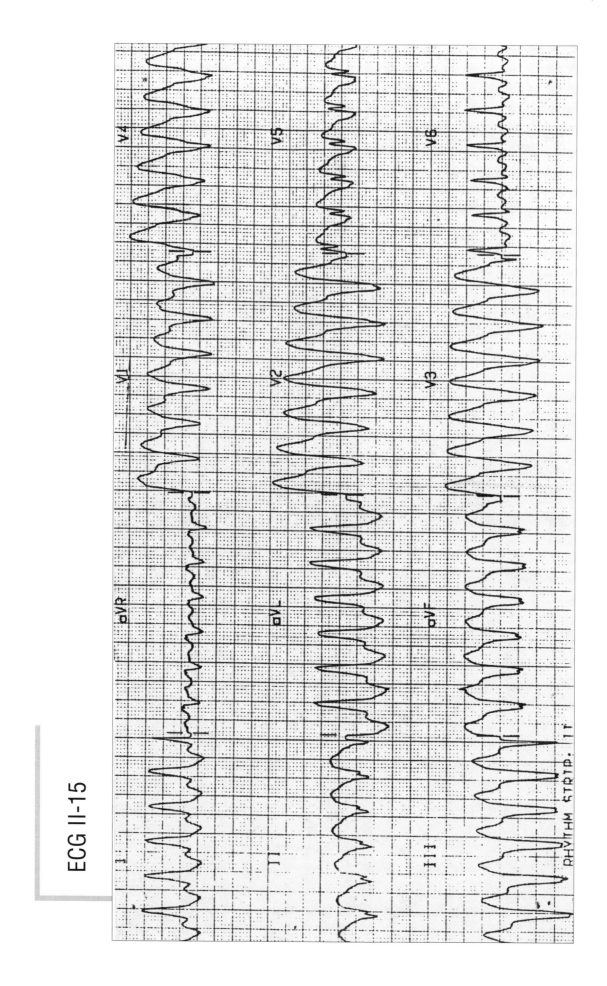

ECG II-15

Diagnoses

Right ventricular tachycardia (rate about 160/min)

Clinical Data

Unknown

Comments

Features in this tracing that are clues to ventricular ectopy are:

- QRS duration > 0.14 s (here 0.17 s)

- Delayed QS nadir in V1 reached in 0.08 s

- Delayed QRS peak in V6 reached only after 0.11 s

- Marked left axis with no R waves in leads 2, 3, and aVF (a pattern commonly seen in a known ectopic rhythm: right ventricular pacing).

ECG II-16

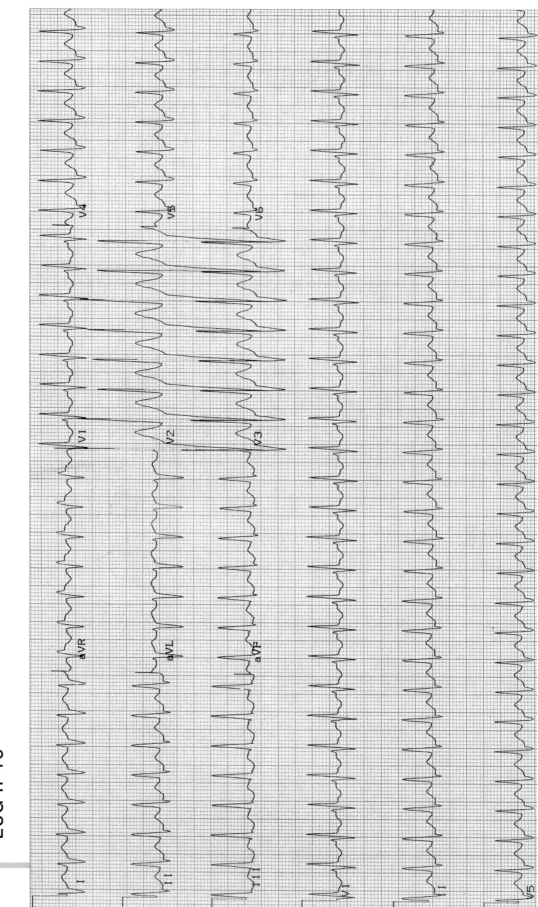

Diagnoses

ECG II-16

1. Supraventricular tachycardia (rate = 180/min), probably AV nodal reentrant tachycardia

2. Incomplete right bundle-branch block (QRS interval is 0.09 s)

3. Right axis deviation (+115 degrees)

Clinical Data

77-year-old woman

Comments

• The absence of any recognizable sign of atrial activity in all leads makes AV nodal reentrant tachycardia the most likely diagnosis.

• The rSR′ pattern in V1 is the unmistakable hallmark of RBBB.

ECG II-17

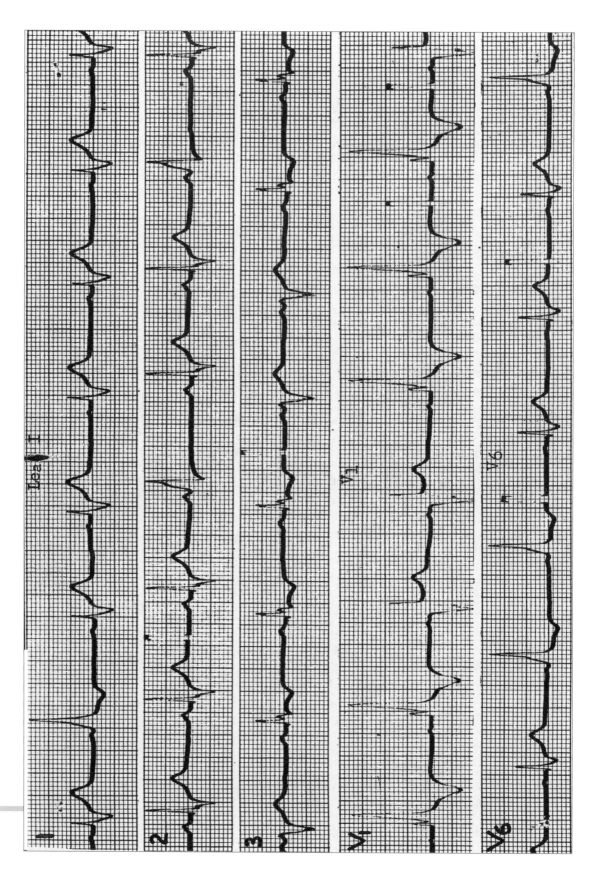

Diagnoses

ECG II-17

1. Sinus rhythm (rate = 60/min)

2. Right bundle-branch block

3. Intermittent preexcitation, WPW type

4. Possible right ventricular hypertrophy

Clinical Data

Unknown

Comments

• The 18-mm amplitude of the delayed R wave in the RBBB beats in V1 suggests RVH.

• Note the wide Q wave and elevated ST segment in the WPW beats in V1—a good example of how preexcitation can mimic the changes of myocardial infarction.

• The intermittent WPW is unexplained; it does *not* appear to be cycle (rate) related.

ECG II-18

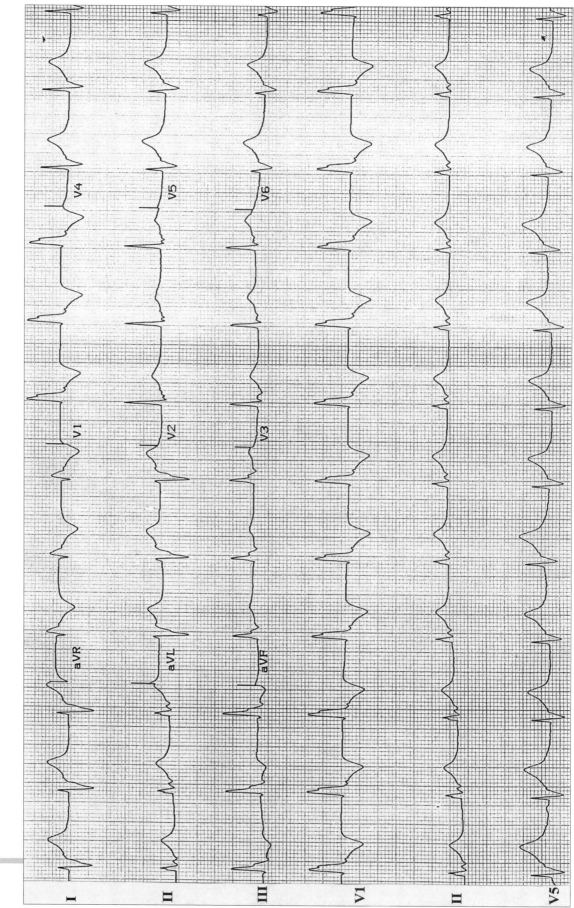

Diagnoses   **ECG II-18**

1. Accelerated idioventricular rhythm from LV (rate = 74/min) with . . .

2. . . . retrograde conduction to atria (retrograde P waves best seen in lead 2 [inverted] and V1 [upright])

Clinical Data

67-year-old man complaining of pulsations in neck

Comments

• The right axis deviation, early peak in V1, and rS shape in V6 all point to an ectopic ventricular rhythm.

• The pulsations were due to the cannon waves that resulted from each atrial contraction (atria contracting while tricuspid valve closed).

ECG II-19

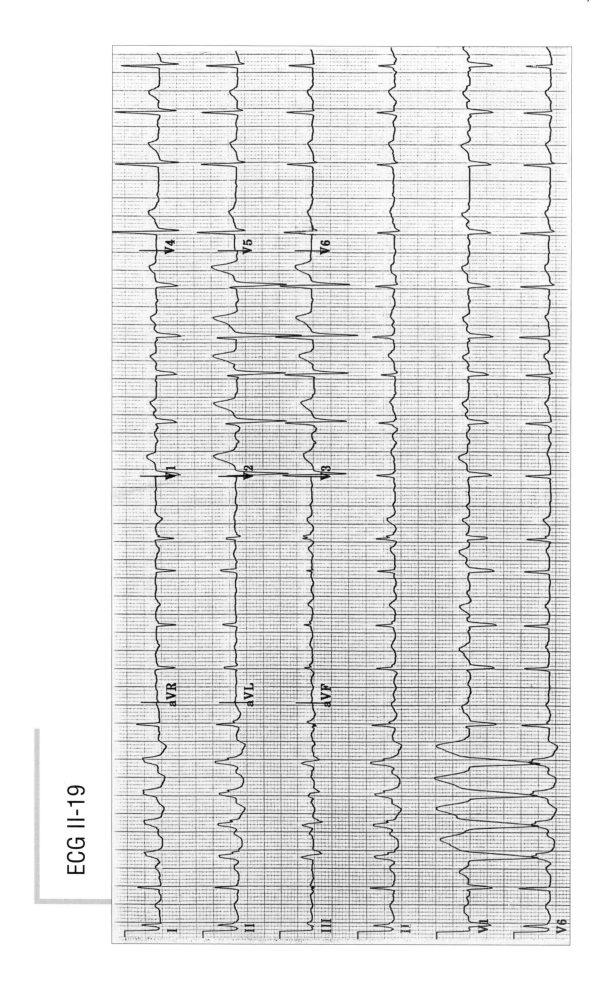

Diagnoses   **ECG II-19**

1. Atrial fibrillation, with rapid ventricular response (average rate about 115/min), including . . .

2. . . . a 4-beat run of LBBB aberration

Clinical Data

76-year-old man

Comment

Of course, you cannot be 100% sure that the run of wide QRSs is aberrant, but with a QRS interval of only 0.12 s, *with the QS nadir in V1 reached in only 0.04–0.05 s,* and with the normal frontal plane axis, ventricular ectopy is most unlikely.

ECG II-20

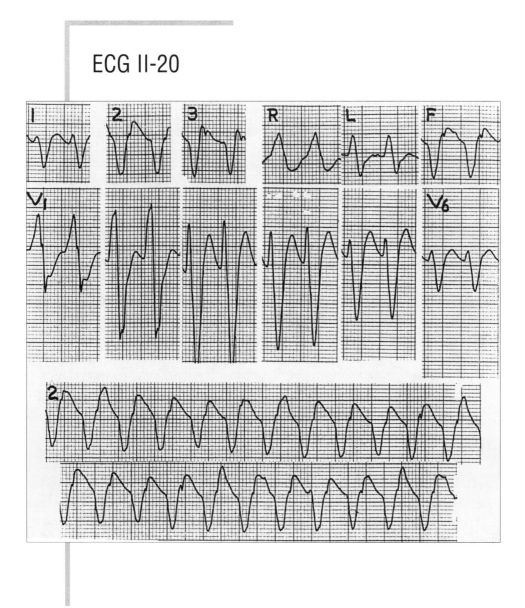

Diagnoses   ECG II-20

1. Ventricular tachycardia (rate = 150/min), dissociated from . . .

2. . . . sinus tachycardia at 120/min

Clinical Data

70-year-old man with palpitations and history of previous myocardial infarction

Comments

The features that favor the diagnosis of VT are:

- Axis in "no-man's land" (about −120 degrees)

- RS in V1

- rS in V6

- "Wide-wide" QRS (QRS interval 0.19 s)

- Dissociated atrial activity (arrows in strip of lead 2)

- Interval from beginning of QRS to nadir of S wave in any V lead > 0.10 s (here 0.17 s in V1)

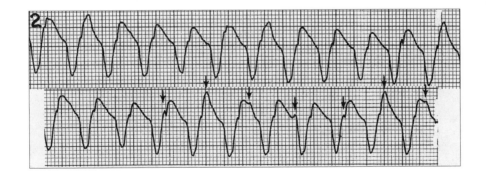

ECG II-21

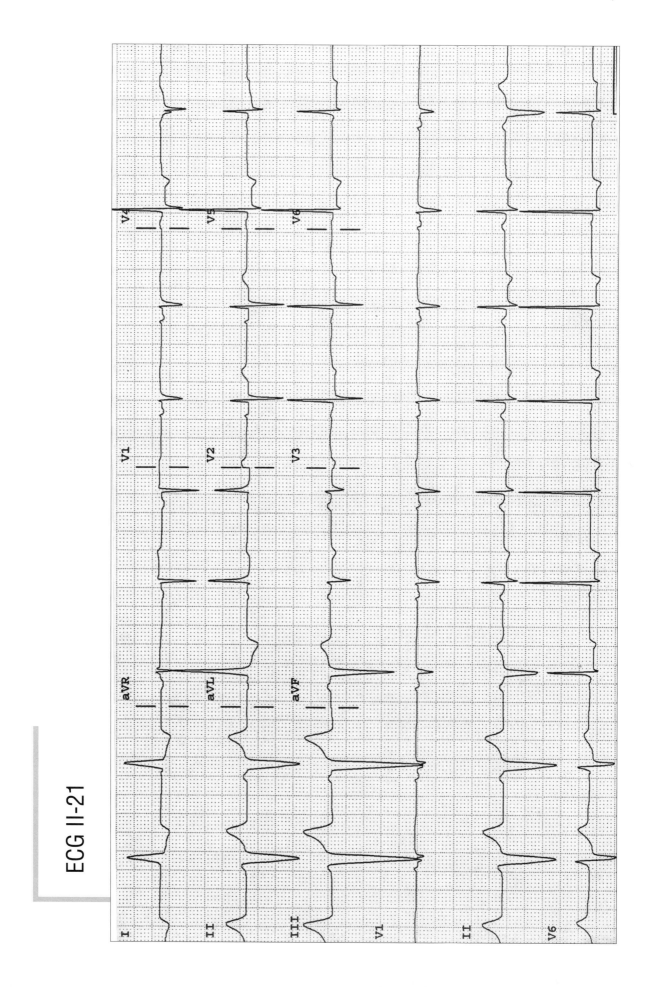

Diagnoses   **ECG II-21**

1. Accelerated idioventricular rhythm (rate = 60/min) competing with . . .

2. . . . sinus rhythm (rate also = 60/min) producing isorhythmic AV dissociation

3. Two fusion beats (3rd and last beats)

4. Left axis deviation of AIVR beats

5. QRS voltage in V6 (rhythm strip) suggests LVH

6. Nonspecific ST-T abnormalities in sinus beats suggest ischemia or may be secondary to LVH

Clinical Data

83-year-old woman with no complaints

Comment

Note QS (no initial R wave) complexes in the inferior leads, common in ectopy (see ECGs II.13 and II.15).

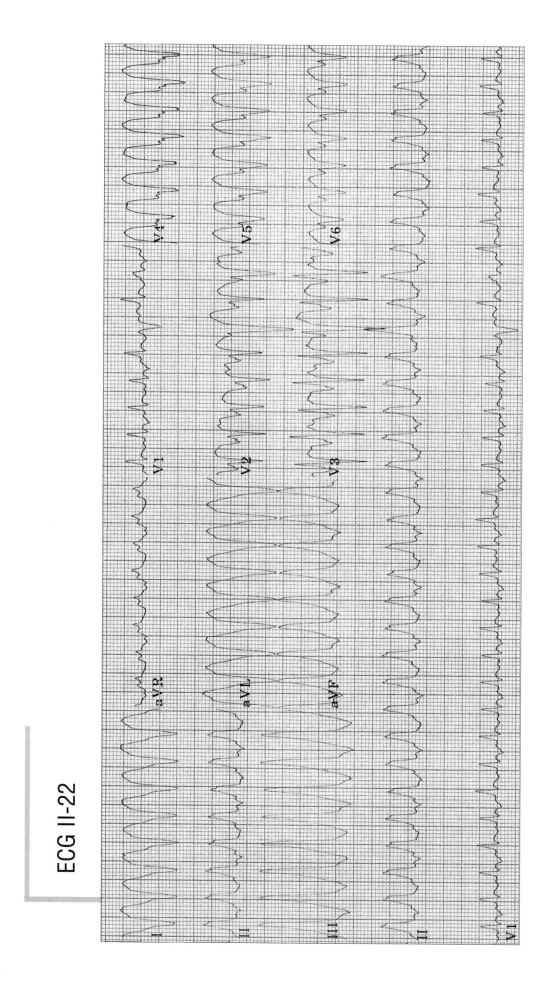

ECG II-22

Diagnoses   **ECG II-22**

1. Ventricular tachycardia (rate = 208/min) with . . .

2. . . . 2:1 retrograde conduction

3. One ventricular premature beat

Clinical Data

43-year-old man

Comments

Clues that favor VT are the right axis deviation, the 2:1 retrograde conduction, and the QS pattern in V6. Preexcited tachycardia is excluded by the negative complexes in V4–6; atrial and orthodromic tachycardias with aberration are excluded by the fewer P waves than QRS complexes.

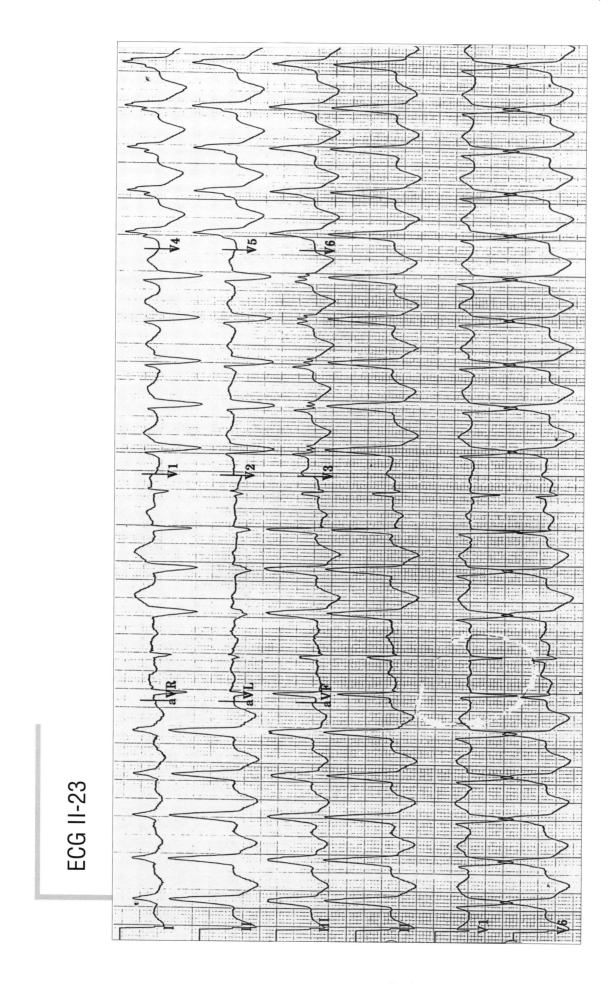

ECG II-23

Diagnoses

ECG II-23

1. Ventricular tachycardia, rate 130/min . . .

2. . . . dissociated from an atrial tachyarrhythmia, with . . .

3. . . . ventricular fusion and capture beats

Clinical Data

51-year-old man who woke with rapid heart beat; history of hypertrophic cardiomyopathy, ventricular tachycardia, and implanted defibrillator (which the rate of 130 was too slow to trigger)

Comments

• A normal QRS axis is unusual in VT.

• The only morphological clue to the diagnosis is the wide (> 0.04s) initial R wave in V1—typical of RV ectopy.

• Beats 6 and 10 are fusion beats (see ECG below, *F*), and 7 and 11 are capture beats (*C*) (or fusions?). Because each pair (6 and 7, 10 and 11) represents a rate faster than the ventricular rate, you can deduce that the dissociated atrial rhythm must be a faster tachycardia than the ventricular— perhaps atrial flutter at a rate slightly more than double the VT rate (say, 275/min) with 2:1 conduction, or perhaps atrial fibrillation. (After conversion, next day's tracing showed atrial fibrillation.)

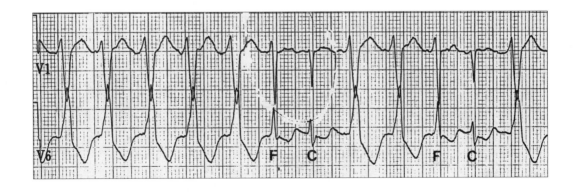

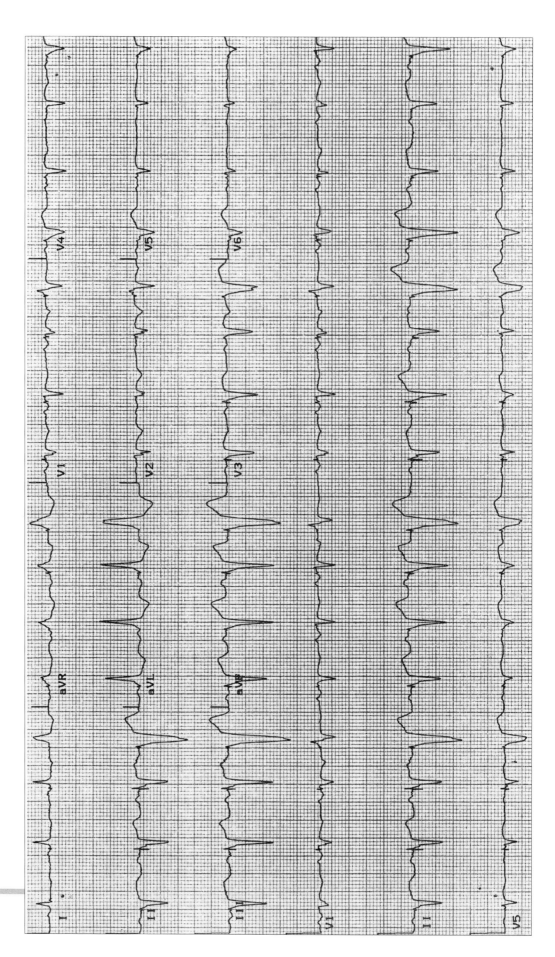

ECG II-24

Diagnoses   **ECG II-24**

1. Sinus rhythm with . . .

2. . . . electronic pacemaker in atrial-tracking mode

3. Numerous atrial premature beats

4. Varying degrees of ventricular fusion

Clinical Data

74-year-old woman

Comments

Note that the only fully paced ("captured") beats are three of the atrial prematures; all the other beats are fusion beats with varying contributions from the sinus impulse. The reason for this is that the earlier (premature) atrial impulses are conducted with more delay (RP/PR reciprocity, the hallmark of type I AV block; see Section V), and therefore the paced impulse has more time available to spread through the ventricles without interference from the atrial impulse.

ECG II-25

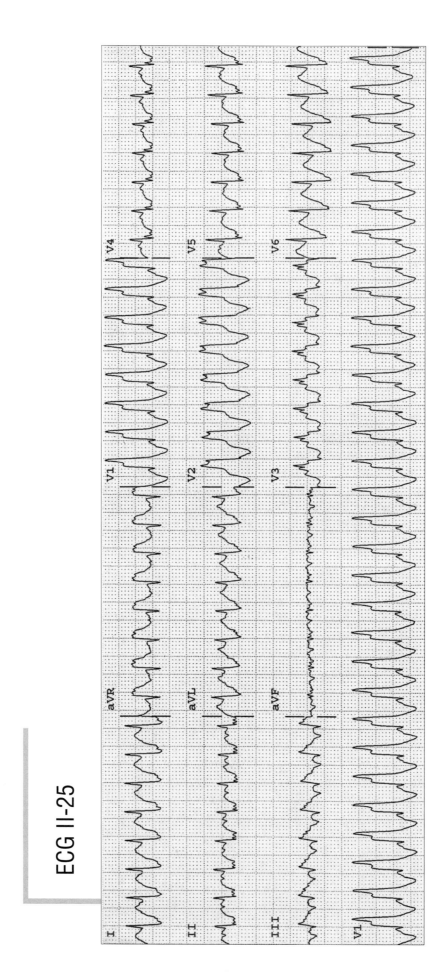

Diagnoses

1. Supraventricular tachycardia (rate = 188/min)—mechanism uncertain

2. Right bundle-branch block

Clinical Data

32-year-old woman with Ebstein's anomaly; converted with adenosine to sinus rhythm with RBBB

Comment

Inverted P waves, with RP > PR, are evident in the inferior leads, suggesting as the mechanism either "fast-slow" AV nodal reentrant tachycardia, or orthodromic tachycardia with slow-conducting accessory pathway.

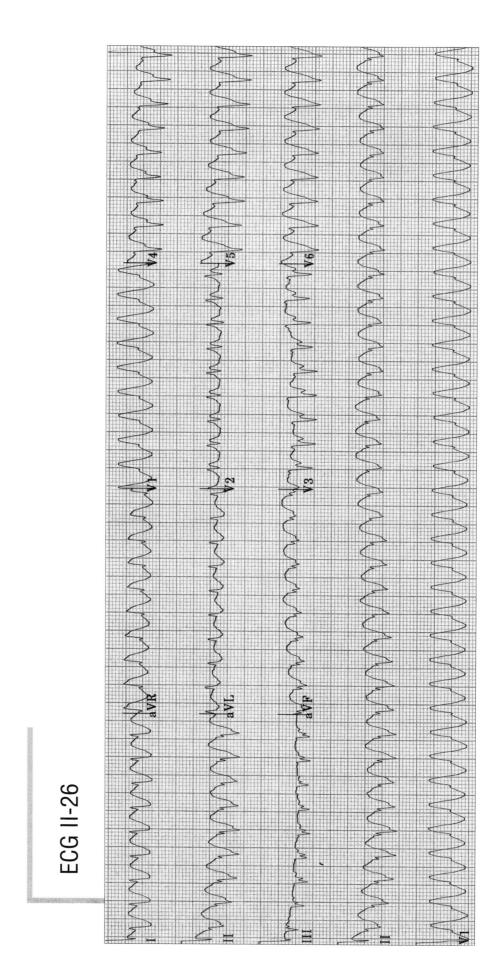

ECG II-26

Diagnosis   **ECG II-26**

Left ventricular tachycardia or SVT with aberration (rate = 222/min)

Clinical Data

42-year-old man, no history of heart attack or disease; tachycardia failed to respond to lidocaine, promptly converted with adenosine. Computer interpretation: atrial flutter.

Comments

Clues favoring VT are: (a) axis in upper right quadrant ("no-man's land"), (b) single peak in V1, and (c) rS configuration in V6. The first is a potent clue; the other two are relatively weak.

But the patient's age, lack of cardiac history (except for five paroxysms of tachycardia in the past 3 years), and response to adenosine all argue for supraventricular tachycardia.

- Which is it?

  Answer: SVT with aberration. A previous tracing shows an unmistakable SV tachy at about the same rate. Its lead V1 shows alternation (see ECG below). Therefore, the most likely mechanism is orthodromic tachycardia.

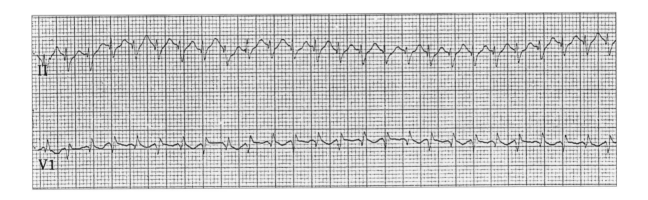

ECG II-27

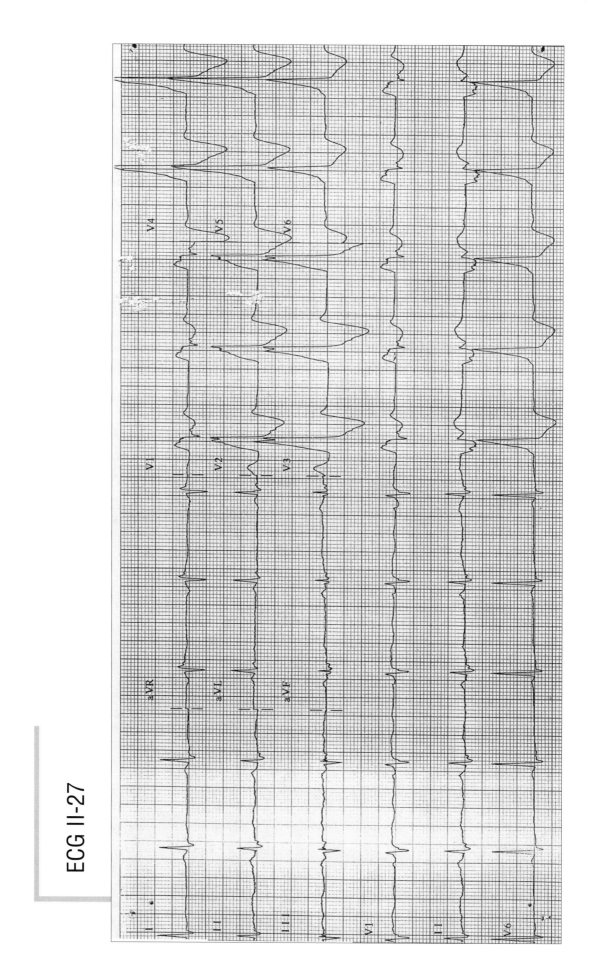

Diagnoses   **ECG II-27**

1. Sinus rhythm (rate = 62/min) interrupted by . . .

2. . . . accelerated idioventricular rhythm (rate = 61/min) with . . .

3. . . . retrograde conduction to atria

4. Nonspecific ST-T abnormalities

Clinical Data

70-year-old man with recent-onset angina

Comments

Note:

• Characteristic morphologic features of left ventricular ectopy: early peak in V1 and positive concordance V1–6

• The AIVR begins with a *premature* beat, which is unusual and should make you think of a possible parasystolic mechanism.

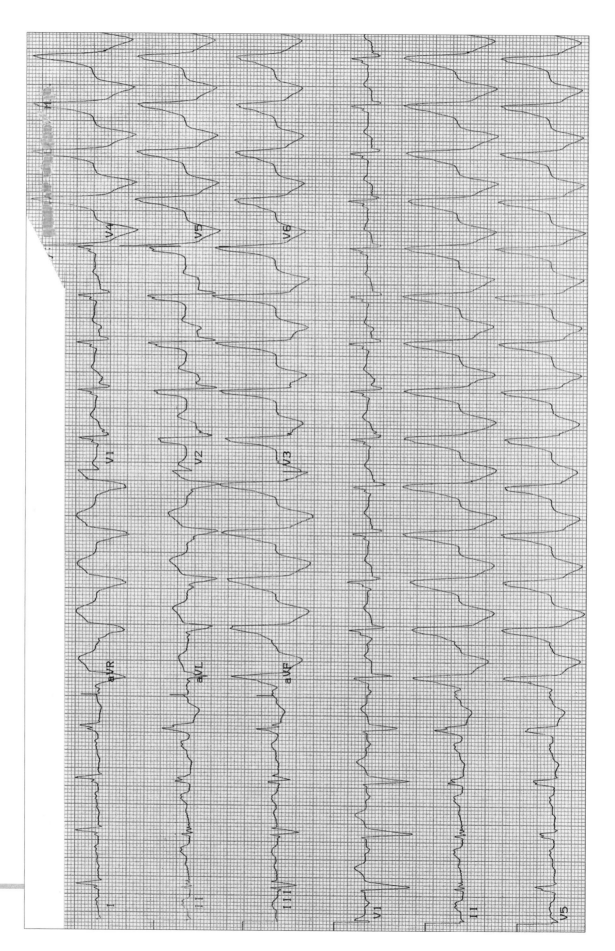

ECG II-28

Diagnoses   **ECG II-28**

1. Left atrial abnormality/intra-atrial block

2. Ventricular tachycardia (rate = 112/min) dissociated from . . .

3. . . . sinus tachycardia (rate = 105/min) producing . . .

4. . . . three fusion beats (beats 3, 4, and 5)

5. Left bundle-branch block with left axis deviation

Clinical Data

65-year-old man

Comment

P waves are wider than 0.11 s and are notched with peaks > 0.04 s apart; also, the P-terminal force in V1 is > 0.04 mm/s.

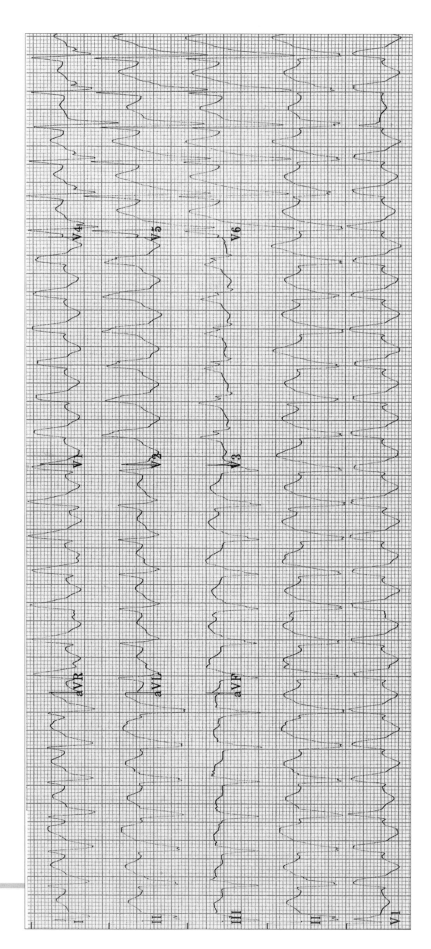

ECG II-29

Diagnoses   **ECG II-29**

1. Left ventricular tachycardia (rate = 156/min), dissociated from . . .

2. . . . sinus tachycardia (rate = 102/min) with . . .

3. . . . occasional capture (see ECG below, *C*) and fusion (*F*) beats

Clinical Data

75-year-old man with severe three-vessel disease and congestive heart failure

Comments

The clues that make the diagnosis of VT virtually certain from the ECG are:

- The axis in the right upper quadrant

- The independent atrial activity (best seen in lead 2), with capture and fusion beats (best seen in lead V1)

- Other helpful, but less powerful, clues in V6 are the RS (no q) pattern and the negative (S) deflection > 15 mm.

- The ST elevation in the capture beat in V1 suggests underlying anteroseptal injury.

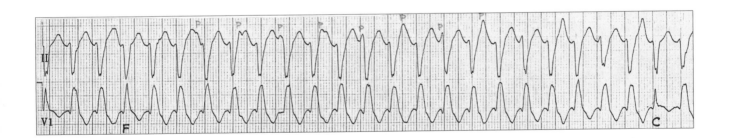

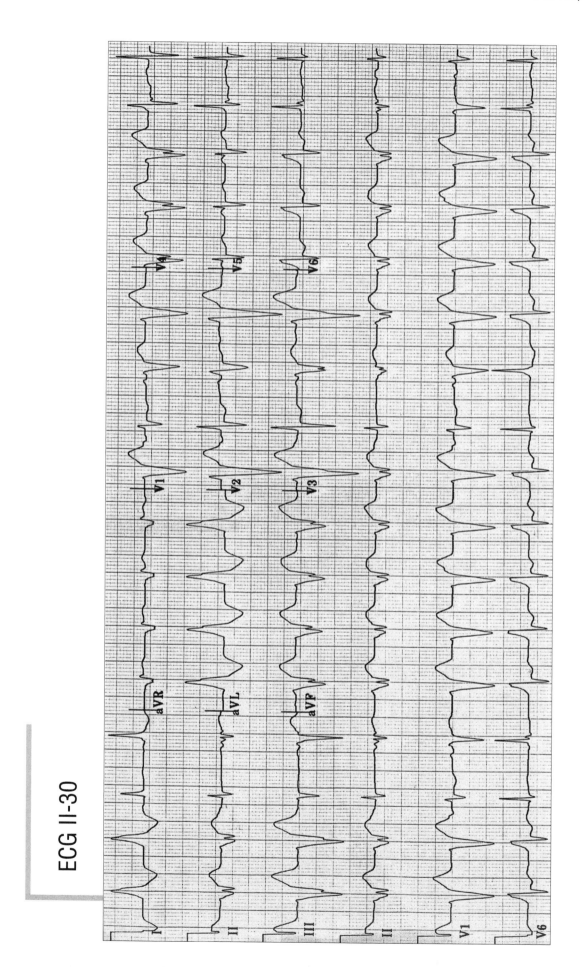

ECG II-30

Diagnoses   **ECG II-30**

1. Ventricular tachycardia (rate = 101/min) dissociated from . . .

2. . . . sinus rhythm (rate = 85/min)

3. Beats 3, 10, and 17 are ventricular captures (conducted sinus beats), but you cannot exclude a little fusion.

4. Beats 4, 11, and 16 are ventricular fusion beats.

5. Nonspecific ST-T abnormalities in the sinus beats

Clinical Data

72-year-old diabetic woman

Comments

• At a rate of 101/min, should we call it VT or AIVR?

• If there were any thought that the wide-QRS mechanism might be junctional with aberration, the three points that substantiate the diagnosis of ventricular ectopy are the delayed QRS nadir (0.09 s) in V1, delayed QRS peak (0.11 s) in V6, and the fusion beats.

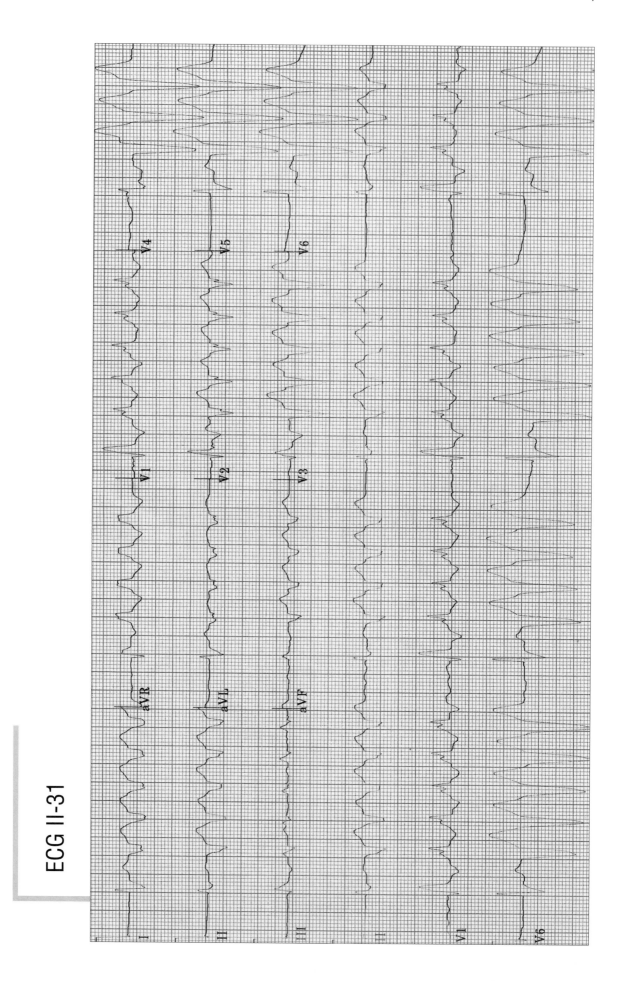

ECG II-31

Diagnoses   **ECG II-31**

1. Atrial fibrillation with . . .

2. . . . RBBB, interrupted by . . .

3. . . . four and five-beat runs of left ventricular tachycardia

4. The conducted beats show evidence of possible old inferior infarction and of current lateral ischemia.

Clinical Data

82-year-old man

Comments

Clues that indicate ventricular tachycardia include:

- The axis in "no-man's land"

- The QS complex in V6

- The negative QRS of more than 15-mm depth in V6.

The negative QRS (QS) complexes in V4–6 also serve to exclude accessory pathway conduction.

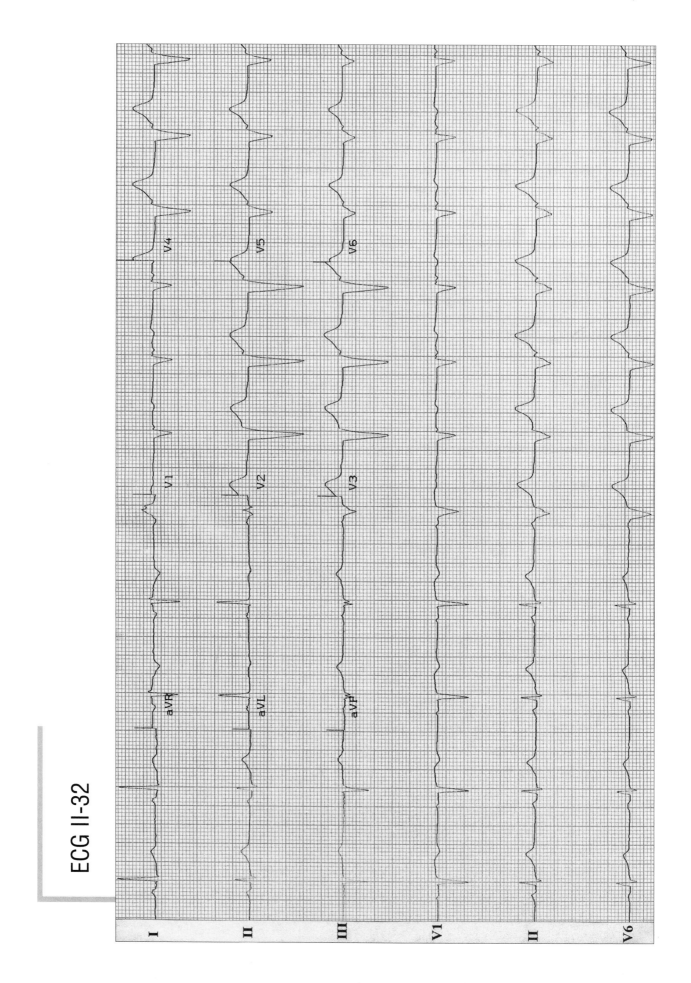

ECG II-32

Diagnoses   **ECG II-32**

1. Sinus rhythm (rate = 60/min) interrupted by . . .

2. . . . accelerated idioventricular rhythm at rate 75/min with . . .

3. . . . retrograde conduction to atria beginning with 3rd beat

4. T-wave abnormality

Clinical Data

40-year-old woman

Comments

The first beat of the AIVR shows minimal fusion; the second is dissociated; and retrograde atrial activation begins with the third beat.

The T wave is abnormally inverted in aVL, with a QRS-T angle of about 75° (the upper normal limit is about 45°). The QRS axis is about $-10°$, with the T wave axis about $+65°$.

Note the negative concordance of the ectopic rhythm, typical of right ventricular ectopy (e.g., see most paced rhythms).

ECG II-33

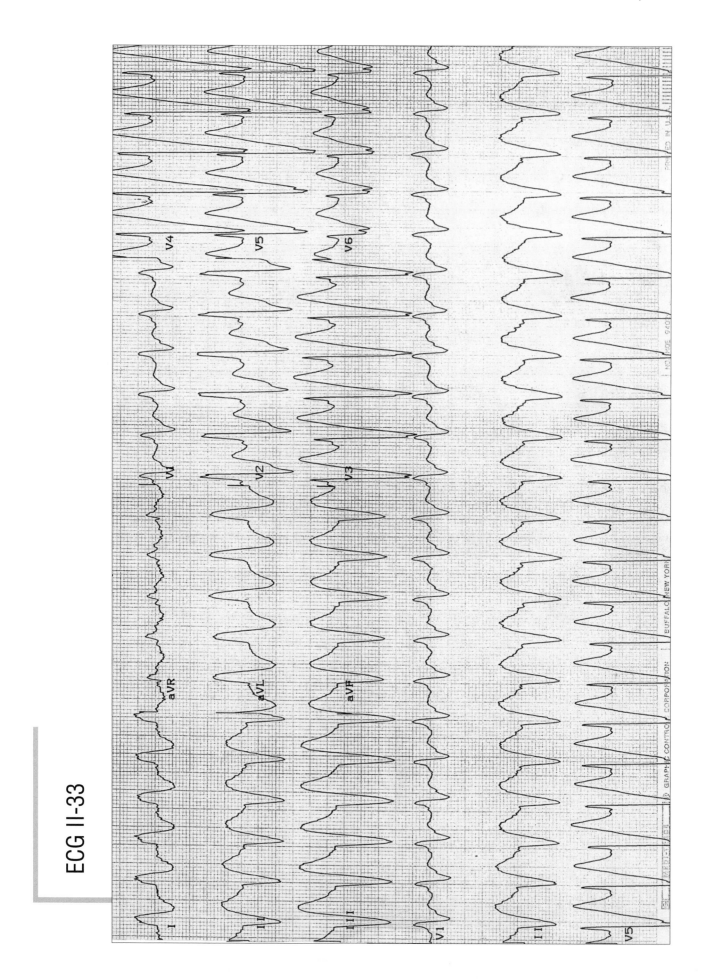

Diagnoses

1. Probable ventricular tachycardia, rate 134/min with . . .

2. . . . probable 1:1 retrograde conduction to atria

Clinical Data

84-year-old man with dyspnea and chest pain

Comments

Nothing is 100%, but the following clues give us about a 90% probability of VT:

- The interval from beginning of QRS to nadir of S wave in V1 is 0.12 s (i.e., > 0.10 s).

- There is an rS complex in V6.

- The left axis has monophasic complexes in 1, 2, 3, and aVF. Preexcitation is excluded by the negative QRSs in V4–6.

There appear to be P waves in a 1:1 relationship to the QRSs (best seen in lead 2); therefore, if this *is* VT, they must be retrograde. (Retrograde conduction to the atria occurs in about 50% of VTs.)

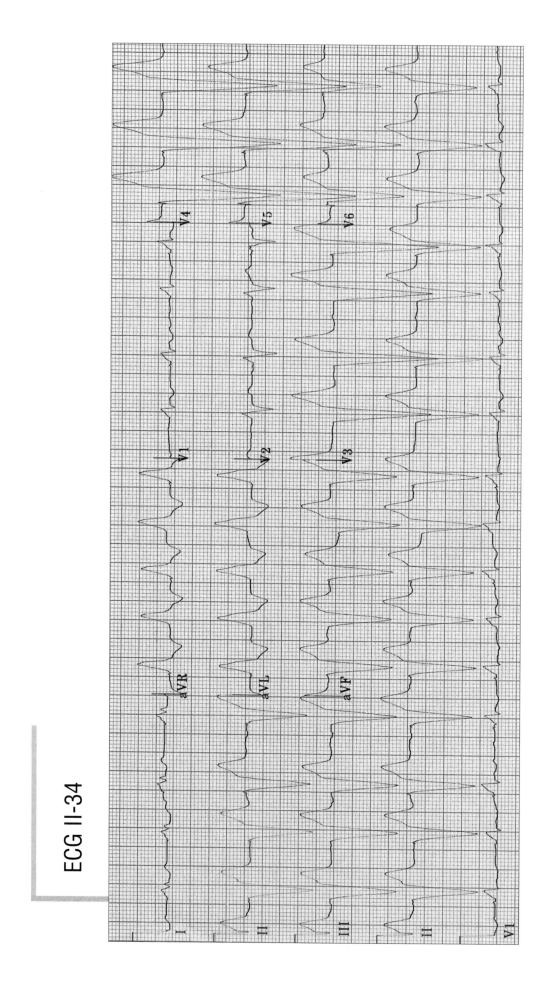

ECG II-34

Diagnoses   **ECG II-34**

1. Atrial fibrillation

2. Atrial-tracking electronic pacemaker

Clinical Data

80-year-old man

Comments

The computer diagnosed sinus rhythm with right bundle-branch block, and inferior and possibly antero-lateral infarcts of uncertain age.

Pacemaker blips are almost impossible to recognize except with the first beat in V4–6 and in one or two other isolated spots.

Section III

Supraventricular Arrhythmias

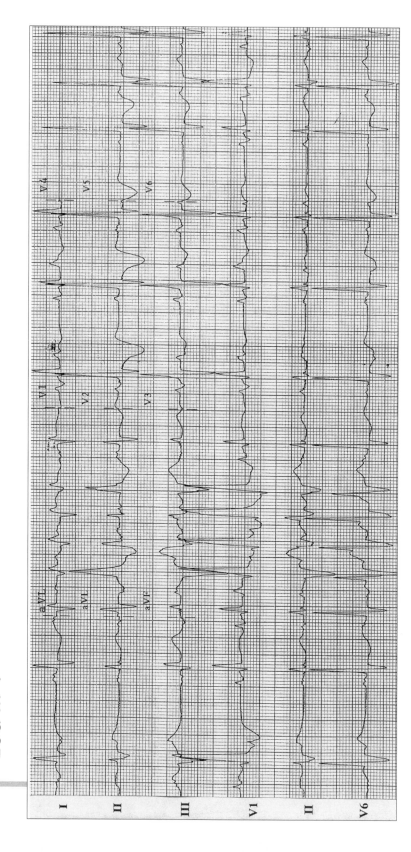

ECG III-1

Diagnoses   **ECG III-1**

1. Atrial premature beats and short bursts of irregular atrial tachycardia (several nonconducted beats)

2. Incomplete RBBB in conducted sinus beats

3. Complete RBBB and left anterior hemiblock aberration of several beats ending the shorter cycles

4. ? Right atrial enlargement (prominent positive P deflections in sinus beats in leads V1–3); also cannot exclude biventricular hypertrophy (tall RV2, high voltage V5–6)

5. ST-T abnormalities suggesting significant anterior ischemia

Clinical Data

66-year-old man complaining of shortness of breath and palpitations

Comments

None

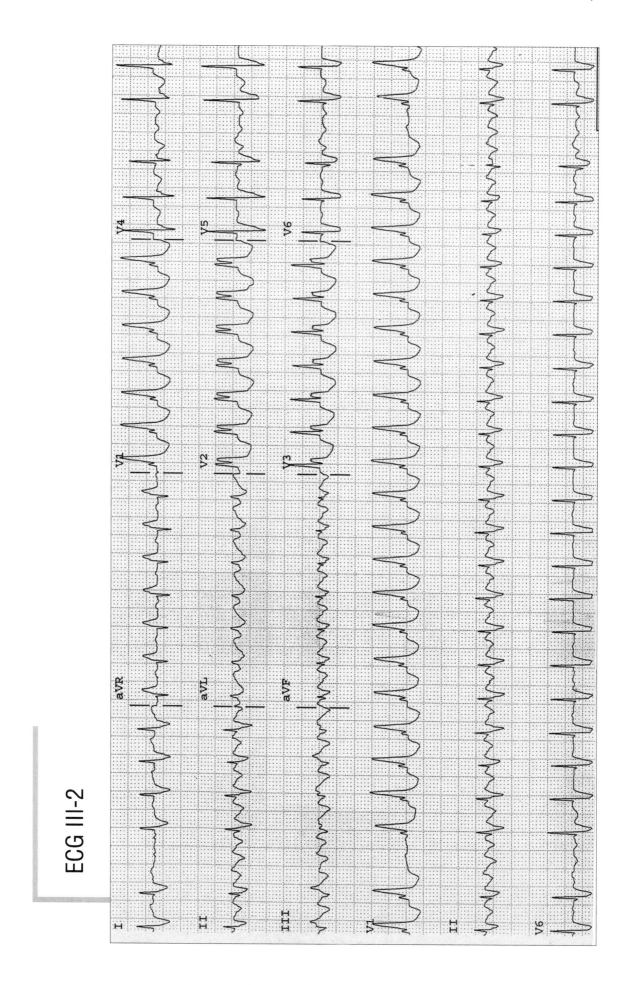

ECG III-2

Diagnoses   **ECG III-2**

1. Atrial flutter (atrial rate = 330/min) with mostly 2:1 AV conduction (4:1 on two occasions)

2. Right bundle-branch block

Clinical Data

56-year-old man

Comments

None

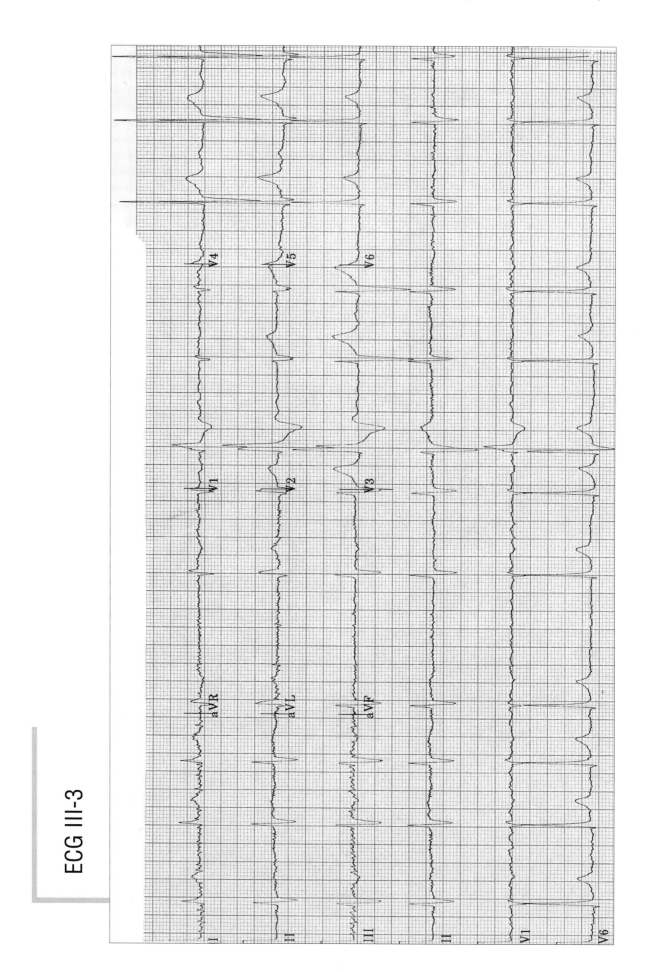

ECG III-3

Diagnoses

ECG III-3

1. Atrial fibrillation with moderate ventricular response (ventricular rate = 65–70/min)

2. Left axis deviation (axis −50°, ? left anterior hemiblock)

3. One aberrantly (RBBB) conducted beat

4. Probable left ventricular hypertrophy

5. Significant concealed conduction into the AV node (accounting for the controlled rate and cycle of 1.4 s)

Clinical Data

83-year-old man

Comments

The aberrant beat, ending a cycle of 0.47 s, shows that the AV node is capable of conducting at a rate well over 100/min; but bombardment and unpredictable partial penetration of the node ("concealed conduction") by the fibrillating impulses keeps it somewhat refractory and accounts for the normal ventricular rate and the varying cycle length, including the occasional long cycle. *Clinically,* this is the most practical aspect of concealed conduction.

Tall, pointed T waves associated with increased QRS voltage in V5–6 suggest LV *diastolic* overloading—? mitral regurgitation.

ECG III-4

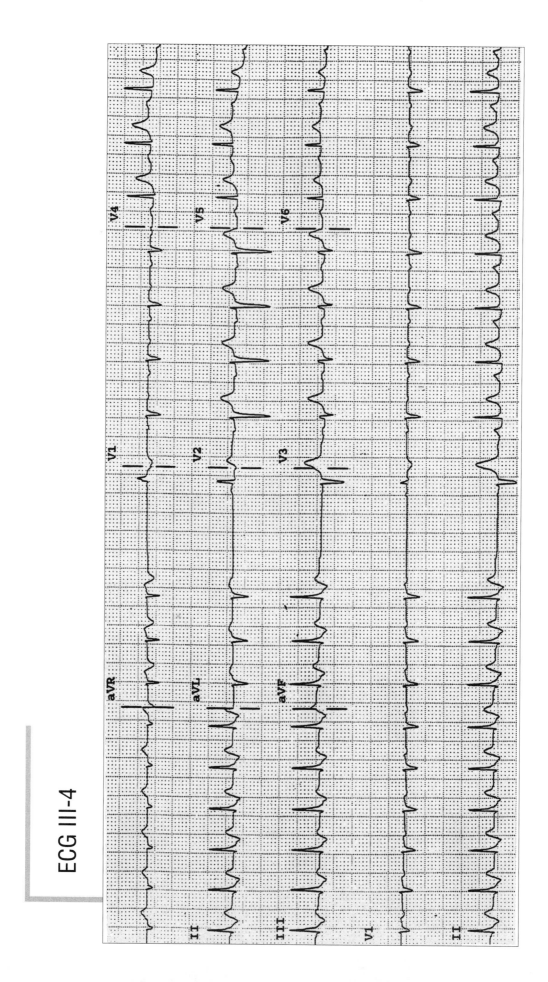

Diagnoses   **ECG III-4**

1. Orthodromic tachycardia (rate = about 135/min), terminating in the anterograde limb of the reentrant circuit

2. Atrial escape with ventricular aberration

3. Sinus tachycardia (rate = 102/min)

4. Vertical QRS axis (about +95 degrees)

Clinical Data

30-year-old woman with WPW syndrome

Comments

• "Orthodromic" = down the AV junction and up an accessory pathway—the most common SVT in the WPW syndrome.

• It may be useful to note the "weak link" in the reentrant circuit, because if prophylactic therapy is an option, it makes sense to attack the weakest limb of the circuit. Here it is the anterograde path (i.e., the AV node) because, when the paroxysm ends, the final event inscribed is the retrograde P wave; thus, a beta-blocker would be a reasonable choice.

• Note that the cycle of the orthodromic tachycardia is gradually lengthening (from 42 to 47) as the AV node "tires" before finally blocking and interrupting the circulating wave.

ECG III-5

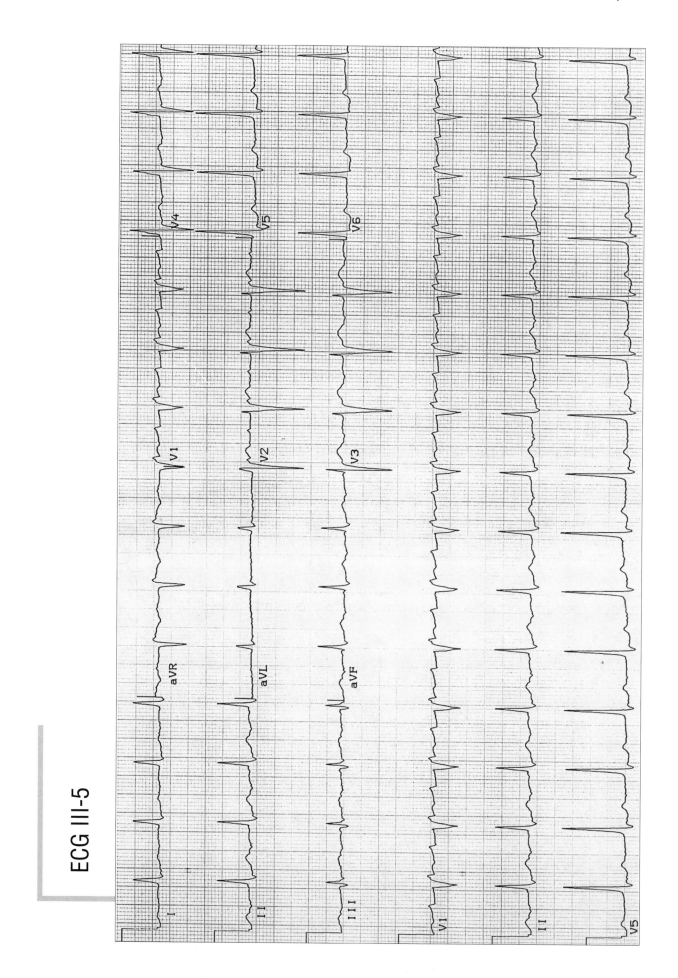

Diagnoses   **ECG III-5**

1. Atrial tachycardia (rate = 188/min) with 2:1 AV conduction

2. ST-T abnormalities in leads 1, 2, V5, and V6

Clinical Data

74-year-old woman complaining of palpitations and pulsations in her neck

Comment

Note that the only leads from which you can be sure of the arrhythmic diagnosis are V1 and V2, while lead 2 is virtually useless.

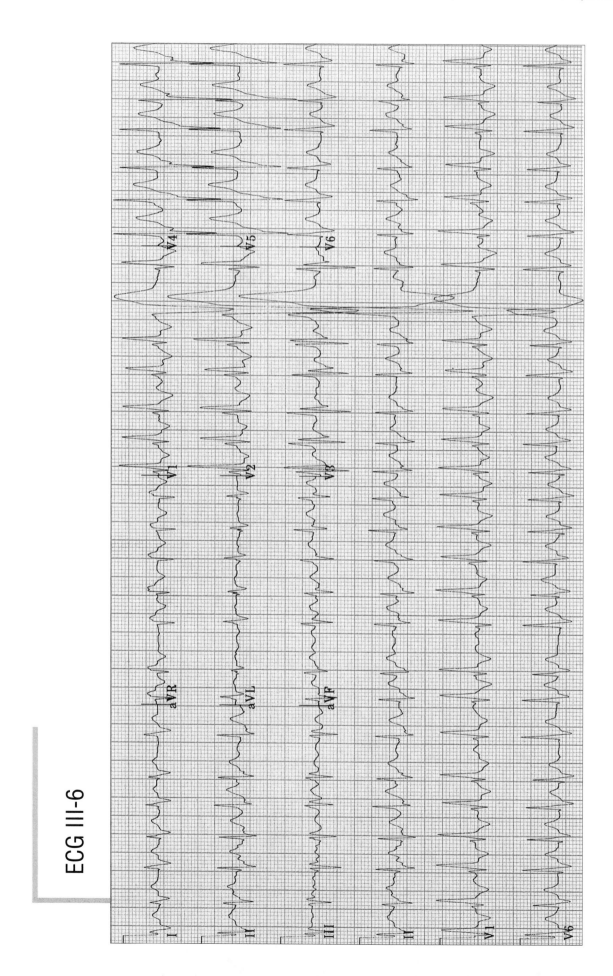

ECG III-6

Diagnoses   **ECG III-6**

1. Atrial fibrillation with rapid ventricular response (rate = about 165/min)

2. Right bundle-branch block

3. One right ventricular extrasystole

Clinical Data

89-year-old woman

Comments

• In the presence of atrial fibrillation, you don't know when to expect the next beat, so it makes no sense to call ectopic ventricular beats "premature"; it is more appropriate to fall back on the tongue-twisting "extrasystole."

• Note that this RV ectopic, as usual, takes > 0.07 s (here about 0.09 s) to reach its nadir in V1 and its peak in V6—helpful clues in differentiating RV ectopy from LBBB.

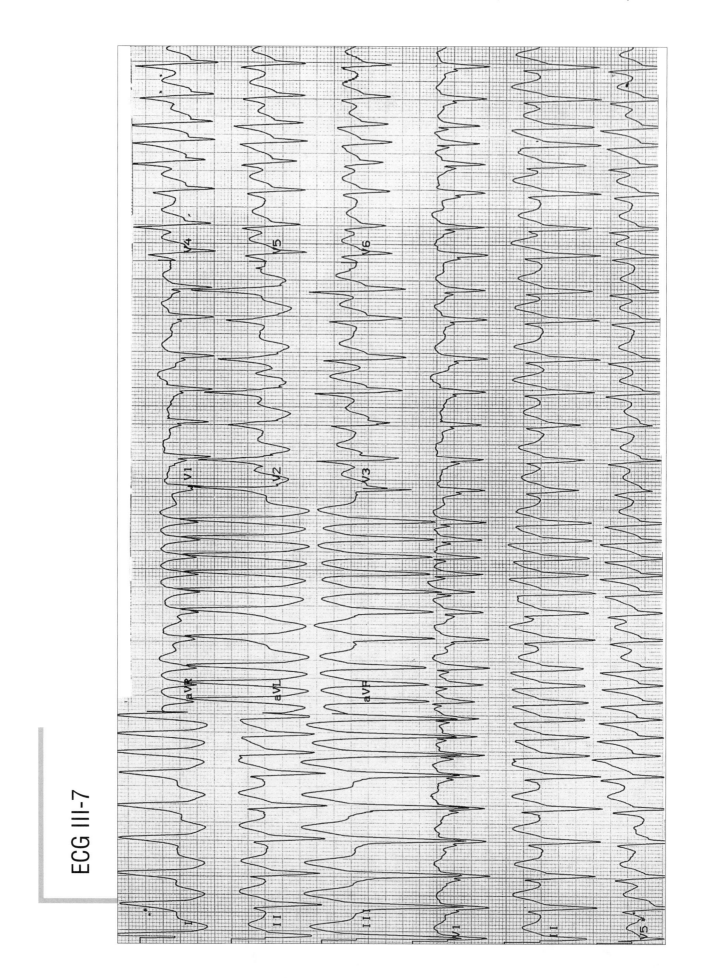

ECG III-7

Diagnosis   **ECG III-7**

Atrial fibrillation with AV conduction via an accessory pathway (WPW syndrome)

Clinical Data

39-year-old man with palpitations

Comments

Between 1940 and 1970, these types of ECGs often were diagnosed and published as ventricular tachycardia—part of the reason VT got the reputation for being irregular. Clues to the correct diagnosis here are:

• The extreme irregularity (making VT unlikely)

• The fact that some cycles represent a rate over 300/min (a rate rarely seen in VT, and much more likely to be due to accessory pathway conduction).

Below are this patient's chest leads during sinus rhythm, documenting preexcitation.

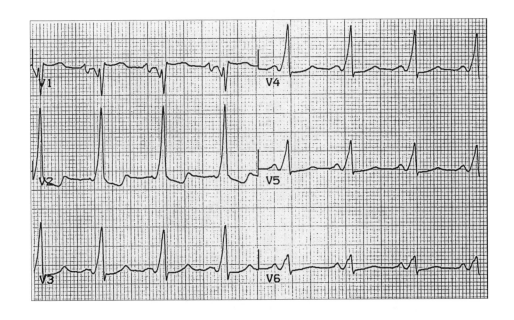

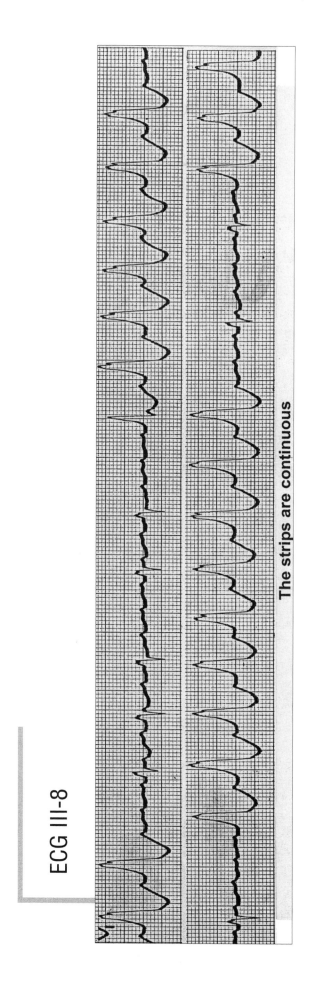

ECG III-8

The strips are continuous

Diagnoses   ECG III-8

1. Atrial tachycardia (? flutter) (rate = 230/min) with . . .

2. . . . bilevel pattern of conduction in junction: 2:1 conduction at upper level and 4:3 and 3:2 Wenckebachs at lower level (see laddergram below)

3. Ventricular tachycardia (rate = 115/min); paroxysm begins with fusion beat in middle of top strip

Clinical Data

Unknown

Comments

• As is often the case with atrial flutter and varying conduction, there is physiological 2:1 "filtering" of
the atrial impulses at an upper level in the junction, with Wenckebach conduction lower down from the
beats that pass the "filter."

• Although the diagnosis of VT is definite, 2 to 1 conduction with ventricular aberration must be
considered because the rate of the anomalous tachycardia is exactly half the atrial rate; and because
aberration can begin, rarely and paradoxically, with a late beat. However, the points defining VT are
strong: (a) the QRSs have a taller left peak, (b) the first beat of one run is a fusion beat, and (c)
aberration is much more likely to begin with a shorter, not longer, cycle.

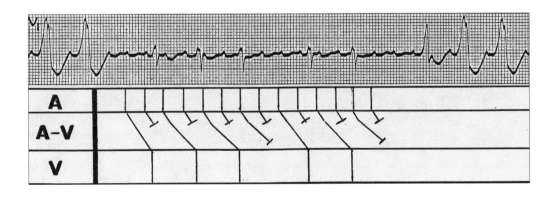

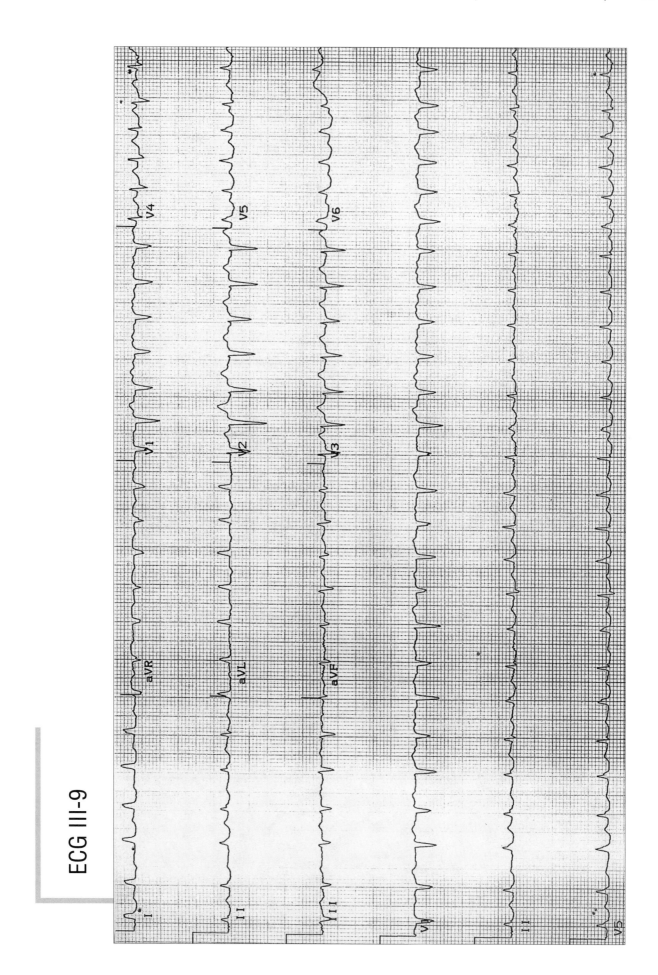

ECG III-9

Diagnoses   **ECG III-9**

1. Atrial fibrillation with rapid ventricular response (rate = 165/min)

2. Low voltage throughout

3. Tendency to QRS alternation (best seen in V1 rhythm strip)

4. Nonspecific ST-T abnormalities

Clinical Data

74-year-old woman with breast carcinoma and malignant pericardial effusion with tamponade

Comment

Note that the tendency to electrical alternans (often seen with pericardial effusion) is apparent, especially in lead V1, despite the ventricular irregularity from the atrial fibrillation.

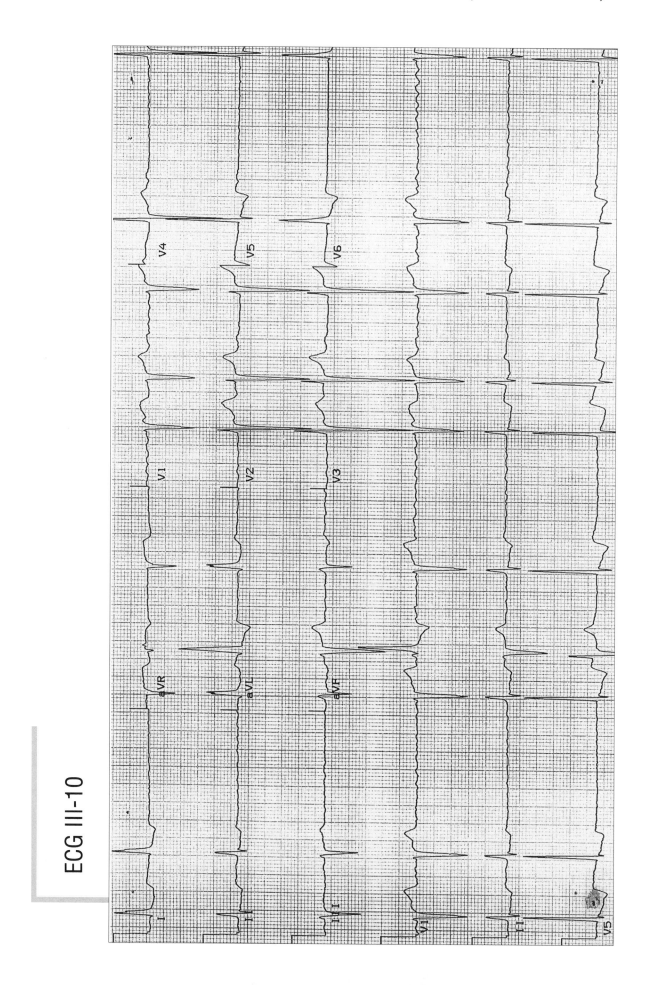

ECG III-10

Diagnoses   ## ECG III-10

1. Atrial fibrillation with slow to moderate ventricular response (50–60/min) and marked irregularity, its cycle rates ranging from 32/min to 125/min owing to the variable effect of concealed conduction

2. One aberrantly (RBBB + LAHB) conducted beat

3. Left ventricular hypertrophy with borderline left-axis deviation

Clinical Data

53-year-old man, hypertensive, short of breath, and aware of irregular heart beat

Comments

The diagnoses are relatively easy, but the importance of **concealed conduction** in clinical decision-making is often overlooked. The aberrantly conducted beat and the 7th beat show that his AV junction has no difficulty in conducting at rates well over 100/min. His long cycles are therefore due to the effect of superimposed concealed conduction into the junction and *not* to significant AV block. Unfortunately, those long cycles are likely to generate the urge to implant a pacemaker. This patient could be converted to sinus rhythm, thereby eliminating the frenetic atrial activity and the concealed conduction that goes with it. The shorter cycles make it clear that he is capable of AV conduction at rates over 100/min. A pacemaker is clearly not indicated—until and unless a trial of restored sinus rhythm has been undertaken and found wanting.

ECG III-11

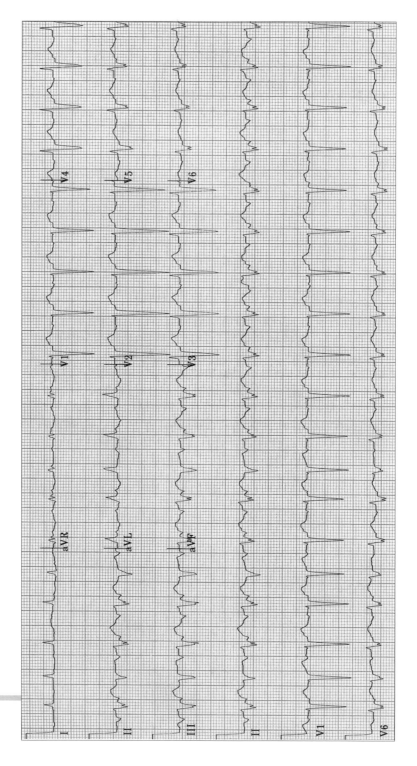

Diagnoses

ECG III-11

1. Atrial tachycardia (rate = 212/min) with alternating 2:1 and 3:2 (Wenckebach) AV conduction (see laddergram below)

2. Left axis deviation ($-60°$)

3. Nonspecific ST-T abnormality

Clinical Data

65-year-old man

Comments

• You cannot exclude anterior hemiblock, but the appropriate increased QRS voltage is lacking.

• Although the ST-T is somewhat distorted by the atrial activity, these T-wave abnormalities are evident: low/diphasic T in lead 1, inverted T in aVL, TV1 taller than TV6.

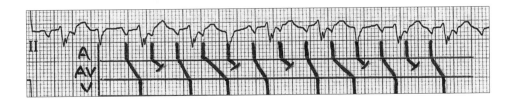

ECG III-12

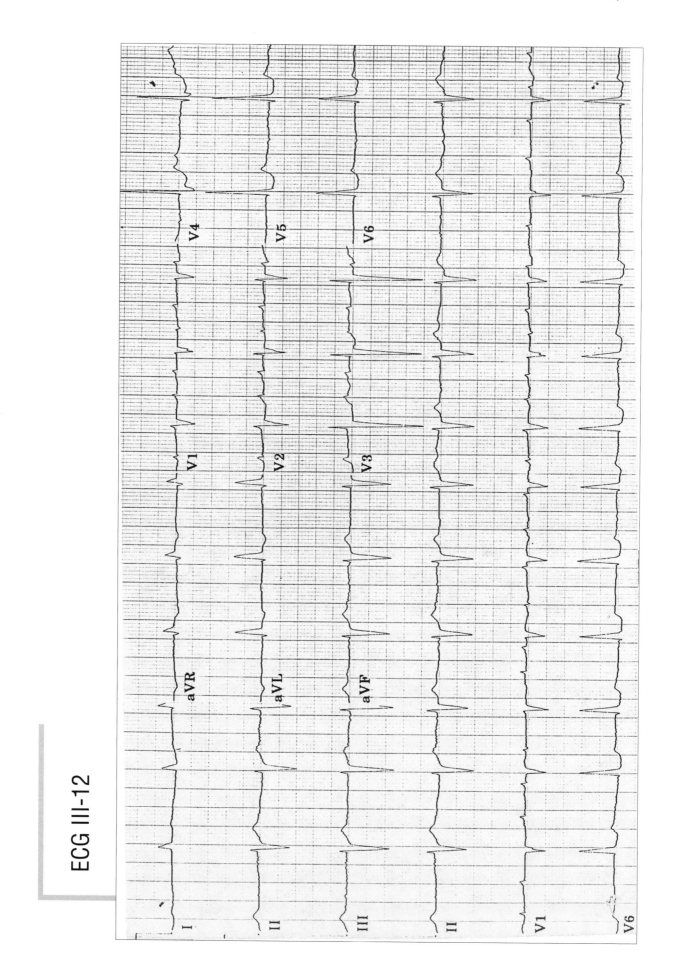

Diagnoses   **ECG III-12**

1. Irregular atrial tachycardia (rate = about 165/min) with . . .

2. . . . varying AV block and resulting ventricular rate of 75/min

3. Probable digitalis effect and intoxication

4. Left anterior hemiblock (axis about $-70°$)

5. Possible LVH

Clinical Data

86-year-old man on prednisone, aspirin, and digoxin

Comments

The computer and overreader interpreted this rhythm as atrial fibrillation. However, the ST-T configuration in V4–6 suggests digitalis effect, while the arrhythmia ("PAT with block") points to intoxication—neither of which are likely to be recognized if the rhythm is mistaken for atrial fibrillation!

ECG III-13

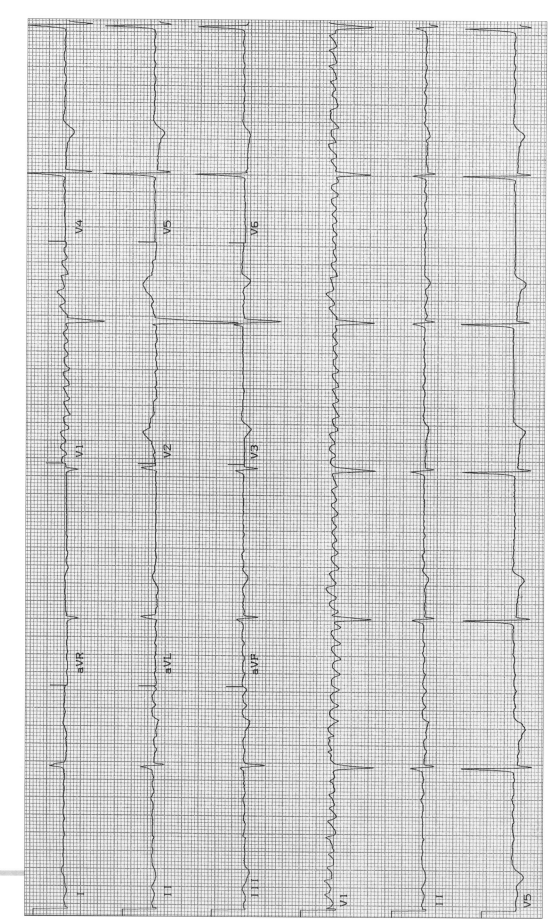

Diagnoses   **ECG III-13**

1. Atrial fibrillation

2. Complete AV block

3. Junctional escape rhythm (rate = 36/min)

4. ST-T abnormalities and prolonged QT interval

Clinical Data

92-year-old woman complaining of "lightheadedness"

Comments

• As here, atrial fibrillation often shows up best in V1, and sometimes is well seen *only* in V1.

• Always keep in mind that, in the presence of atrial fibrillation, block may not be as bad as it looks—because of the contribution of concealed conduction of innumerable impulses into the AV node keeping it refractory. It is always possible that sinus impulses at a reasonable rate could be conducted.

• The QT interval measures 0.60–0.64 s, yet at this slow rate of 36/min in a woman, the upper limit of normal is about 0.52 s.

ECG III-14

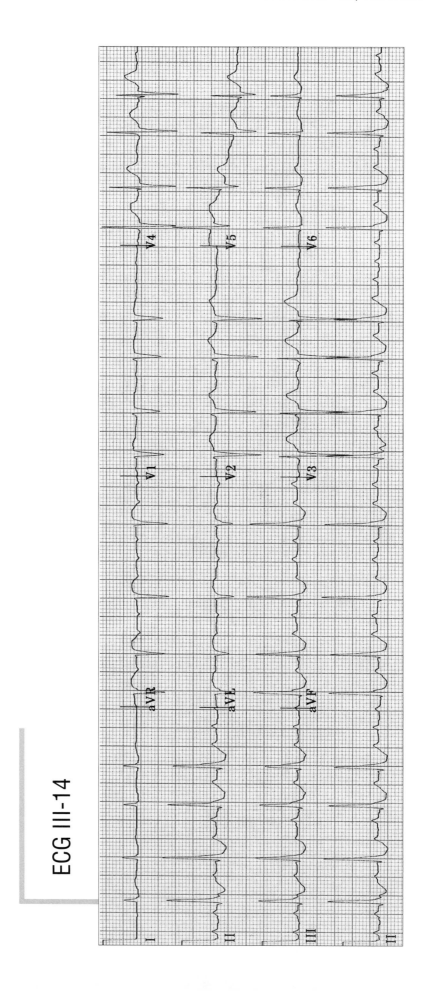

Diagnoses ECG III-14

1. Atrial flutter (rate = 299/min) with varying AV conduction (2:1, 3:1, 4:1, and 5:1)

2. Digitalis effect (suggested by sagging STs in all leads with positive QRSs)

Clinical Data

Not available

Comments

Although in this case there is a good mix of odd and even ratios, it is worth noting that as a *sustained* ratio the odd numbers are really rare, i.e., 2:1 and 4:1 are far more common conduction ratios in atrial flutter than 1:1, 3:1, and 5:1.

Note also that the usual "sawtooth" waves of atrial flutter are not seen in the inferior leads—the flutter waves look like discrete P′ waves with an isoelectric baseline between them.

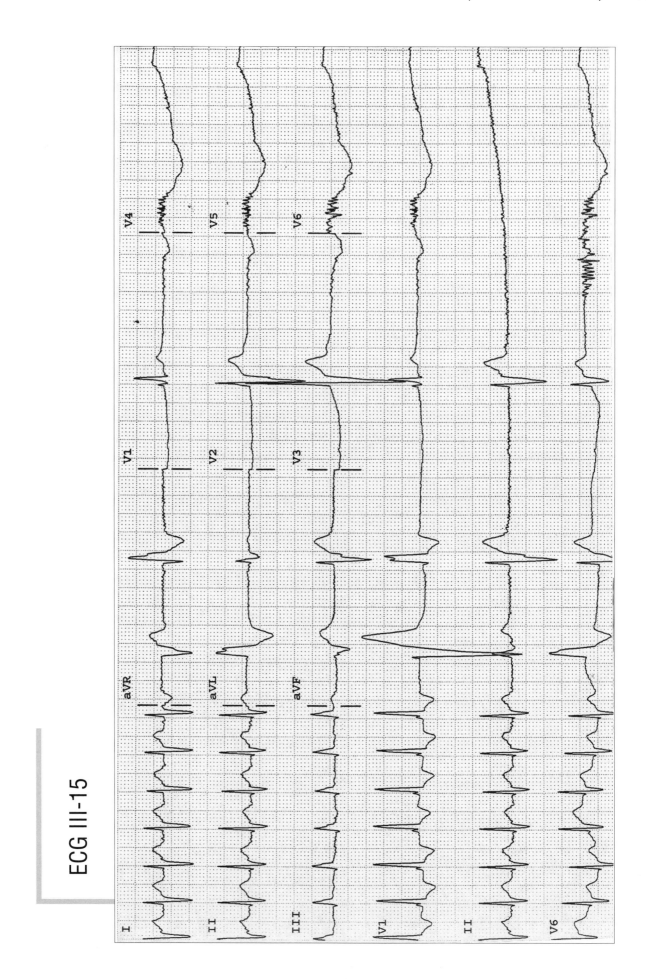

ECG III-15

Diagnoses   **ECG III-15**

1. End of paroxysm of supraventricular tachycardia (response to adenosine 6 mg), probably AV nodal reentrant with incomplete RBBB aberration

2. Returning beats are either ventricular escapes or junctional with aberration

3. Ventricular asystole for several seconds

Clinical Data

24-year-old man, i.v. drug addict; mitral valve replaced due to bacterial endocarditis with severe mitral regurgitation

Comments

The source of the escaping beats is uncertain, but morphologic evidence points to junctional with aberration.

  • The first reaches its S-wave nadir in V1 in 0.04 s and therefore presumably represents LBBB in a junctional beat rather than ventricular ectopy.

  • The second is probably junctional with RBBB aberration.

  • The third, with its rsR's' configuration, also is almost certainly junctional with RBBB.

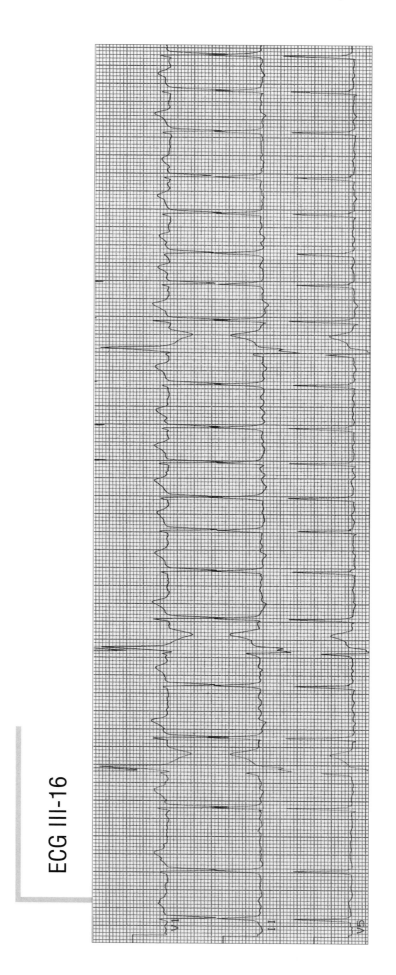

ECG III-16

Diagnoses

ECG III-16

1. Atrial fibrillation with rapid ventricular response (about 140/min)

2. Intermittent RBBB + left anterior hemiblock aberration

3. Probable LVH with secondary ST-T changes

Clinical Data

21-year-old man, cocaine addict; in acute alcoholic intoxication

Comment

The pattern of LVH may be related to the repeated hypertensive crises induced by cocaine.

ECG III-17

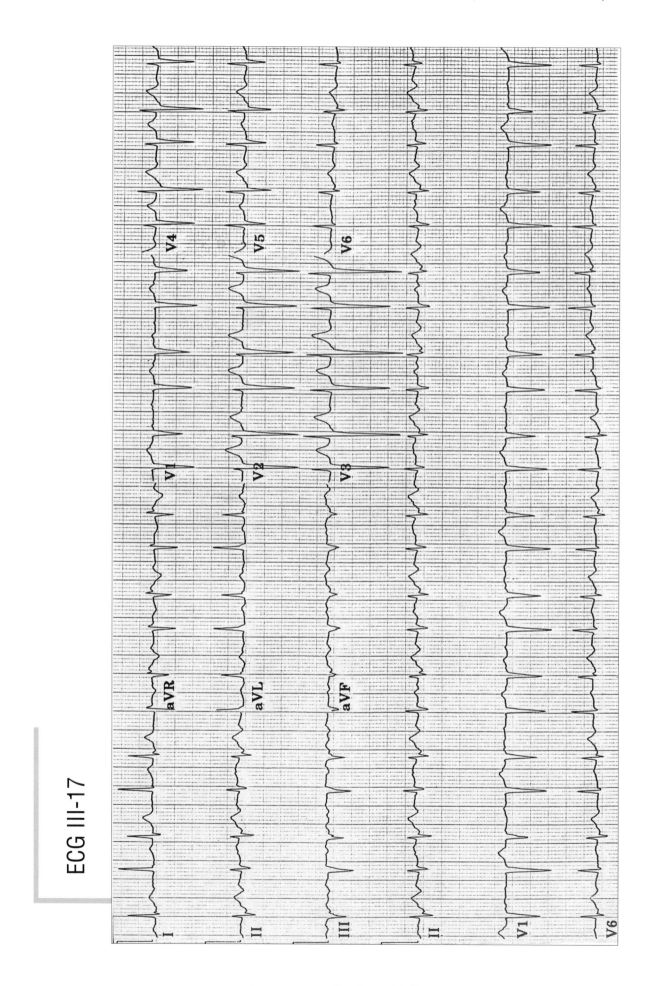

Diagnoses   **ECG III-17**

1. Atrial flutter with 4:2 AV (Wenckebach) conduction, with . . .

2. . . . minor aberration of the beats ending the shorter ventricular cycles

3. Left axis deviation

Clinical Data

70-year-old man

Comments

This is a tricky one. The computer called it "sinus tachycardia with atrial bigeminy." A few clues to the right diagnosis:

- There are no clearly recognizable, normally directed P waves in any lead.

- Careful scrutiny reveals small, regular, inverted waves in the inferior leads and upright ones in V1 at rate 280/min.

- When like, supraventricular beats are seen in pairs, a 3:2 Wenckebach is always suspect.

This diagnosis is confirmed when sinus rhythm is restored and normal P waves are sizeable; with sinus tachycardia, normal P waves tend to get larger and would have been easily visible.

The alternating amplitude of the QRS complexes (well seen in V1) is probably owing to mild aberration from minor delay in the RBB in the beats ending the shorter cycles.

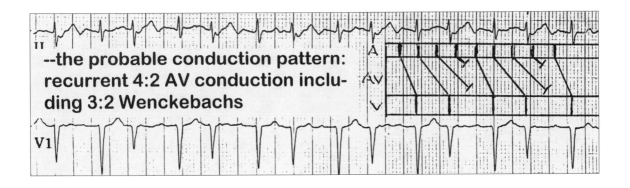

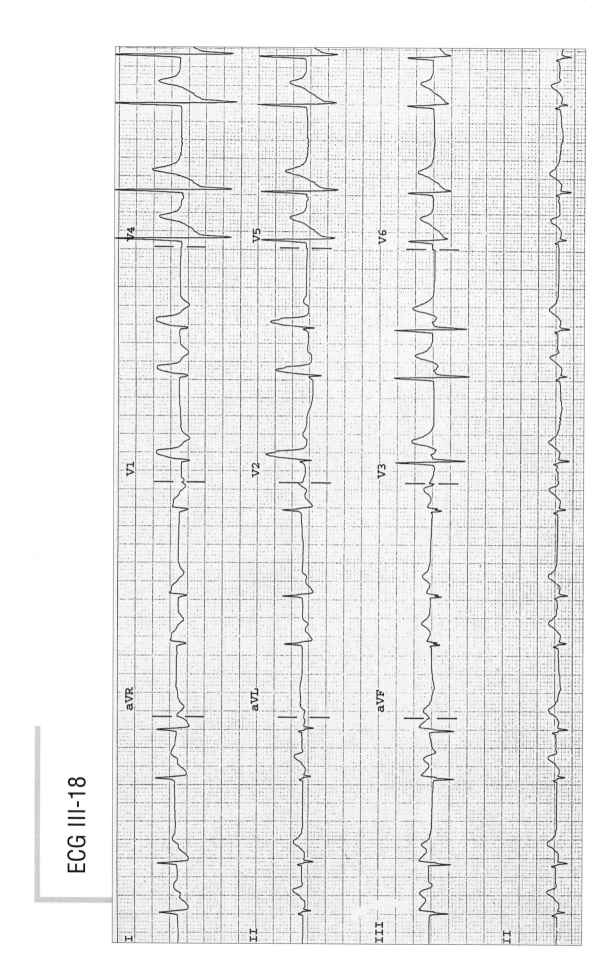

ECG III-18

Diagnoses   **ECG III-18**

1. Acute inferior myocardial infarction

2. Junctional ectopic tachycardia (rate = 123/min) with . . .

3. . . . 3:2 Wenckebach conduction below junctional pacemaker (see laddergram) reducing ventricular rate to 82/min

4. Right bundle-branch block

Clinical Data

85-year-old man with rheumatoid spondylitis; fell and injured neck, producing compression of cord with consequent quadriparesis. Died 2 days later.

Comment

Paired, like beats should always lead you to suspect a 3:2 Wenckebach.

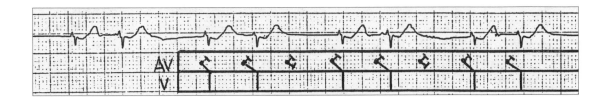

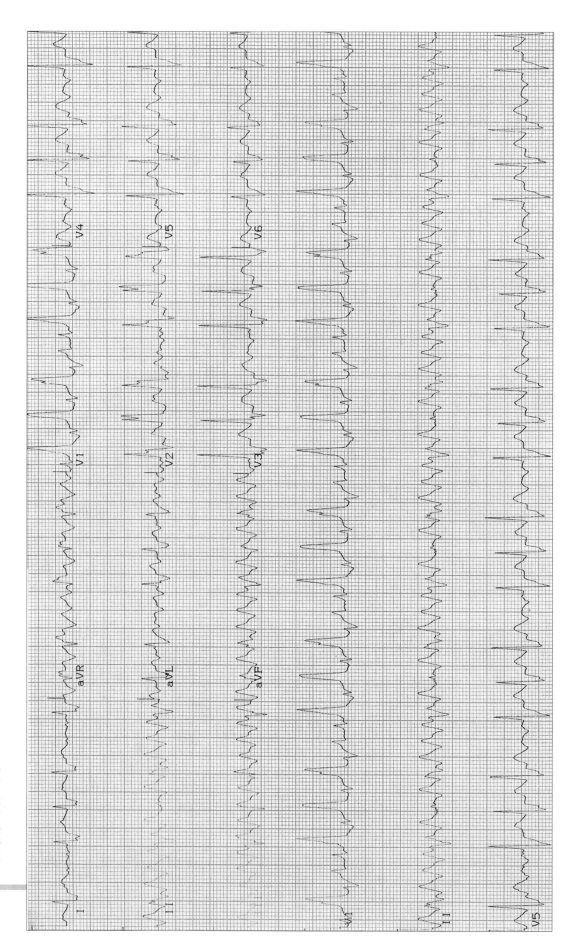

ECG III-19

Diagnoses   **ECG III-19**

1. Atrial flutter (rate = 336/min) with 2:1 and 4:1 AV conduction

2. Right bundle-branch block

Clinical Data

Unknown

Comments

• **Group beating** during atrial flutter (as seen here with the ventricular complexes grouped in trios) is almost always due to bi-level patterns of conduction in the junction—2:1 "filtering" at the upper level with Wenckebach (here 4:3) conduction at the lower level of the beats that get through the "filter" above.

• In the groups of three beats, it looks (best seen in V1) as though the QRS is changing shape from beat to beat. This is *not* because of any intrinsic QRS change, but is due to the changing relationship of the large, superimposed flutter (F) waves—as the Wenckebach develops and the FR interval lengthens—to the QRS complexes.

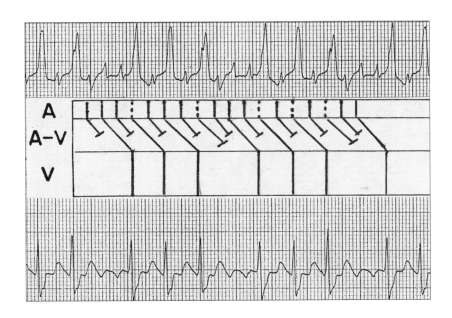

ECG III-20

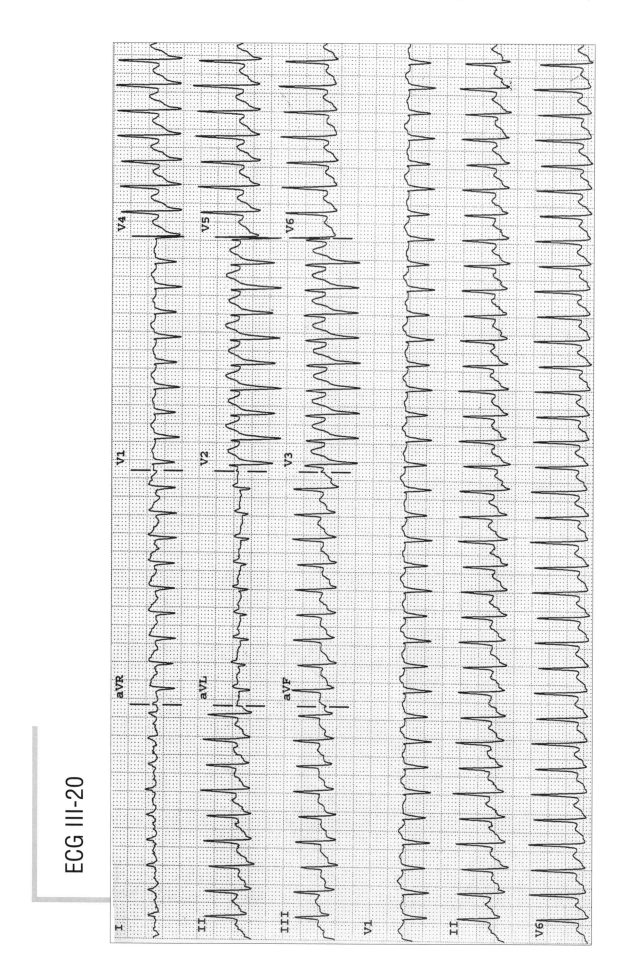

Diagnoses   **ECG III-20**

1. Supraventricular tachycardia (rate = 216/min), most likely orthodromic

2. Secondary ST-T changes

Clinical Data

61-year-old woman in emergency department with palpitations

Comments

The mechanism of the SVT obviously cannot be determined with certainty from the clinical tracing, but statistically the rate (over 200/min) and the QRS alternation (well seen in leads V1, V2, and V6) make orthodromic tachycardia probable.

ECG III-21

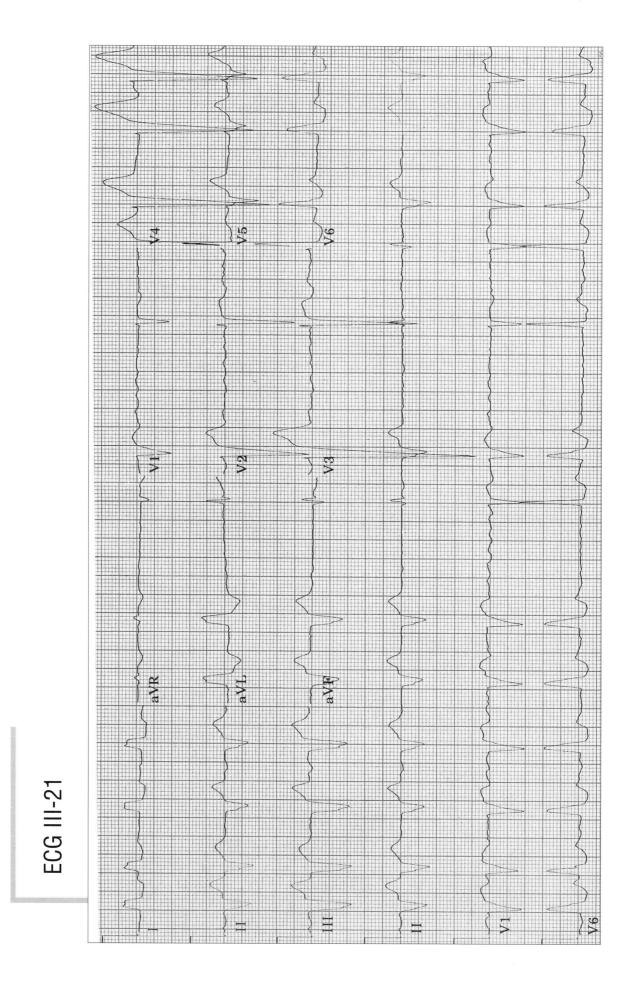

Diagnoses   **ECG III-21**

1. Atrial fibrillation with moderate ventricular response and . . .

2. . . . rate-dependent LBBB

3. Left axis deviation (axis about −60 degrees)

4. Consider old inferior infarct

Clinical Data

83-year-old man

Comments

• It is noteworthy that the beats ending the shortest cycles (see ECG below, *X*) are conducted with somewhat narrower complexes, implying a lesser degree of LBBB than other beats, and this requires explanation. There seem to be two possibilities:

(a) The atrial impulse slips through during the supernormal phase of LBB conduction; or
(b) The early impulse encounters delay in the *right* BB which, by balancing delay in the LBB, somewhat normalizes the QRS complex. (This is the more likely possibility, because "supernormal" conduction is a refuge of the diagnostically destitute—and there's usually another explanation.)

• Q waves in leads 2 and aVF are significant and probably indicative of old inferior infarction.

• **Concealed conduction** is, as usual, responsible for the marked variation in cycle length—representing rates from 36 to 148/min.

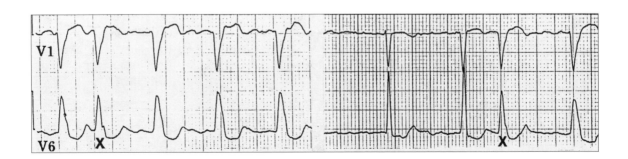

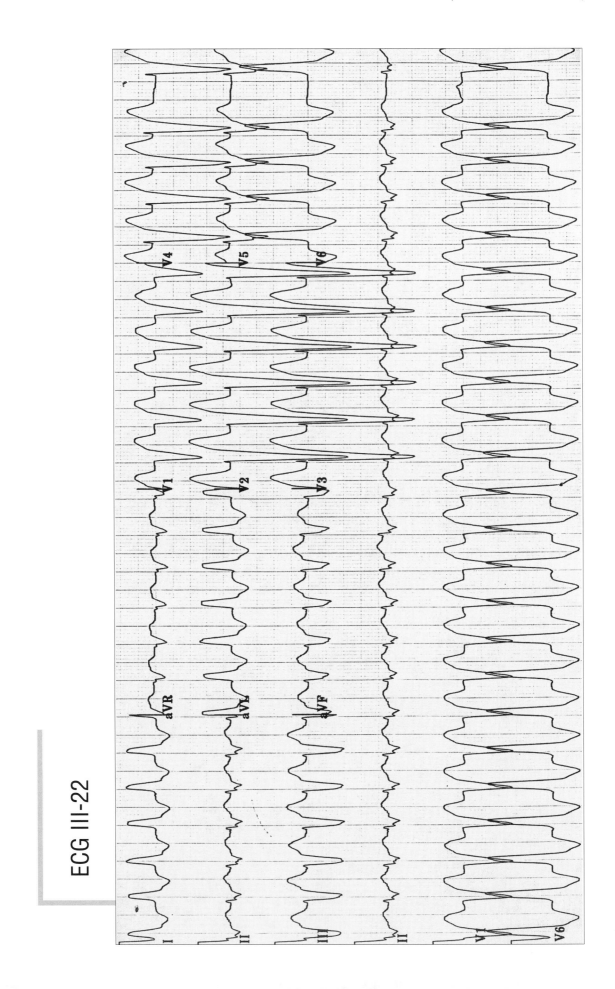

ECG III-22

Diagnoses   **ECG III-22**

1. Atrial flutter with 2:1 AV conduction (and one 3:1 cycle)

2. Left bundle-branch block and LAD (−45 degrees)

Clinical Data

89-year-old woman with ulcerative colitis; feeling weak and dizzy for past week

Comments

At this ventricular rate of 148/min, you should always think of, and look for evidence of, atrial flutter with 2:1 conduction. Here, as is so often the case, the break in the rhythm (at the end of the strip) affords a clue: A single atrial wave is visible, and there is a subtle change in direction on the downslope of the previous T wave, which, if it represents atrial activity, indicates a rate of about 300/min—just right for flutter.

Sure enough, an hour after treatment with diltiazem and digoxin, the flutter waves were obvious (see ECG below). Note in this case that, unlike most flutters, lead 2 is useless for recognizing the atrial activity.

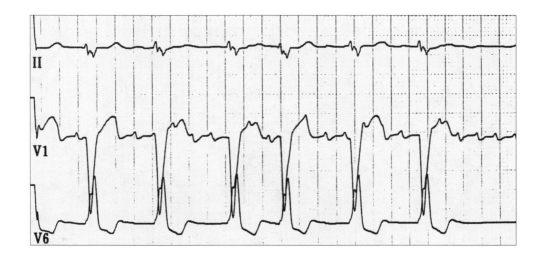

ECG III-23

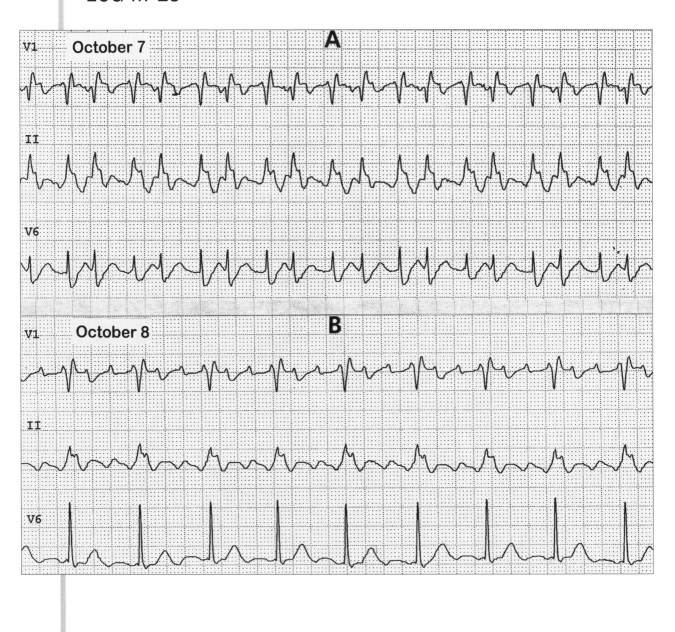

Diagnoses   **ECG III-23**

1. ECG *A* shows atrial flutter (rate = 246/min) with 3:2 AV conduction (ventricular rate = 156/min).

2. ECG *B* shows atrial flutter (rate = 228/min) with 3:1 AV conduction (ventricular rate = 77/min).

3. An underlying RBBB is present in both tracings.

Clinical Data

46-year-old woman with mitral stenosis and history of rheumatic fever

Comment

B is an example of the uncommon odd-number-to-one (3:1) ratio of AV conduction in flutter.

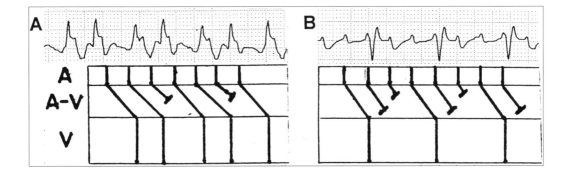

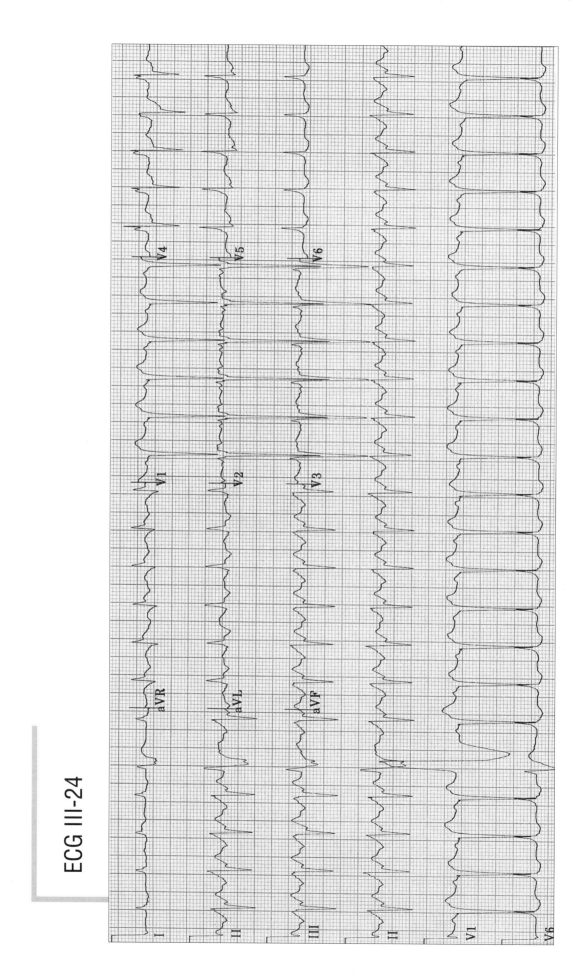

ECG III-24

Diagnoses   ECG III-24

1. Atrial flutter (rate = 284/min) with 2:1 AV conduction

2. One LV extrasystole

3. Left anterior hemiblock

4. Probable LVH

5. ST depression in leads 1, V4–6

Clinical Data

76-year-old man

Comments

• Note the classic morphology in the LVPB: tall R in V1, rS in V6, and frontal plane axis in "no-man's land."

• The deeply negative complexes in V1–2 favor the diagnosis of LVH because LAHB, although it increases the QRS voltage in the limb leads, does not do so in the V leads.

• From lead V1, you might be tempted to diagnose *sinus* tachycardia; the two-per-cycle atrial waves are distinctly seen only in the inferior leads and in V2 and V3.

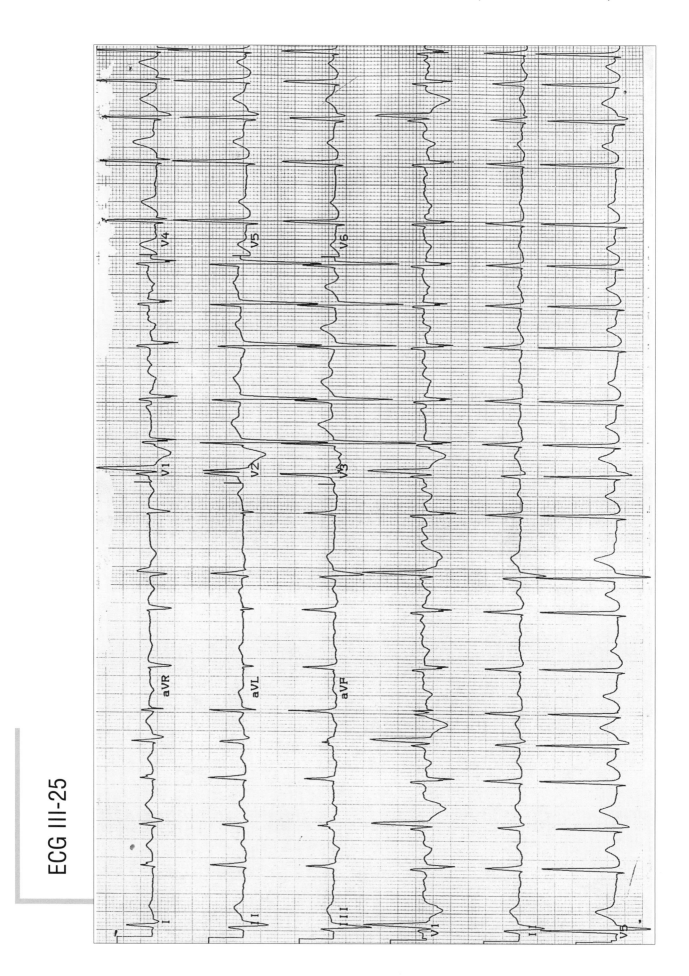

ECG III-25

Diagnoses **ECG III-25**

1. Atrial fibrillation with rapid ventricular response (rate = about 125/min)

2. RBBB aberration of occasional beats, especially when a longer than average cycle is followed by a shorter cycle (Ashman phenomenon)

3. Borderline-high QRS voltage (? LVH)

4. T-wave abnormality

5. Pulmonary embolism should be excluded.

Clinical Data

64-year-old man with chest pain and shortness of breath

Comments

The combination of inverted T waves in inferior leads (here in lead 3) and V1, especially with an atrial tachyarrhythmia, should always make you think of and exclude pulmonary embolism.

Note that the Ashman phenomenon is evident where the 9th beat shows bifascicular—LAHB as well as RBBB—aberration.

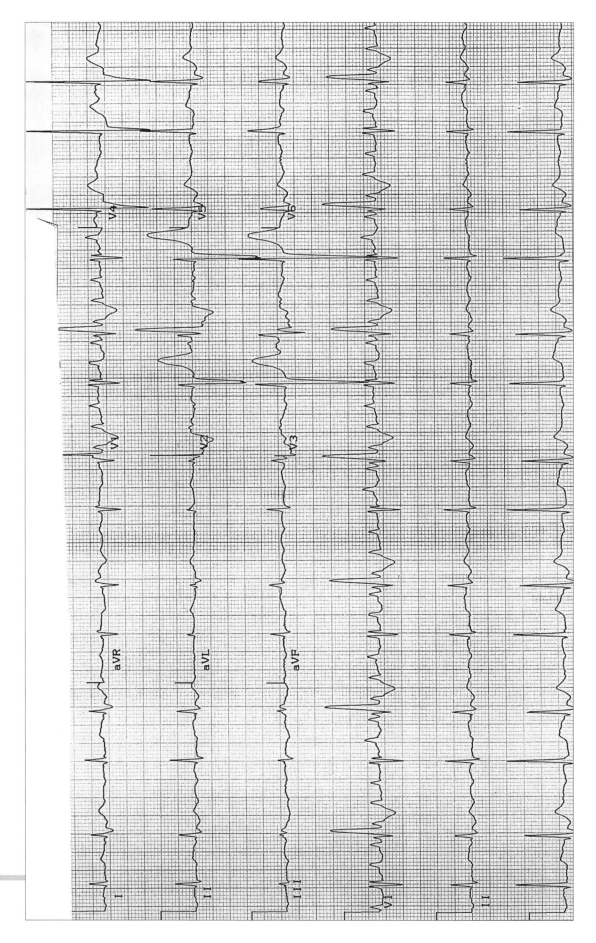

ECG III-26

Diagnoses   ECG III-26

1. Atrial flutter (rate = 262/min) with alternating 2:1 and 4:1 AV conduction

2. Right bundle-branch block aberration of the conducted beats ending the shorter cycles

3. Probable left ventricular hypertrophy

Clinical Data

83-year-old man complaining of shortness of breath and palpitations

Comments

The alternating cycle lengths are the result of conduction failure at *two* levels in the AV junction—2:1 conduction at an upper level, and a 3:2 Wenckebach (of the beats that get through the 2:1 filter) at a lower level (see laddergram below). This is a phase that most patients go through if their 2:1 flutter is treated with digitalis, verapamil, or propranolol, etc. If the patient is receiving digoxin and the aberration is mistaken for ventricular ectopic bigeminy, digoxin intoxication is likely to be diagnosed and the drug stopped when more is needed. Here the beats in question have a classic rsR′ configuration and are not likely to be mistaken for ventricular ectopics.

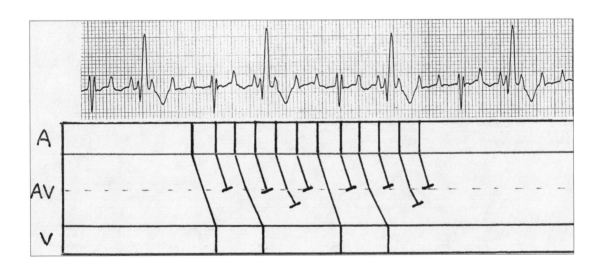

ECG III-27

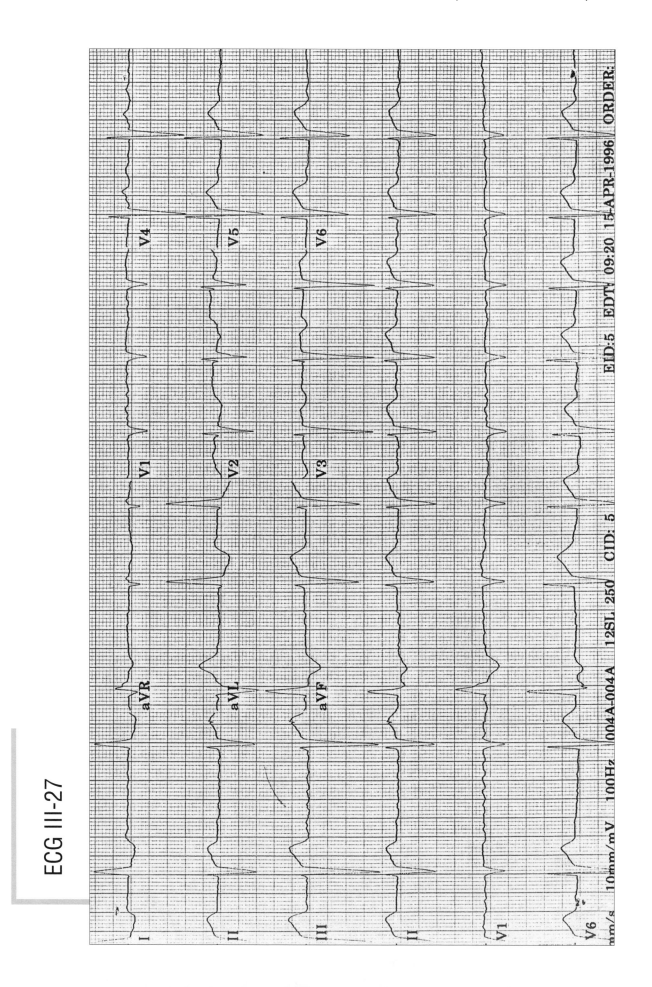

mm/s 10mm/mV 100Hz 004A-004A 12SL 250 CID: 5 EID:5 EDT: 09:20 15-APR-1996 ORDER:

Diagnoses   ECG III-27

1. Atrial fibrillation with controlled ventricular response

2. One left ventricular extrasystole

3. Left anterior hemiblock (axis about $-60°$)

Clinical Data

Unknown

Comments

• Note the positive concordance in this extrasystole (positive in V1 and V6 and presumably in all leads between); this is seen in about 30% of left ventricular ectopic rhythms and has to be distinguished from some type A preexcitations.

• The Q waves in V2–3 are probably due to the hemiblock alone and are not evidence of an old anteroseptal infarct.

• Note that beats 4 to 10 are remarkably regular at 78/min—presumably an accelerated junctional rhythm that eludes the atrial bombardment and usurps control for a few beats.

ECG III-28

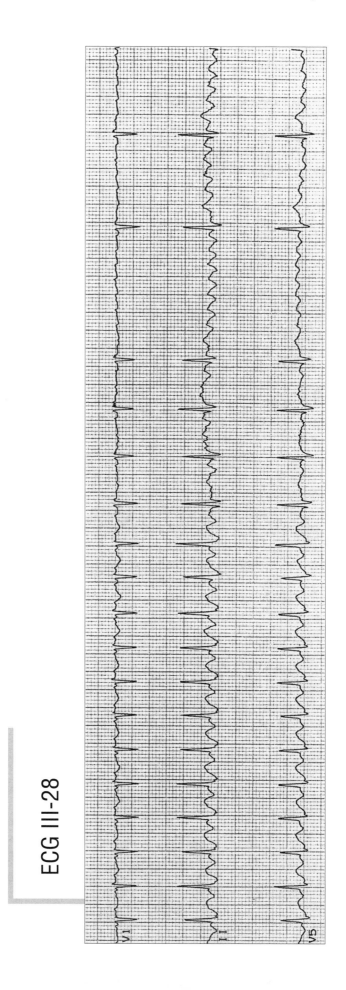

Diagnoses

ECG III-28

1. Atrial flutter (rate = 312/min) with 2:1 AV conduction in first half of strip . . .

2. . . . with superimposed concealed conduction and increasing atrial rate (to 360/min) in second half of strip markedly reducing ventricular response

Clinical Data

55-year-old man complaining only of palpitations; has normal 12-lead tracing

Comments

This case illustrates the *clinically* most important aspect of **concealed conduction,** i.e., *simulating* significant AV block in the presence of atrial flutter or fibrillation. In this tracing there is *no* evidence of *any* AV block: the 2:1 conduction at an atrial rate of over 300 is due to normal AV nodal refractoriness; while the further ventricular slowing at the faster atrial rate (simulating significant AV block) is the result of partial penetration (concealed conduction) into the node by some of the atrial impulses. After cardioversion 6 minutes later, conduction is normal (see rhythm strip below).

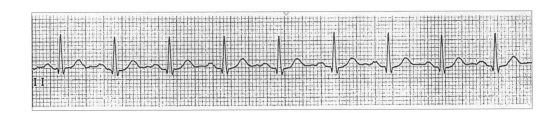

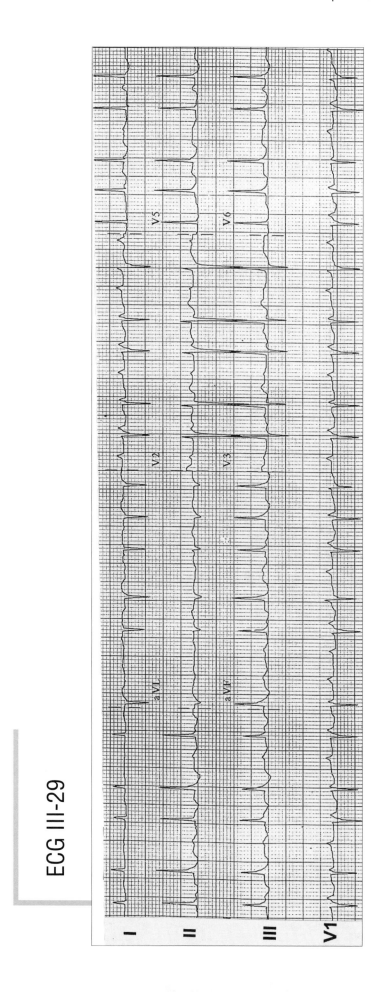

ECG III-29

Diagnoses   **ECG III-29**

1. Atrial tachycardia (rate 200/min) with . . .

2. . . . sagging STs and short QT interval suggesting digitalis effect

Clinical Data

Unknown

Comment

Note the several conduction ratios: 4:3, 4:2, 3:2, and 2:1 (see laddergram).

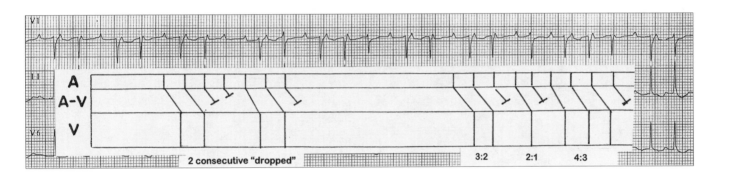

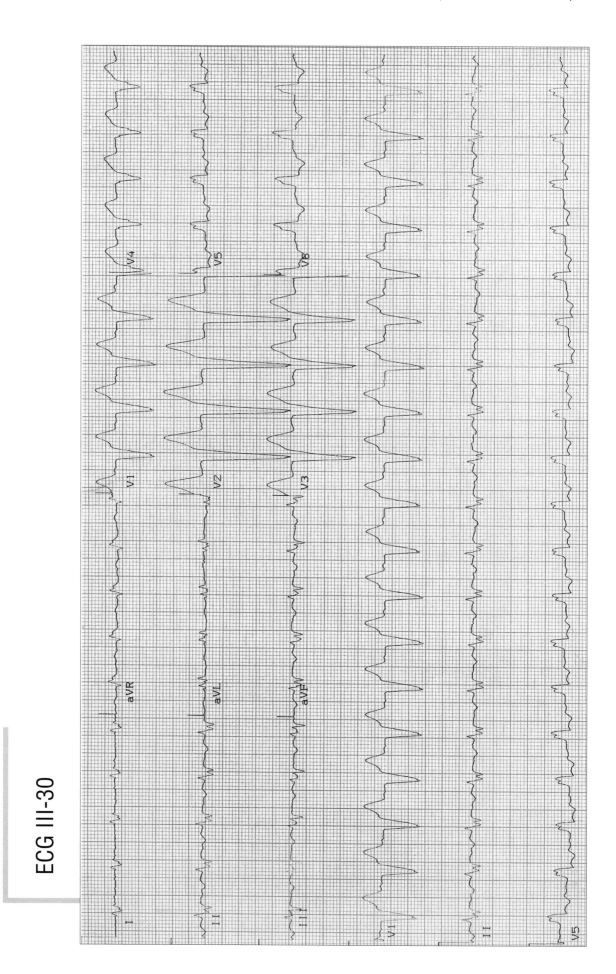

ECG III-30

Diagnoses   **ECG III-30**

1. Atrial flutter/tachycardia (rate = 230/min) with 2:1 AV conduction

2. Left bundle-branch block

3. Low voltage in limb leads and axis in "no-man's land" (upper right quadrant)

Clinical Data

81-year-old man in congestive heart failure

Comments

• Atrial flutter with 2:1 AV conduction is often recognized less by sight than by smell! Here it is easy to suspect, but impossible to be sure of. Below is a rhythm strip of lead 2 a few weeks later revealing the flutter waves in some 3:1 cycles.

• The low voltage and bizarre axis suggest a cardiomyopathy.

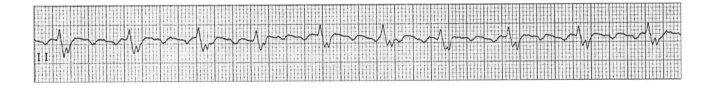

ECG III-31

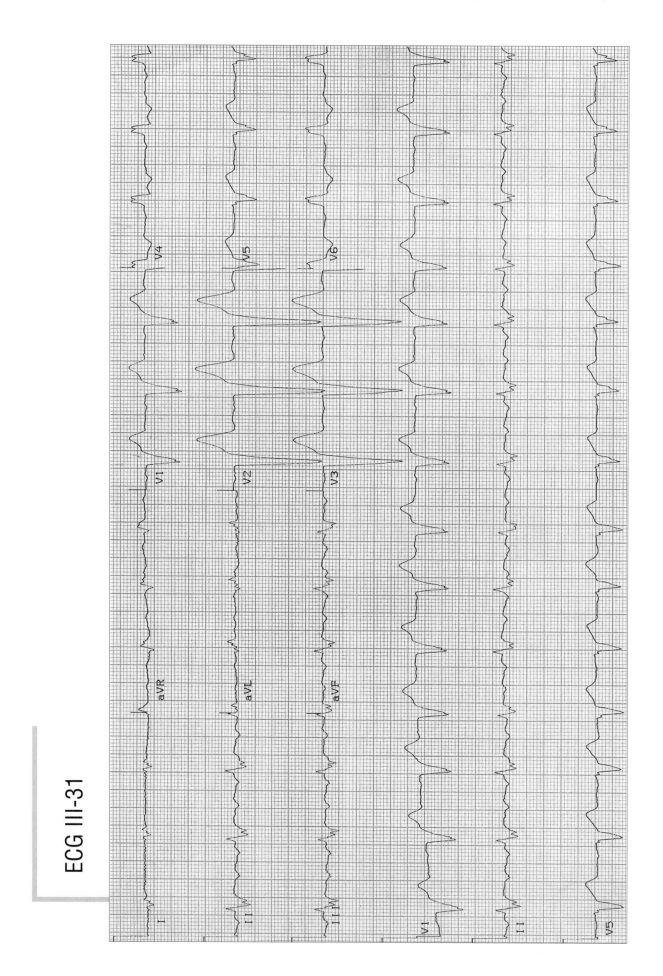

Diagnoses

ECG III-31

1. Atrial flutter (rate = 228/min) with varying 2:1 and 3:1 conduction

2. Left bundle-branch block

3. Bizarre axis, about −95 degrees

4. Leads V4 and V5 are switched.

Clinical Data

82-year-old woman in congestive heart failure

Comments

• The bizarre axis—just reaching into "no-man's land"—should lead you to consider a congestive cardiomyopathy.

• Did you spot the confused leads?

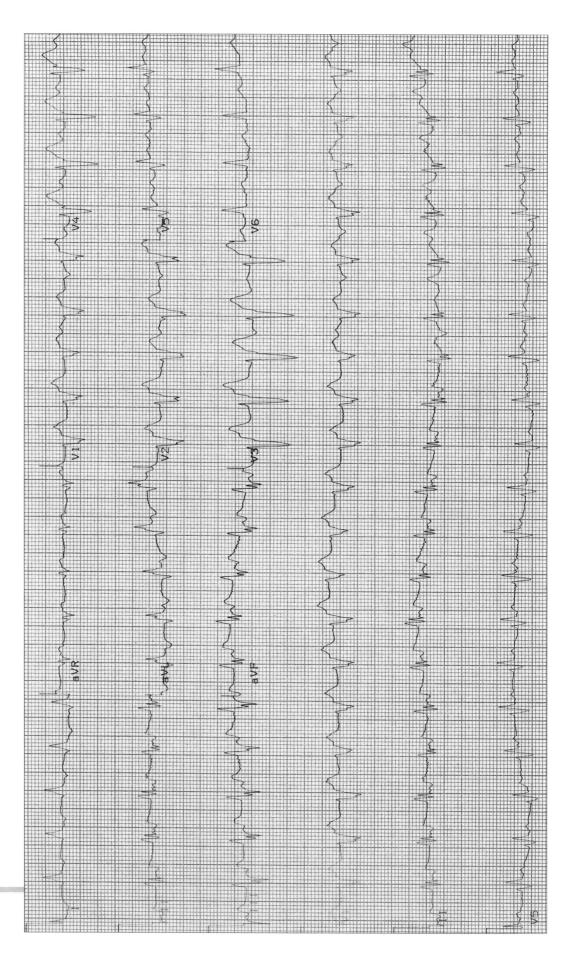

ECG III-32

Diagnoses   **ECG III-32**

1. Junctional tachycardia (possibly orthodromic; rate = 125/min) with retrograde conduction giving place to sinus tachycardia (rate = about 115/min)

1. Left atrial enlargement (increased PTF-V1)

2. Incomplete LBBB (QRS interval = 0.11 s)

3. High lateral infarction, probably recent

Clinical Data

50-year-old man with severe retrosternal pain

Comments

• Note that the RP′ interval suddenly lengthens just before the sinus takes over, and in the next cycle the retrograde P wave is missing. It is this failure of retrograde conduction that gives the sinus its opportunity, and it *escapes*—it does not *usurp* control.

• The significant Q waves and inverted T waves in leads 1 and aVL make infarction probable.

ECG III-33

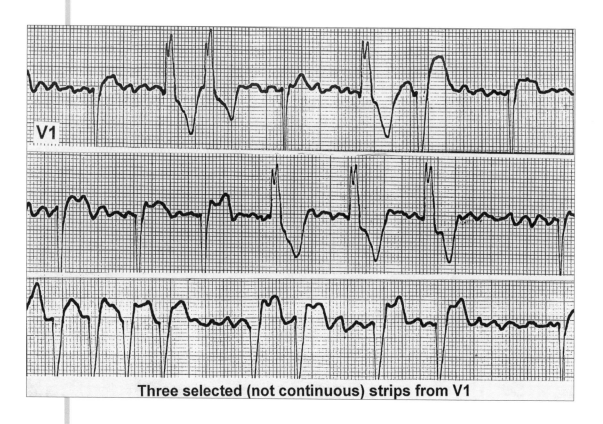

Three selected (not continuous) strips from V1

Diagnoses   ECG III-33

1. Atrial fibrillation

2. Intermittent RBBB and LBBB aberration

Clinical Data

83-year-old man

Comments

The LBBB beats have already been established as rate-dependent LBBB. The only question is:

• What are the RBBB-like beats? Are they ectopic? They appear to be unrelated to cycle length, and they have a taller right peak, which puts them in the ballpark for RBBB aberration.

Answer: the only interpretation that seems to explain all features of this arrhythmia is bilateral aberration due to the unpredictability of **concealed conduction** into each bundle branch: With atrial fibrillation, you never know when an impulse will be conducted to the ventricles or when it will get only as far as into one of the bundle branches. Thus, both AV *and* IV conduction may be totally unpredictable, which seems to be the situation here.

ECG III-34

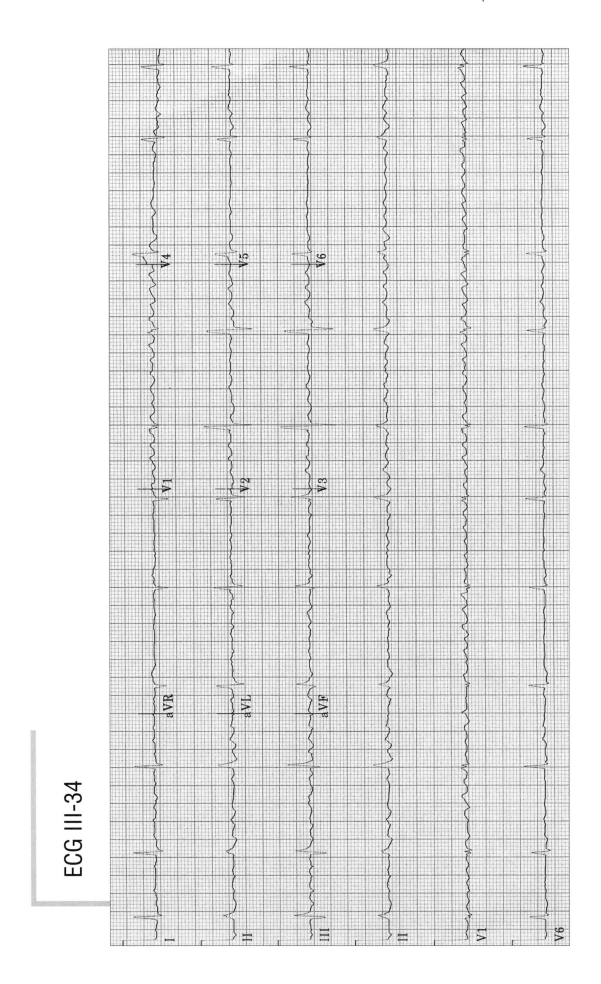

Diagnoses   **ECG III-34**

1. Atrial fibrillation with controlled ventricular response (rate = about 60/min)

2. Possible old inferior infarction

3. Low-voltage T wave throughout, without significant ST depression—must consider hypothyroidism

Clinical Data

61-year-old woman in hospital with pneumonia

Comment

V1 is undoubtedly the best *single* lead for constant monitoring because it produces such characteristic QRS shapes. But there are glaring exceptions, and this is one—a good example of a V1 that is virtually useless as a QRS monitor.

Section IV

Intraventricular Blocks

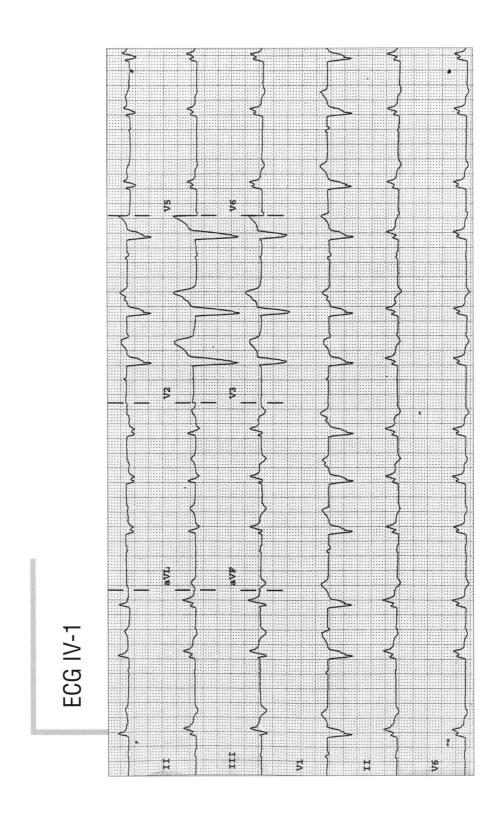

ECG IV-1

Diagnoses   **ECG IV-1**

1. Sinus tachycardia (rate = 104/min) with . . .

2. . . . type I AV block with 3:2 and 4:3 Wenckebachs

3. Left bundle-branch block

4. Evolving, acute, inferolateral myocardial infarction

Clinical Data

80-year-old woman

Comment

Once upon a time it used to be said that it was difficult or impossible to diagnose acute myocardial infarction from the ECG in the presence of LBBB. The truth is that it can be easy, as in this case, if you concentrate on the ST-T.

ECG IV-2

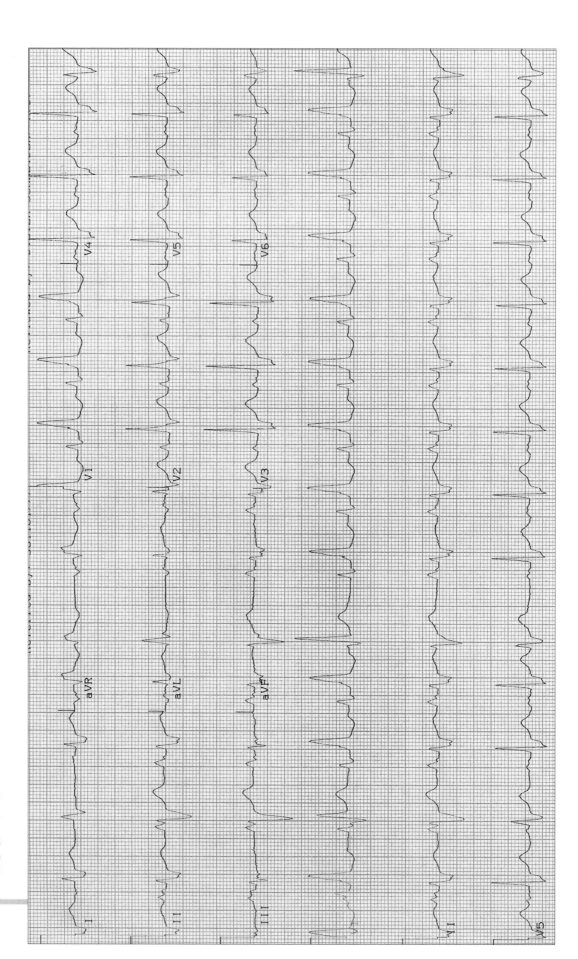

Diagnoses   **ECG IV-2**

1. Sinus rhythm (rate = 86/min) with biatrial enlargement

2. Right bundle-branch block

3. Three premature ventricular beats with varying coupling, but that do not measure for parasystole

4. Probable right ventricular hypertrophy

5. Borderline AV conduction (PR = 0.20 s)

Clinical Data

68-year-old man with no clinical complaints; persistent splitting of S2

Comments

None

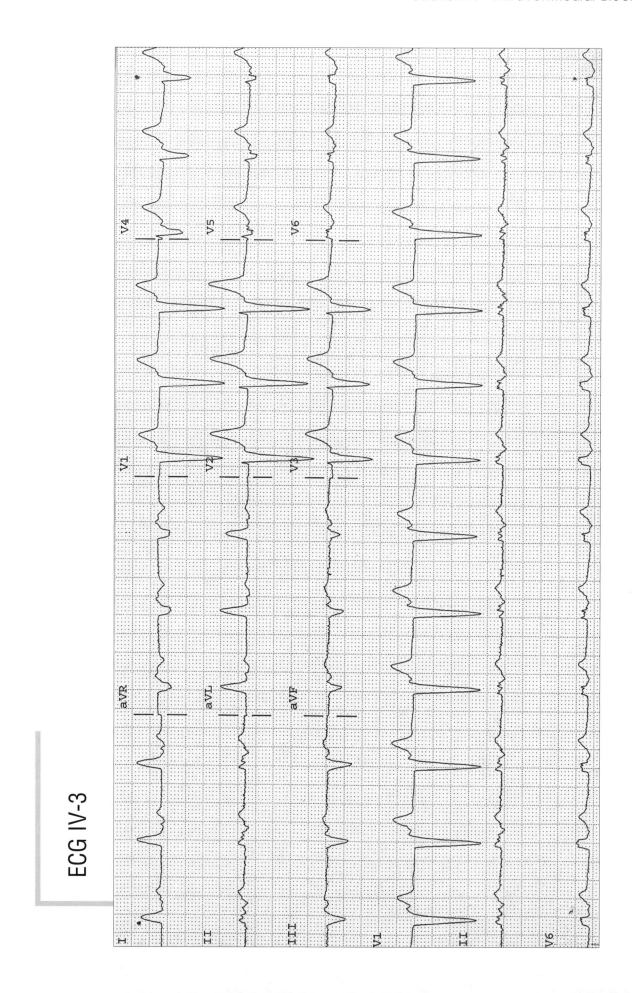

ECG IV-3

Diagnoses   **ECG IV-3**

1. Accelerated junctional rhythm (rate = 74/min) with . . .

2. . . . retrograde conduction to atria

3. Left bundle-branch block

Clinical Data

Unknown

Comment

You must consider accelerated idioventricular rhythm here, but in V1 the QRS nadir is reached in 0.05 s, which makes LBBB more likely than ventricular ectopy, and therefore implies a junctional pacemaker (i.e., accelerated junctional rhythm).

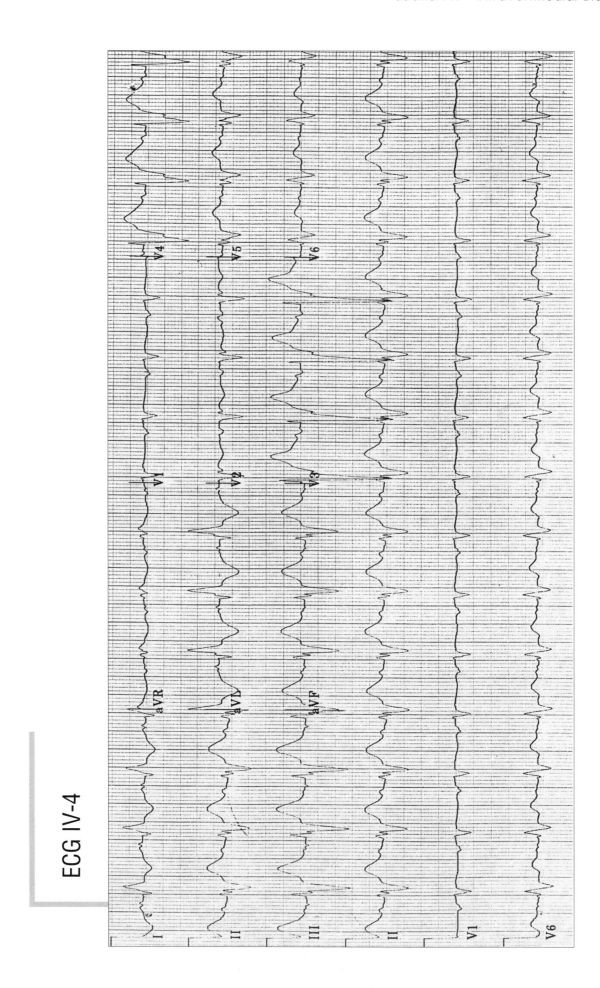

ECG IV-4

Diagnoses   **ECG IV-4**

1. Sinus rhythm (rate = 90/min) with intra-atrial block and left atrial enlargement

2. Atypical left bundle-branch block with left axis deviation

3. Old anterior myocardial infarction (Q waves 1, aVL, V6)

Clinical Data

Unknown

Comment

Decades ago at the Mayo Clinic, an autopsy series demonstrated that patients with LBBB and Q waves in *lateral* leads had *anteroseptal* infarcts. (See Rhoades DV, et al: The electrocardiogram in the presence of myocardial infarction and intraventricular block of the left bundle-branch block type. Am Heart J 62:78, 1961.)

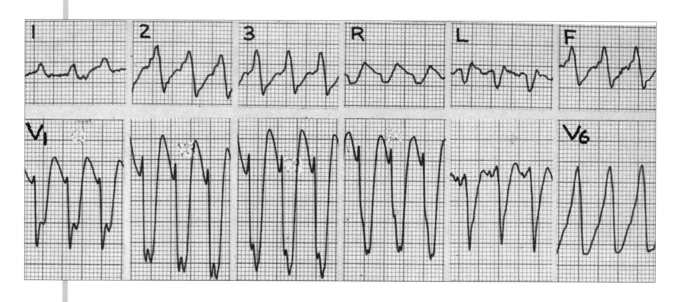

Diagnoses   **ECG IV-5**

1. Supraventricular tachycardia (rate = about 185/min) with . . .

2. . . . left bundle-branch block

Clinical Data

Patient cardioverted in emergency department after futile treatment for VT with lidocaine

Comments

The only good clue that this is LBBB and not ventricular tachycardia—and it is a very good clue—is in V1: the slick downstroke to early (< 0.07 sec) nadir with notching on the upstroke. Sure enough, after lidocaine had failed to convert, cardioversion restored sinus rhythm *with LBBB.*

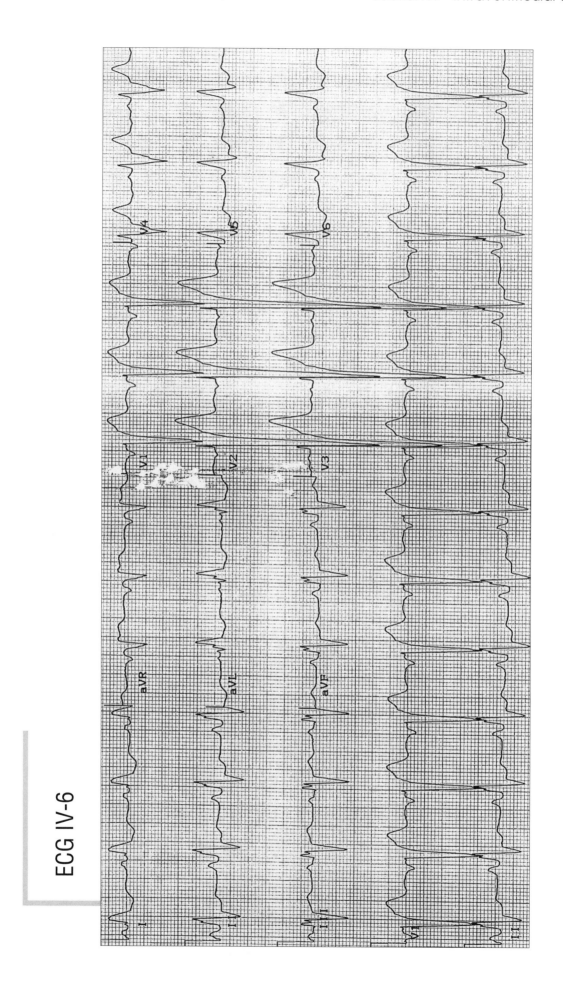

ECG IV-6

Diagnoses   **ECG IV-6**

1. Sinus rhythm (rate = 81/min) with left bundle-branch block

2. Left atrial (perhaps biatrial) enlargement (P-terminal force in V1 = 0.16 mm/s)

3. Probable lateral wall ischemia

Clinical Data

58-year-old man, no cardiac symptoms

Comments

None

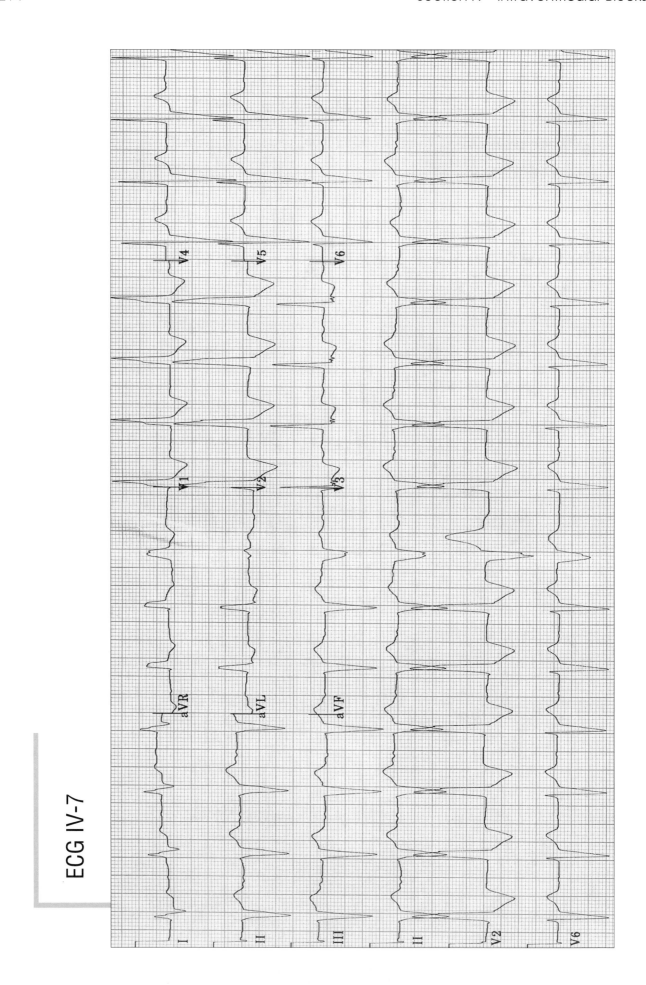

ECG IV-7

Diagnoses   **ECG IV-7**

1. Sinus rhythm (rate = 88/min) with first-degree AV block (PR = 0.30 s)

2. Right bundle-branch block

3. Left anterior hemiblock

4. One right ventricular premature beat

Clinical Data

78-year-old man

Comments

Note:

- The unusually—for RBBB—tall, monophasic QRS in V1 (> 10 mm) suggesting RVH

- In V6, the rS configuration produced by the bifascicular block and mimicking the common pattern of LV ectopy

- The negative concordance of the VPB.

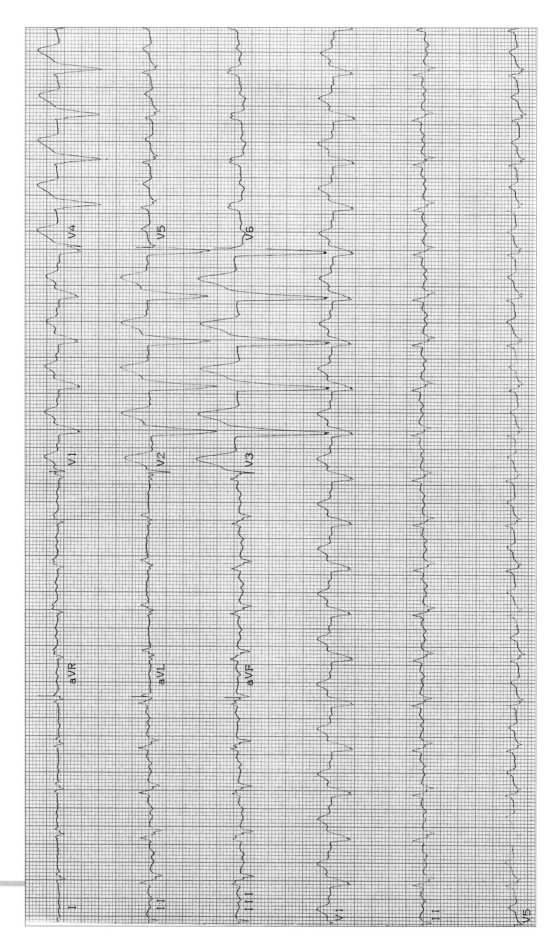

ECG IV-8

Diagnoses

ECG IV-8

1. Atrial flutter (rate = 240/min) with 2:1 AV conduction

2. Left bundle-branch block

3. Low voltage in limb leads with bizarre axis

Clinical Data

81-year-old woman with dilated cardiomyopathy

Comment

The low voltage and unusual axis in association with LBBB should make you think of a cardiomyopathy.

ECG IV-9

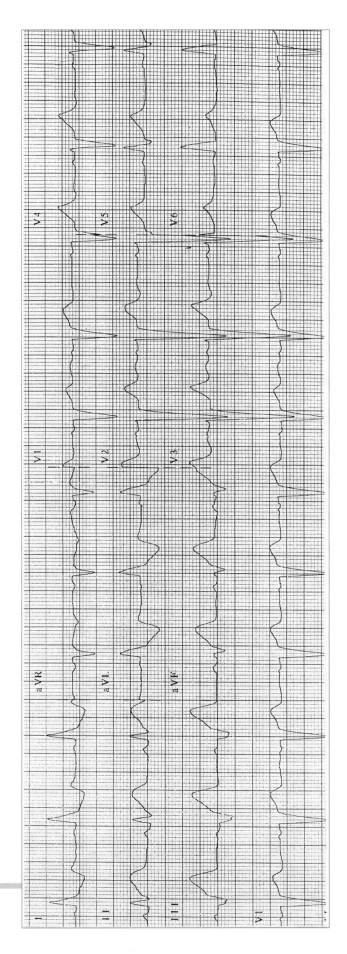

Diagnoses   **ECG IV-9**

1. Sinus rhythm (rate = 65/min)

2. Acute inferior infarction

3. Left bundle-branch block

Clinical Data

83-year-old man with clinical picture of myocardial infarction

Comments

Here is another excellent example of the ease with which acute infarction can be recognized, despite the presence of LBBB, if you focus on the ST-T. Note straightening of the ST and widening of the T wave in indicative leads 2, 3, and aVF, with slight reciprocal depression of the ST take-off in anteroseptal leads where the take-off should be *elevated* secondary to the LBBB. Note also the primary T-wave change in V6—upright where it should be inverted with LBBB.

ECG IV-10

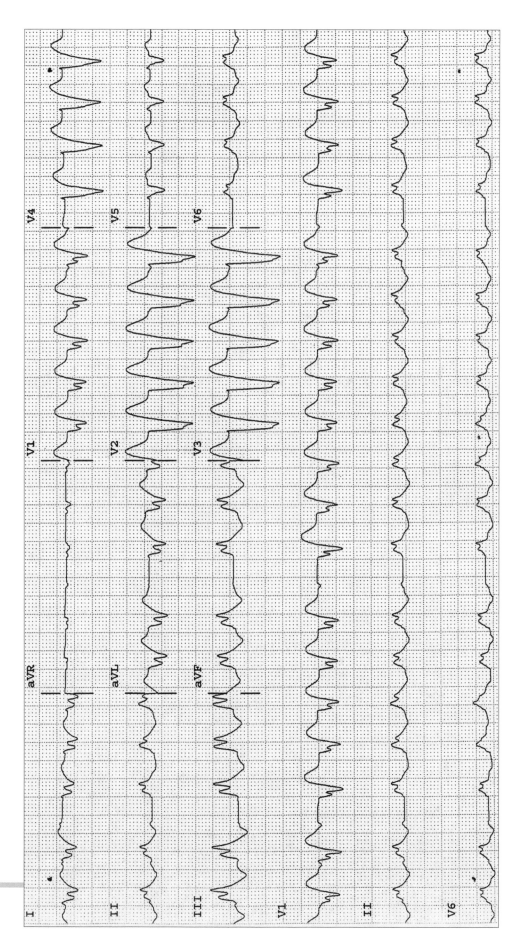

Diagnoses   **ECG IV-10**

1. Sinus tachycardia (rate = 132/min) with . . .

2. . . . 6:5 and 9:8 AV Wenckebach conduction

3. Atypical left bundle-branch block with . . .

4. . . . right axis deviation (+115 degrees)

Clinical Data

64-year-old man with severe ischemic heart disease who died shortly after this recording

Comments

• The LBBB is atypical not only because of the right axis deviation (which suggests a primary cardiomyopathy), but also because of the delayed QS nadir (0.09 s) in V1—usually a cogent clue favoring ventricular ectopy.

• There are only two places where consecutive P waves can be seen (rhythm strip below, *arrows*), but this is enough to establish the atrial rate and the diagnosis of AV Wenckebachs to account for the group beating.

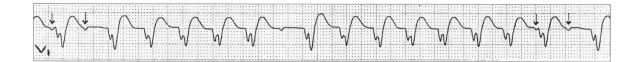

ECG IV-11

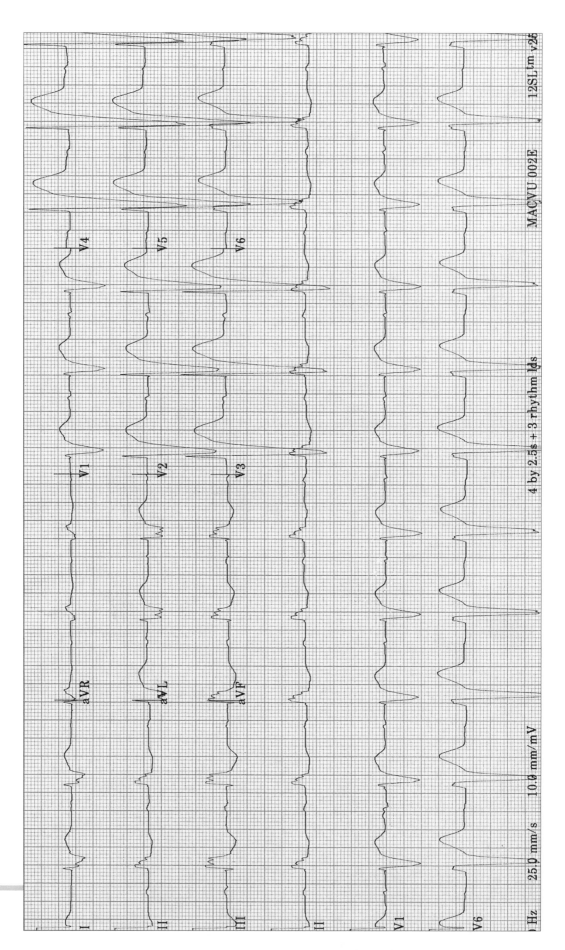

Diagnoses   **ECG IV-11**

1. Sinus rhythm (rate = 66/min) with . . .

2. . . . first-degree AV block (PR = 0.25 s)

3. Left bundle-branch block (QRS interval = 0.20 s) with . . .

4. . . . *right* axis deviation

5. Cannot exclude an acute ischemic episode

Clinical Data

73-year-old woman in congestive heart failure from a primary cardiomyopathy

Comments

• The unusual combination of LBBB with *right* axis deviation strongly suggests a primary cardiomyopathy. (See Nikolic G, Marriott HJL: Left bundle-branch block with right axis deviation: A marker of congestive cardiomyopathy. J Electrocardiol 17:157, 1985.)

• The loss of expected secondary ST concavities should make you question the possibility of acute ischemia/injury.

• Note the most unusual QRS configuration for LBBB in the left precordial leads.

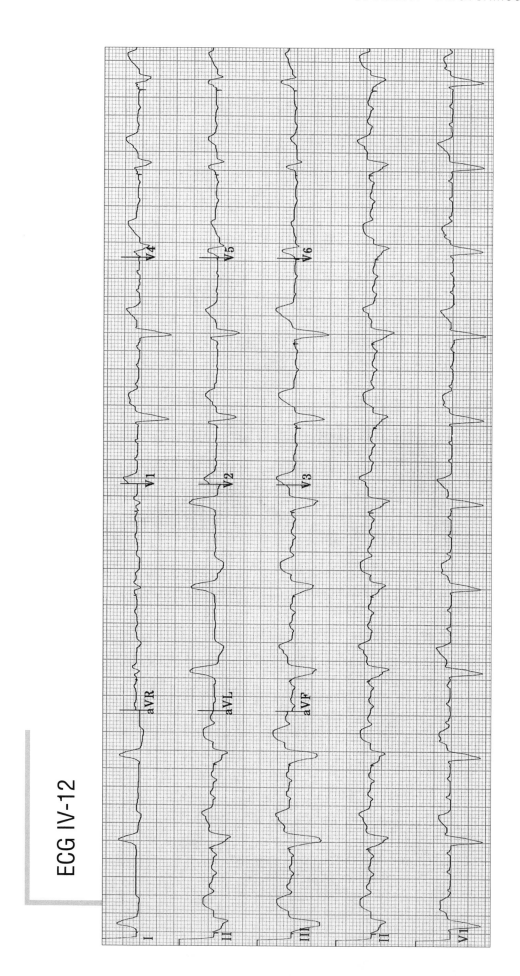

ECG IV-12

Diagnoses   **ECG IV-12**

1. Atrial flutter (rate = 290/min) with . . .

2. . . . *some,* indeterminate degree of AV block and . . .

3. . . . right ventricular paced rhythm, producing . . .

4. . . . complete AV dissociation

Clinical Data

74-year-old man

Comments

• As the relationship of flutter waves to QRSs keeps changing, the AV dissociation is evident.

• The site of the ventricular pacemaker is not so obvious, since the tiny pacemaker stimuli, best seen in V3–5, were missed by the computer and could also be overlooked by the hurried human. This is especially so since at first glance the QRS downstroke in V1 appears to be slick with early nadir, and therefore strongly suggests LBBB rather than ventricular ectopy. But this early nadir is an illusion:

   (a) Lead 2 shows that the paced QRS begins immediately with the pacemaker spike.
   (b) If the timing of the invisible pacer stimulus in V1 is aligned with the visible spike in V3, it becomes obvious that the initial part of the QRS in V1 is isoelectric, and the nadir is therefore late—about 0.09 s—typical of RV ectopy.

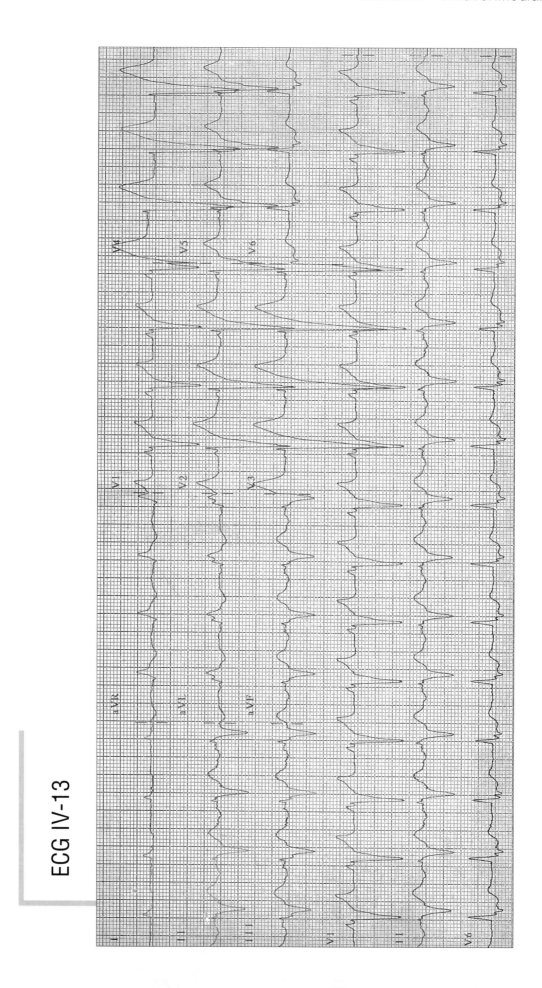

ECG IV-13

Diagnoses   ECG IV-13

1. Atrial tachycardia (rate = 180/min) with . . .

2. . . . 2:12 AV conduction

3. Left bundle-branch block with . . .

4. . . . marked left axis deviation

Clinical Data

Unknown

Comments

• The LBBB is atypical in that V6 is not far enough leftward to show a delayed intrinsicoid deflection; but the pattern is unmistakable in leads aVL and V1–3.

• The alternate, ectopic atrial impulses that are successfully conducted to the ventricles are, of course, those represented by the P′ waves that peak the preceding T waves, with a P′R interval of about 0.40 s.

ECG IV-14

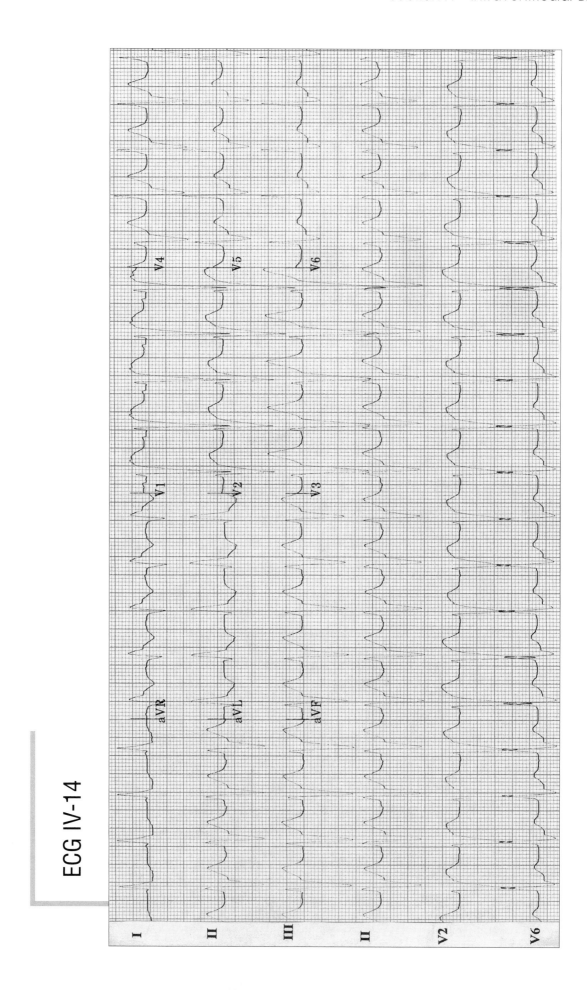

Diagnoses   **ECG IV-14**

1. Atrial tachycardia/flutter (rate = 234/min) with . . .

2. . . . 2:1 AV conduction

3. Left bundle-branch block with . . .

4. . . . left axis deviation (about −60 degrees) and . . .

5. . . . primary ST-T abnormalities

Clinical Data

84-year-old man

Comments

• From several leads, the QRS interval is clearly 0.12–0.13 sec, and therefore a diagnosis of BBB is justified. Although the QRS in V6 is not typical of LBBB, a typical QRS might be obtained by recording V7. Another possible diagnosis for this sort of pattern is incomplete block in the main LBB, with left anterior hemiblock distally.

• The 2:1 AV ratio is best seen in V1. (The computer's misdiagnosis was "sinus tachycardia.")

ECG IV-15

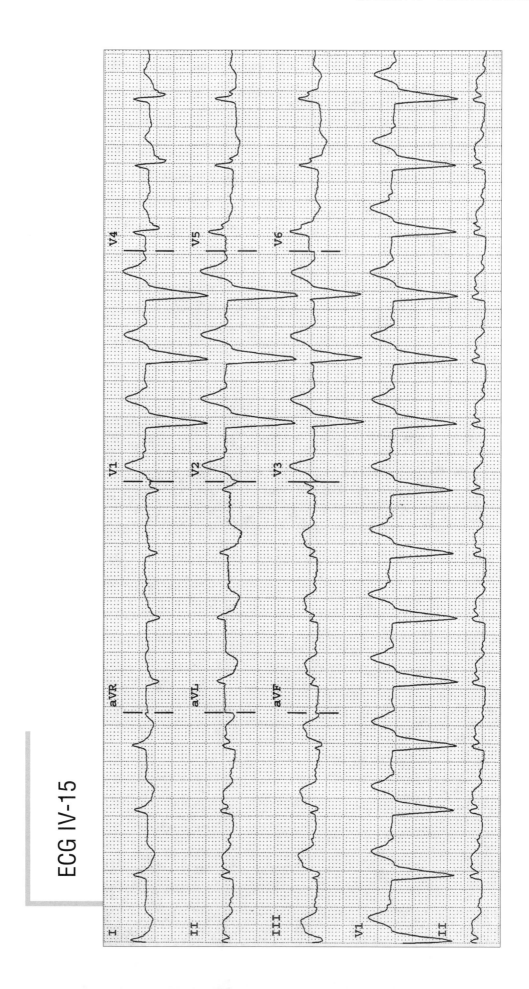

Diagnoses

ECG IV-15

1. Sinus rhythm (rate = 83/min) with . . .

2. . . . intra-atrial block (P waves notched, with peaks > 0.04 s apart, and measure 0.14 s) and . . .

3. . . . first-degree AV block (PR = 0.33 s)

4. Left bundle-branch block

5. Acute inferior infarction

Clinical Data

79-year-old woman

Comments

Note, the slightly depressed ST take-off in V1 and V2 where, in LBBB, it should be slightly elevated. In this tracing, there is obviously no difficulty in diagnosing the acute infarction from the indicative leads, 2, 3, and aVF. However, in some inferior infarctions in the presence of LBBB, the indicative leads may be equivocal, and then an ST take-off in the anteroseptal leads that is below the baseline when it should be above can be invaluable in establishing the diagnosis of acute inferior injury.

ECG IV-16

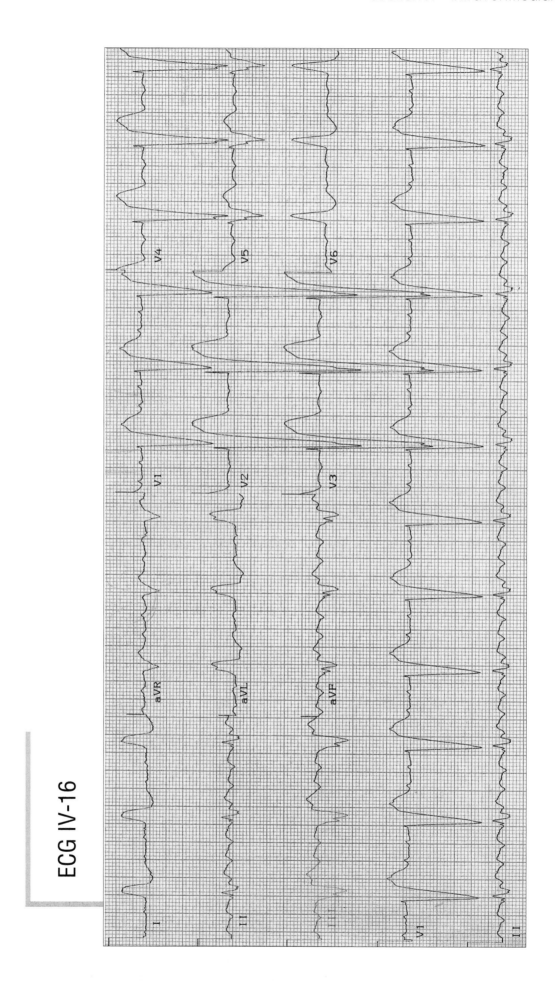

Diagnoses   **ECG IV-16**

1. Atrial flutter (rate = 284/min) with 4:1 AV conduction

2. Left bundle-branch block

3. ? Digitalis effect

Clinical Data

75-year-old man

Comments

The loss of "secondary" upward ST concavity in the V leads demands explanation.

• Is it acute anteroseptal injury or digitalis effect?

Answer: Since the ST in leads 1 and aVL is sagging, and the take-off shows no sign of elevation, digitalis effect is more likely than anterior ischemic injury.

ECG IV-17

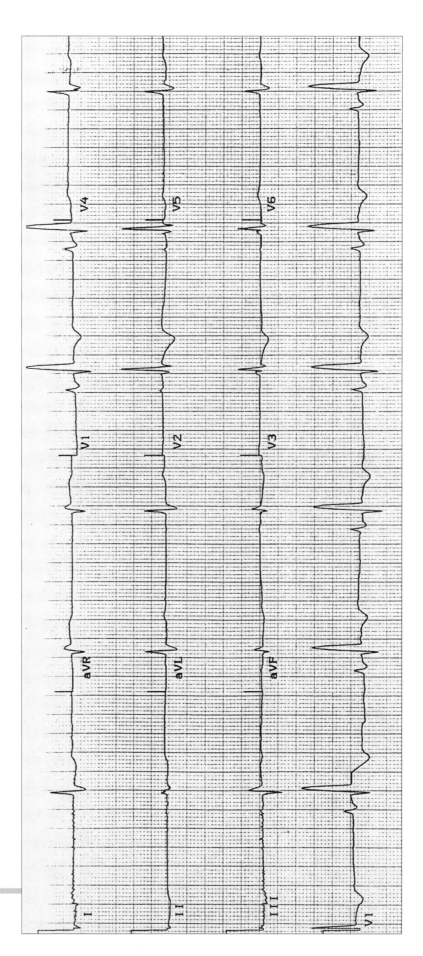

Diagnoses   **ECG IV-17**

1. Sinus bradycardia (rate = 40/min)

2. Right bundle-branch block

3. Probable biatrial hypertrophy

4. Probable old inferior infarction

5. Probable old anteroseptal infarction

Clinical Data

92-year-old woman

Comment

The P waves in V1 are initially 2.5 mm tall, followed by a P-terminal force of about 7 mm/s.

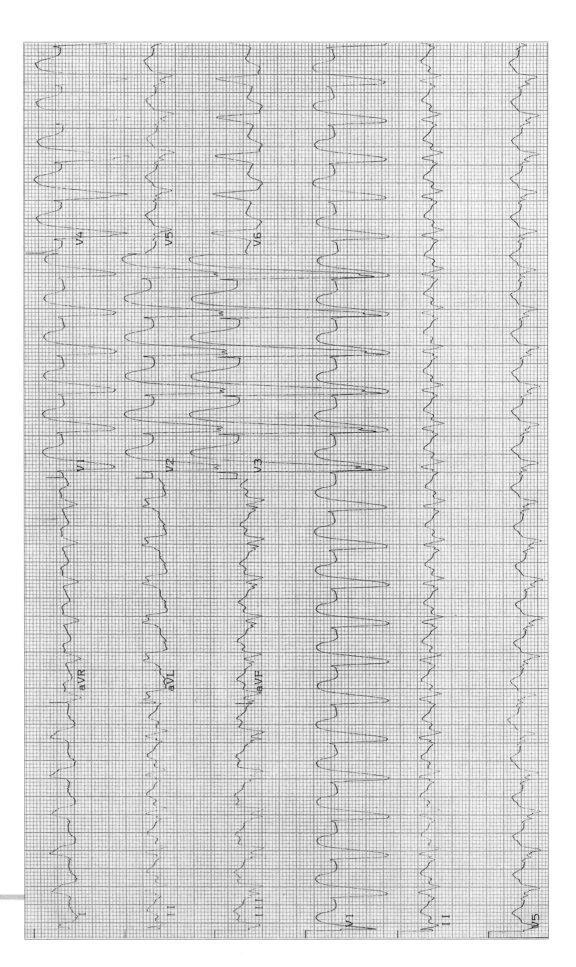

ECG IV-18

Diagnoses   **ECG IV-18**

1. Atrial flutter (rate = 278/min) with 2:1 AV conduction

2. Left bundle-branch block

3. You cannot exclude acute anteroseptal injury ("domelike" ST-Ts in leads V1–4).

Clinical Data

75-year-old man complaining of rapid heart beat and shortness of breath

Comments

None

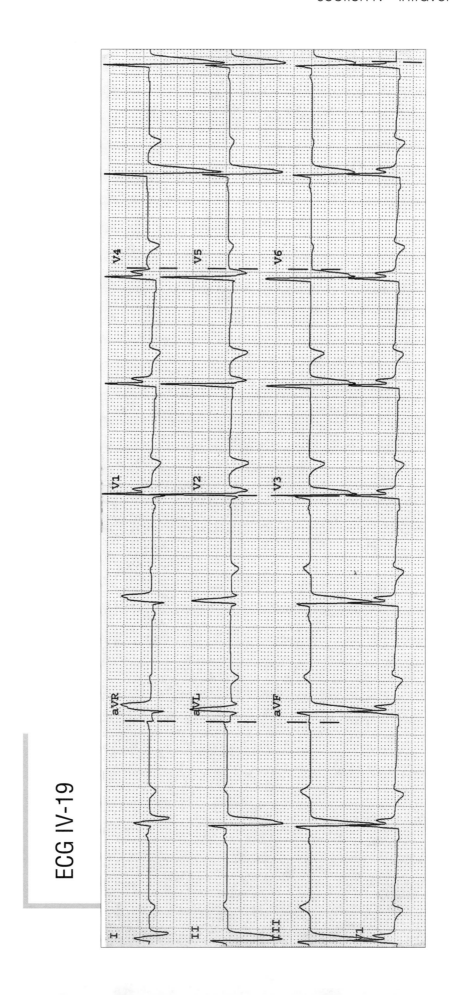

ECG IV-19

Diagnoses   **ECG IV-19**

1. Sinus bradycardia (rate = 48/min), with . . .

2. . . . bifascicular block (RBBB + LAHB)

3. Primary T-wave changes

Clinical Data

Unknown

Comments

• Note how the hemiblock converts the precordial pattern of RBBB to simulate that of left ventricular ectopy, i.e., the taller left peak ("rabbit-ear") in V1 and the absent Q with small R and deeper, wider S wave in V6. The presence of a hemiblock is the most common cause of this deception.

• The primary T wave changes—T waves in *same* (here, negative) direction as the terminal part of the QRS—are well seen in leads 1, aVL, and V2–6. They indicate myocardial disease, presumably ischemic, in addition to the conduction disturbance.

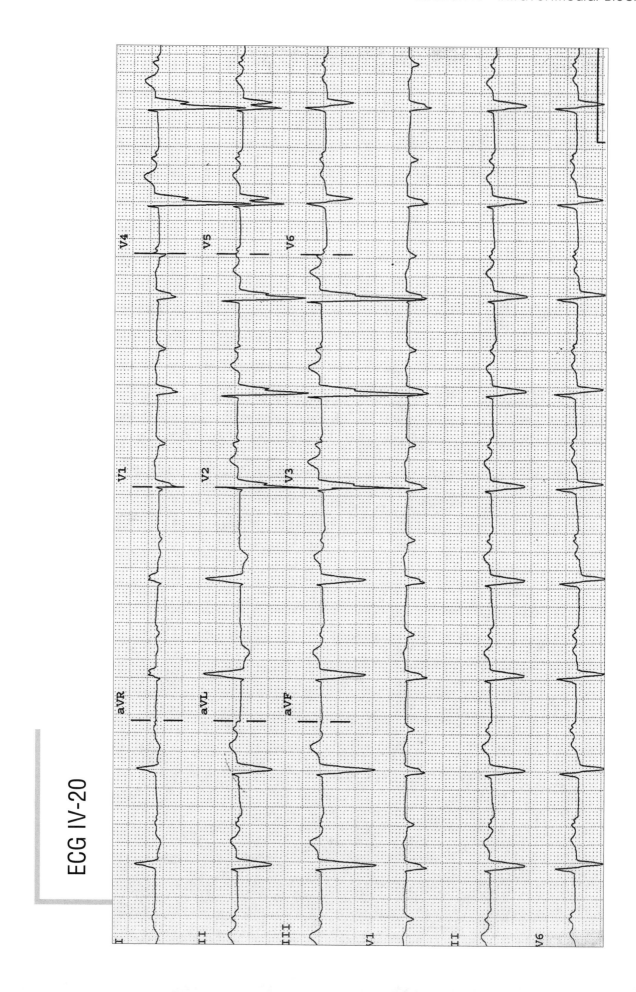

ECG IV-20

Diagnoses **ECG IV-20**

1. Sinus bradycardia (rate = 57/min) with . . .

2. . . . first-degree AV block (PR = 0.56 s)

3. Left bundle-branch block with marked left axis deviation (about −75 degrees)

4. Intra-atrial block (P waves > 0.12 s duration)

5. Left atrial enlargement (P-terminal force in V1 > 0.04 mm/s)

Clinical Data

78-year-old man

Comment

Here the P wave is about 0.15 s wide and notched with peaks more than 0.04 apart in lead 2, and the P-terminal force in V1 is about 0.12 mm/s.

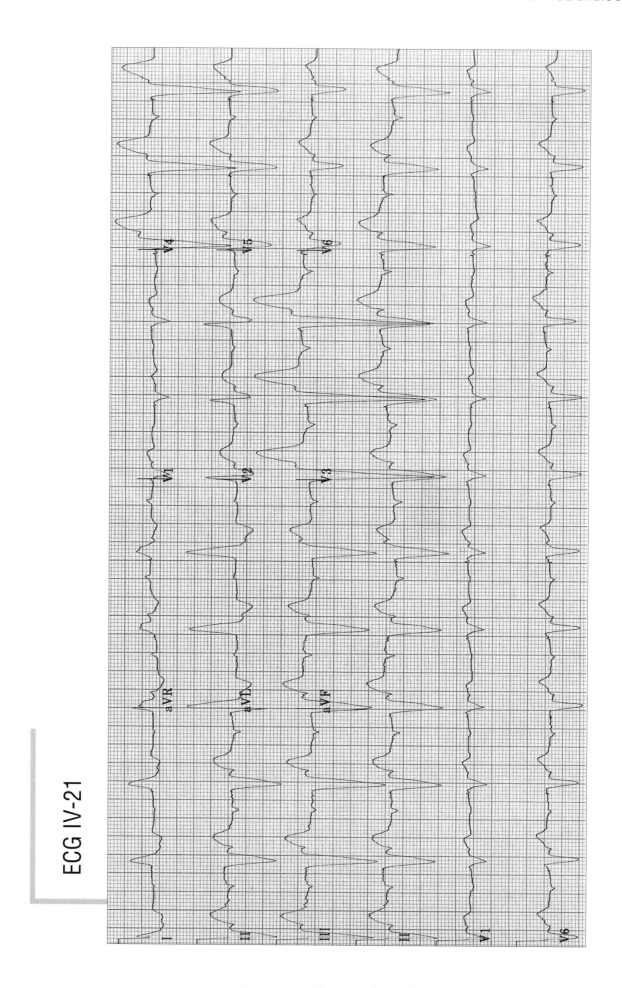

ECG IV-21

Diagnoses   **ECG IV-21**

1. Atrial tachycardia (rate = 142/min)

2. Dual-chambered pacemaker in atrial-tracking mode pacing RV in response to every alternate atrial impulse

Clinical Data

88-year-old man

Comment

This is another good example of lead V2 being "left out in the cold" because of the way we stagger the V leads—the QRS in V2 does not look as though it belongs between V1 and V3 (see ECG III-7)

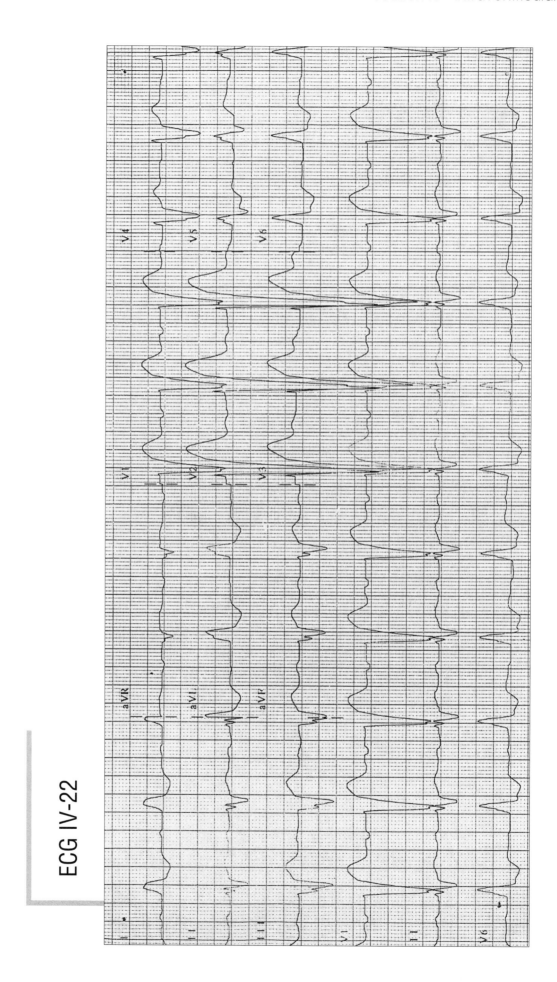

ECG IV-22

Diagnoses   **ECG IV-22**

1. Sinus rhythm (rate = 65/min) with first-degree AV block, PR = 0.32 s

2. Left atrial enlargement (P-terminal force in V1 = 0.09 mm/s)

3. Left bundle-branch block with left axis deviation (−50 degrees)

4. Cannot exclude acute injury (loss of secondary ST-T contours in both anteroseptal and inferior leads)

Clinical Data

80-year-old woman

Comment

None

ECG IV-23

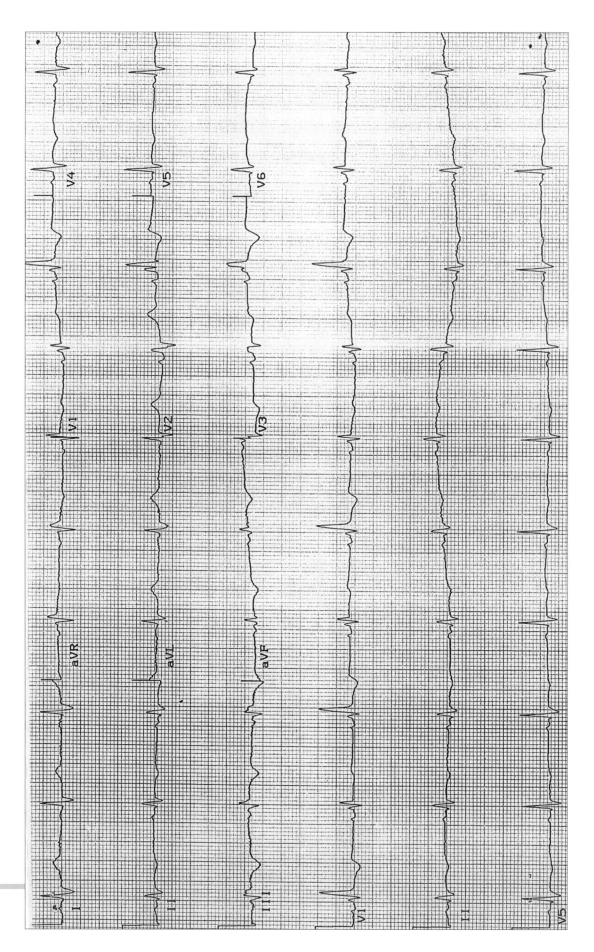

Diagnoses   **ECG IV-23**

1. Probable sinus rhythm (rate = 64/min), but with abnormal P waves (terminally negative in lead 2) and rather short PR (0.12 s)

2. Varying degrees of RBBB

3. Inferior infarction of uncertain date, probably recent

Clinical Data

91-year-old woman

Comment

If you measured the last three cycles, you would say the RBBB is rate-related; but if you then measured the first four cycles, you would find that there is no correlation between cycle length and the pattern of intraventricular conduction.

ECG IV-24

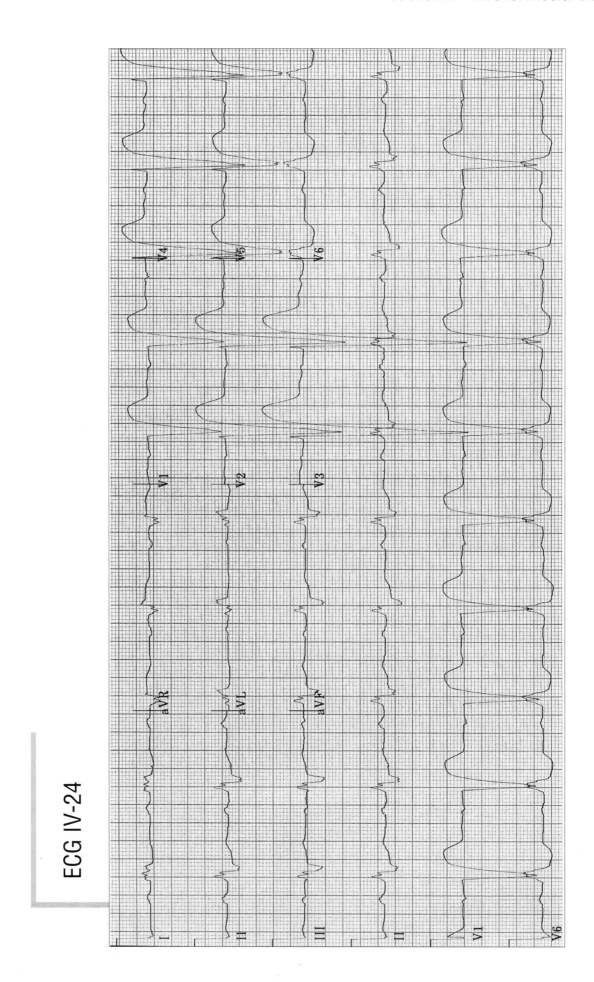

Diagnoses   **ECG IV-24**

1. Sinus rhythm (rate = 61/min) with first-degree AV block (PR = 0.26–27 s)

2. Left bundle-branch block

3. Probably acute anterior infarction

Clinical Data

72-year-old man

Comments

• Note the uncommonly wide QRS (QRS interval = 0.20 s).

• In the presence of LBBB, the loss of the expected, secondary, upward ST concavity in V1–5, with replacement by marked convexity upward (though the degree of ST elevation is only borderline), is extremely suspicious of acute anterior injury/infarction.

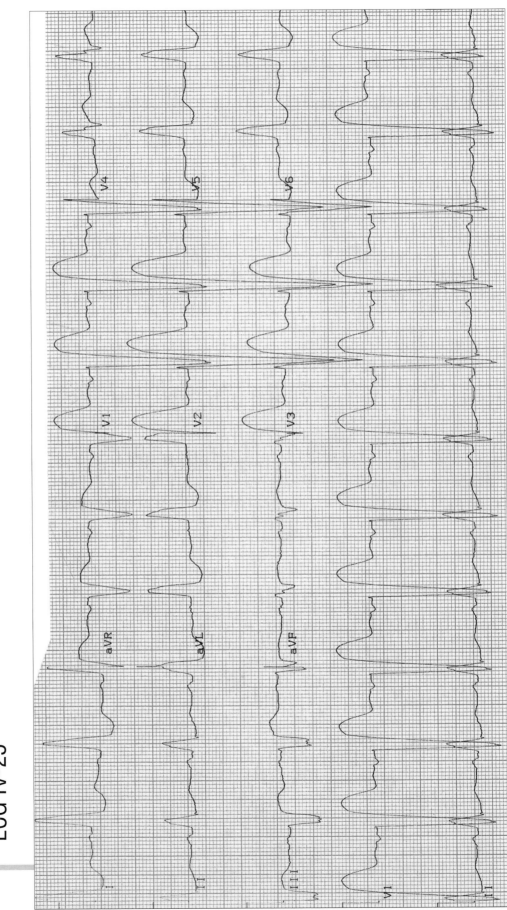

ECG IV-25

Diagnoses   **ECG IV-25**

1. Sinus rhythm (rate = 74/min)

2. Left bundle-branch block

3. Acute anteroseptal infarction

4. Left atrial enlargement

Clinical Data

68-year-old woman

Comments

• Note the disproportionate ST elevation in V1–3 with upward convexity, and the elevated ST in V4 despite the mainly positive QRS—another good example of the ease with which acute infarction can be diagnosed in the presence of LBBB.

• The P wave has a duration of 0.12 s, and the P-terminal force in V1 is 8 mm/sec—about twice the normal maximum, indicating left atrial enlargement.

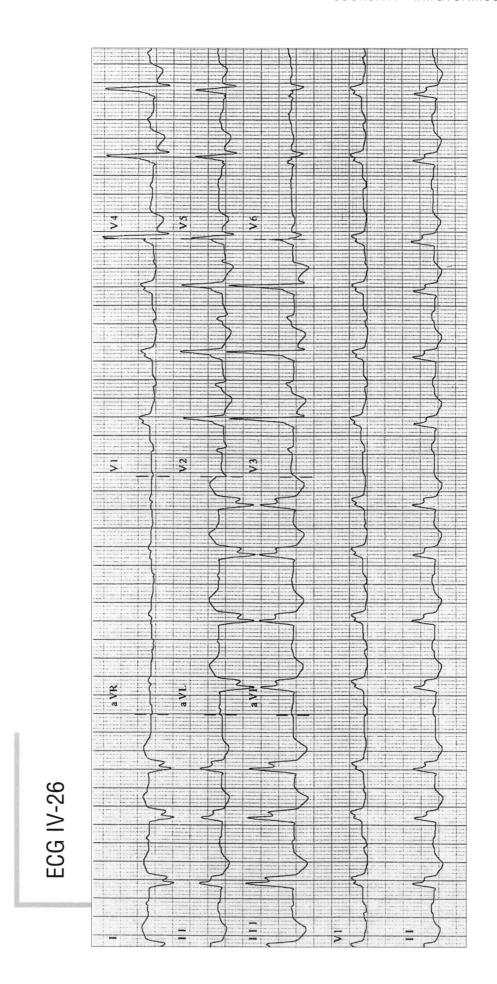

ECG IV-26

Diagnoses   **ECG IV-26**

1. Sinus rhythm (rate = 82/min), with . . .

2. . . . frequent atrial premature beats and . . .

3. . . . first-degree AV block (PR = 0.29 s)

4. Bifascicular block—right bundle-branch block with left posterior hemiblock

5. Left atrial, maybe biatrial, enlargement

Clinical Data

78-year-old man

Comment

Left atrial enlargement is indicated by an abnormal P-terminal force in V1. Right atrial enlargement is demonstrated by the 1.5-mm positive P wave in V2.

ECG IV-27

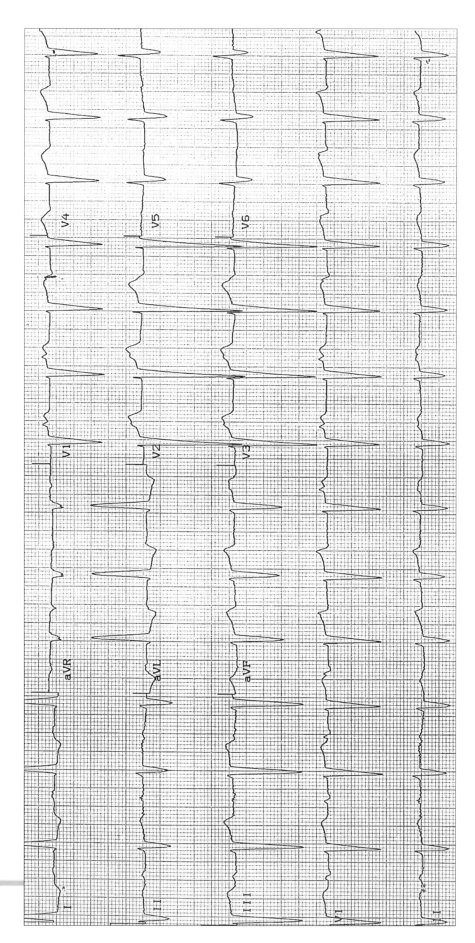

Diagnoses   ECG IV-27

1. Sinus arrhythmia (rate = about 84/min)

2. Left anterior hemiblock, axis −50 degrees

3. First-degree AV block with varying PR interval (0.28–0.52 s)

4. ? Left ventricular hypertrophy

Clinical Data

74-year-old woman

Comments

• A classic example of AV nodal block showing the typical reciprocal RP:PR relationship (the stuff of which Wenckebachs are made). As the atrial rate accelerates and the RP shortens, the PR lengthens; and vice versa. For example, in the second cycle the RP is 57, the PR 29; in the 7th cycle the RP is 25, the PR 46.

• The increased QRS voltage in V2 and V3 probably indicates LVH; but note how the hemiblock, by reducing the R-wave height in V5–6, tends to mask LVH.

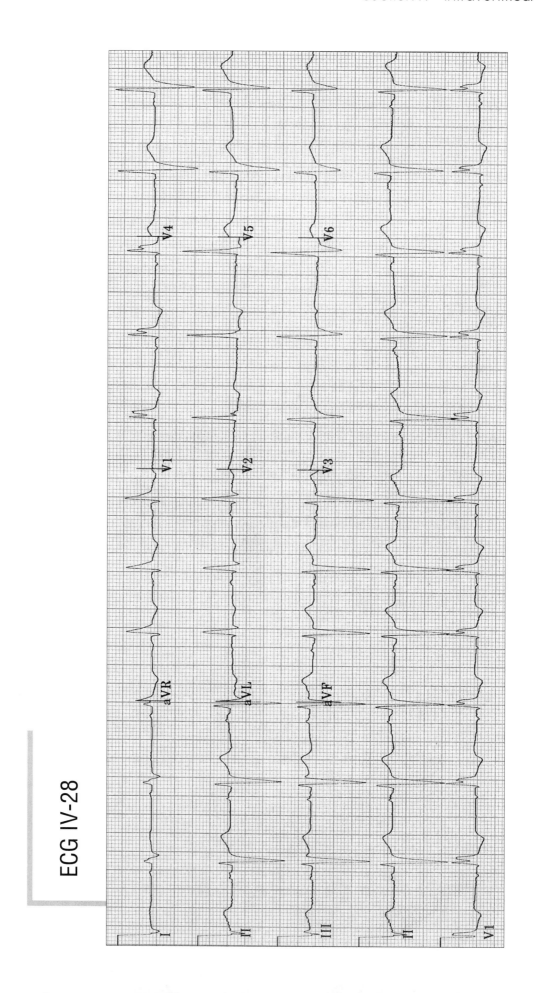

ECG IV-28

Diagnoses   **ECG IV-28**

1. Sinus arrhythmia, average rate 72/min, with . . .

2. . . . bifascicular block (RBBB + left anterior hemiblock)

Clinical Data

92-year-old man

Comment

Note the QRS shape in V1. Usually a taller left peak ("rabbit-ear") in this lead is a valuable clue to ventricular ectopy; but here it is a nice example of the most common exception to this rule: When a hemiblock is associated with RBBB (i.e., in bifascicular block), the left peak of the QRS in V1 is often taller than the right.

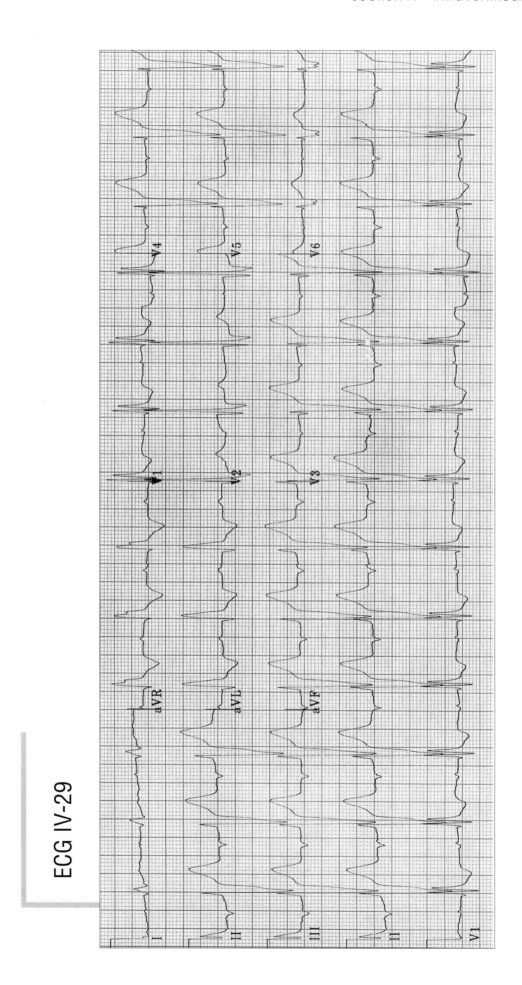

ECG IV-29

Diagnoses   **ECG IV-29**

1. Ectopic atrial rhythm with . . .

2. . . . first-degree AV block (PR = 0.23 s) and . . .

3. . . . bifascicular block (right bundle-branch block + left anterior hemiblock, axis = −85 degrees)

4. Cannot exclude old anteroseptal infarct

Clinical Data

85-year-old man with uremia

Comments

• When sinus P waves are diphasic in V1, they are *positive/negative;* whereas when ectopic and retrograde P waves are diphasic in V1, they are usually *negative/positive* (as here).

• P waves that are inverted in leads 2, 3, and aVF, and negative/positive in V1, *with a more than adequate PR interval,* are more likely ectopic atrial than retrograde from a junctional pacemaker.

• Hemiblock, without infarction, can produce Q waves in anteroseptal leads—but this deep (7 mm in V2)?

ECG IV-30

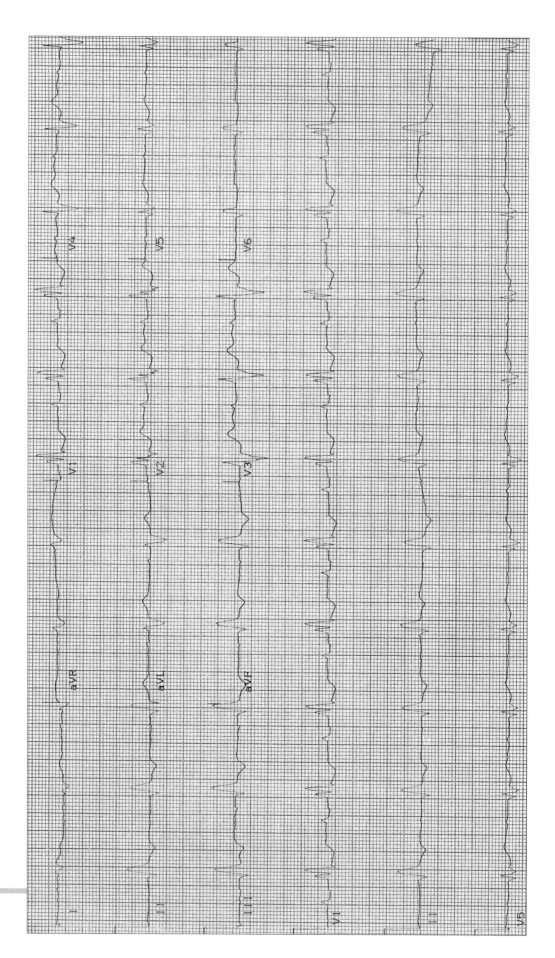

Diagnoses   **ECG IV-30**

1. Probable ectopic atrial rhythm

2. First-degree AV block (PR = 0.28 s)

3. Right axis deviation

4. Right bundle-branch block

5. Inferolateral infarction of uncertain date

Clinical Data

77-year-old man with no cardiac complaints

Comments

• The bizarre P wave probably represents an ectopic atrial focus, but could conceivably represent sinus rhythm with biatrial disease/enlargement.

• In lead 1, the right axis involves only the S wave which represents RV activation; this axis shift, therefore, being unrelated to LV activation, is not due to posterior hemiblock.

Section V

AV Block

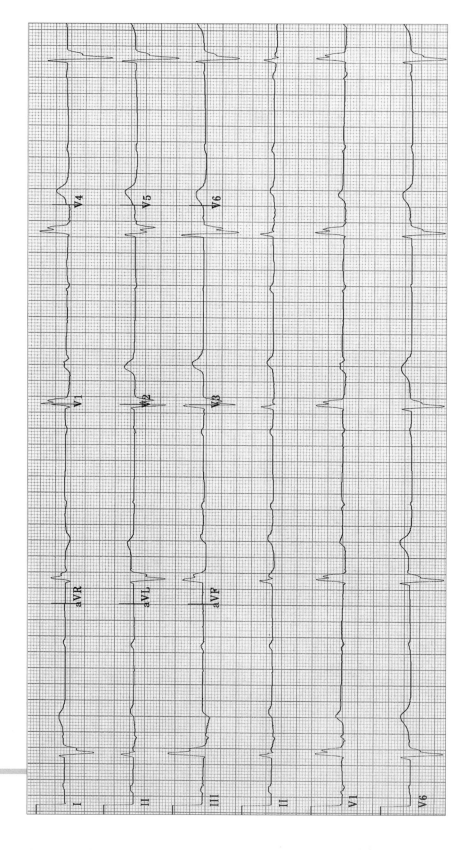

ECG V-1

Diagnoses   **ECG V-1**

1. Sinus rhythm (rate = 66/min) with . . .

2. . . . complete AV block and . . .

3. . . . idioventricular escape rhythm from the LV (rate = 27/min)

Clinical Data

63-year-old man

Comments

The computer's interpretation was "undetermined rhythm" and "RBBB."

• The three criteria for complete AV block are fulfilled: slow enough ventricular rate (< 45/min), enough P waves to probe all phases of the cardiac cycle, and no conduction.

• Note the highly typical features of left ventricular ectopy: rightward axis, qR in V1 with taller left peak ("rabbit-ear"), and rS complex in V6. On the other hand, the QRS pattern is in every way compatible with bifascicular (RBBB + left posterior hemiblock) aberration—remember ECG II-10?

ECG V-2

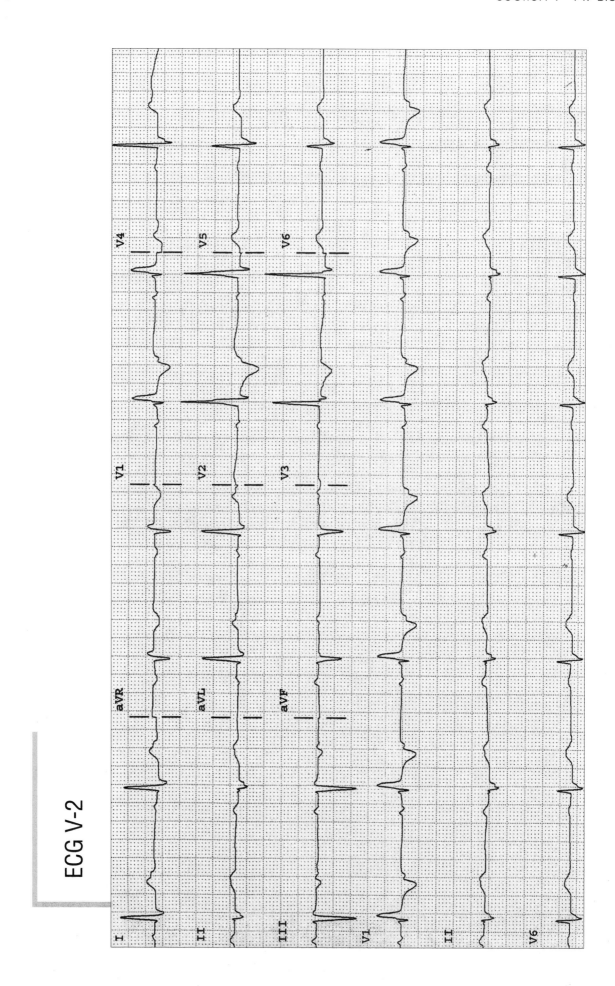

Diagnoses   **ECG V-2**

1. Sinus rhythm with 2:1 type I AV block (PR = 0.24 s)

2. Right bundle-branch block with . . .

3. . . . probable left anterior hemiblock

4. Probable myocardial ischemia

Clinical Data

90-year-old woman

Comments

• The intraventricular blocks (BBB + hemiblock) suggest a type II 2:1 AV block; but the prolonged PR interval makes the far more common form of 2:1 block (AV nodal, i.e., type I) more likely.

• The prolonged, horizontal ST segments in several leads (especially 1, aVL, V4–6) indicate probable ischemia.

ECG V-3

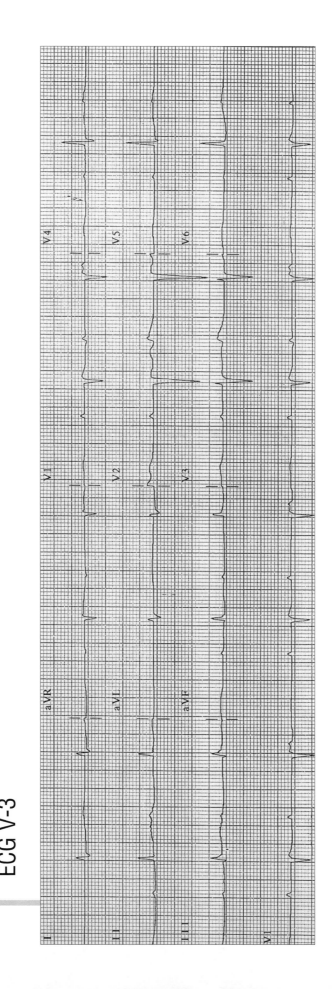

Diagnoses   **ECG V-3**

1. Sinus rhythm (rate = 69/min) with . . .

2. . . . 3:2 AV Wenckebach periods producing a ventricular rate of 46/min

3. Low voltage in limb leads (all under 5 mm)

4. Old anteroseptal infarct cannot be excluded

5. Prominent U waves suggest possibility of hypokalemia, quinidine effect, etc.

Clinical Data

Unknown

Comments

Pairing of like beats immediately suggests a 3:2 Wenckebach. These PR intervals (0.38 and 0.67 s; see rhythm strip below) are longer than usual, but considerably shorter than PRs sometimes stretch (longest PR—so far reported and published—in last conducted beat of a Wenckebach period is 1.04 sec).

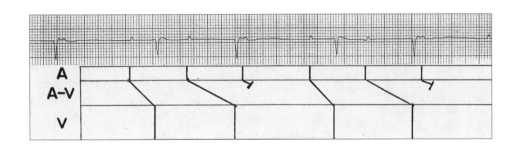

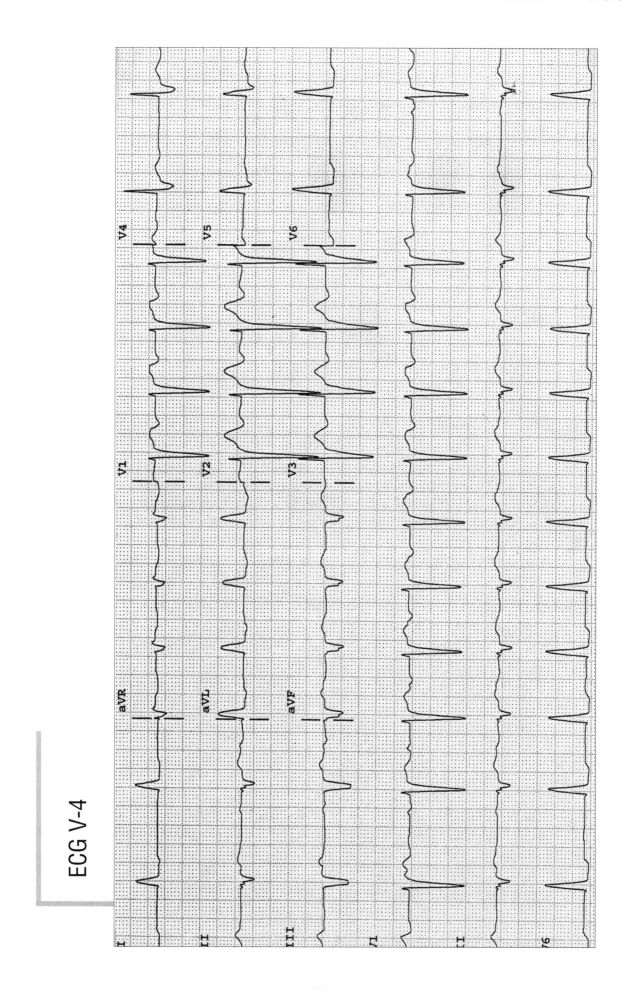

ECG V-4

Diagnoses   **ECG V-4**

1. Sinus rhythm (rate = 86/min) with . . .

2. . . . type I AV block, manifested by an 11:10 Wenckebach

3. Left bundle-branch block, with . . .

4. . . . left axis deviation of −45 degrees

5. Terminal T-wave inversion in V1–3 is suspicious of anterior ischemia

Clinical Data

76-year-old man

Comments

Another simple enough offering, but again too much for the computer, which concluded "accelerated junctional rhythm." Note in the rhythm strip below the paradoxical lengthening of the final PR interval rendering the last ventricular cycle before the dropped beat longer than its predecessors—probably the most commonly encountered deviation from the classic behavior of Wenckebach conduction.

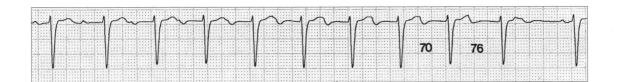

ECG V-5

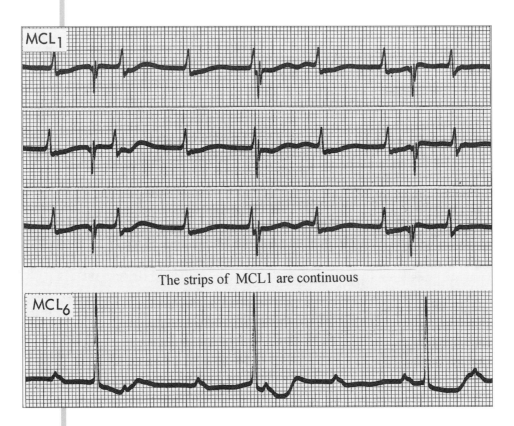

The strips of MCL1 are continuous

Diagnoses

1. Atrial (? sinus) rhythm (rate = 80/min) with . . .

2. . . . high-grade or advanced AV block (probably not complete) permitting . . .

3. . . . junctional escape (rate = 32/min)

4. Probable left ventricular hypertrophy

5. Biatrial enlargement

Clinical Data

31-year-old man with dilated/congestive cardiomyopathy

Comments

• The remarkable P waves in MCL1 look more like ventricular complexes and presumably represent *right* atrial enlargement; in MCL6, the P waves are abnormally broad and presumably reflect *left* atrial enlargement.

• The diagnosis of LVH is perilous from a single lead, but with the high voltage and ST-T changes in MCL6, and the associated biatrial enlargement, LVH is likely (and is certainly consistent with the clinical diagnosis).

• At first glance it looks as though the AV block is complete. But careful measurement of the ventricular cycles reveals that three cycles are 1.81–1.82 s while the rest are measurably shorter (1.61–1.74 s). Whenever the RP is ≥ 1.16 s, the ventricular cycle is < 1.80 s, and one may presume that AV conduction has occurred; but if the RP is as short as 1.00–1.02 s, the impulse is blocked, and the junction escapes at the end of its 1.81–1.82 s cycle.

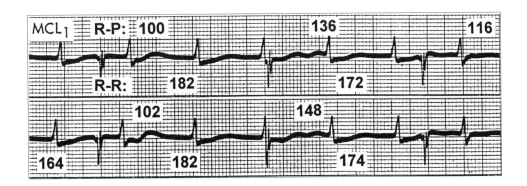

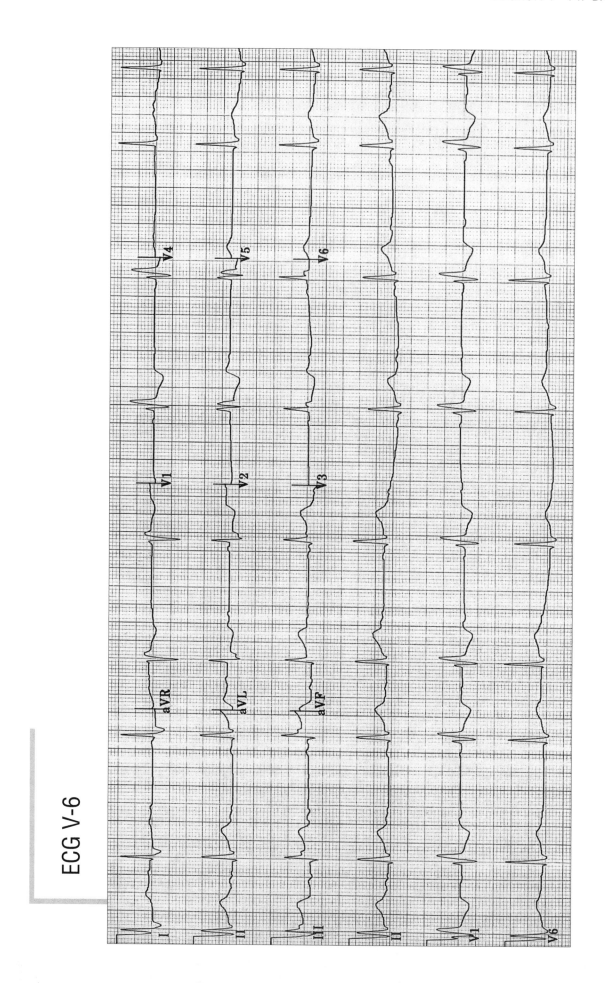

ECG V-6

Diagnoses   **ECG V-6**

1. Sinus rhythm (rate = 83/min)

2. Intra-atrial block (P waves in lead 2 are notched and have duration of 0.16 s)

3. Type I AV block with 2:1 and 3:2 AV conduction

4. Right bundle-branch block

5. Acute inferior infarction

Clinical Data

65-year-old man

Comments

Note that, unlike most type I 2:1 blocks, the PR intervals here are normal during the 2:1 conduction. Thus, if all you had was the 2:1 conduction, the normal PR + BBB would make you suspect type II block; but the 3:2 Wenckebachs here establish the block as type I.

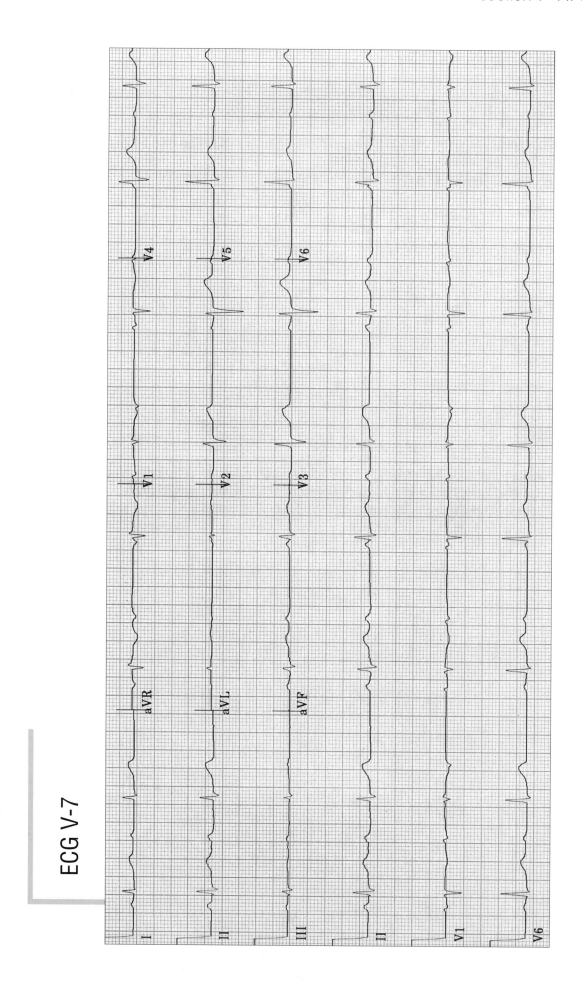

ECG V-7

Diagnoses

ECG V-7

1. Sinus rhythm (rate = 75/min) with . . .

2. . . . some degree of AV nodal (type I) block, resulting in . . .

3. . . . junctional escape at 40/min (producing an allorhythmia [repeated arrhythmic sequence] consisting of two junctional escapes and a ventricular capture)

4. Normal QRS-T

Clinical Data

46-year-old woman with sudden onset of tightness in throat and dizziness; medications are Zoloft, Vistaril, Claritin

Comments

• "Type I" block because there is no bundle-branch block and, in the conducted beats, the PRs are prolonged and are reciprocally related to the associated RPs, confirming the AV nodal level of the block.

• This is the sort of AV block that is often overdiagnosed, even to being called 3rd degree or complete; but the captured beats tell us that if her sinus rate was under 60/min, she would have 1:1 conduction with only first-degree block.

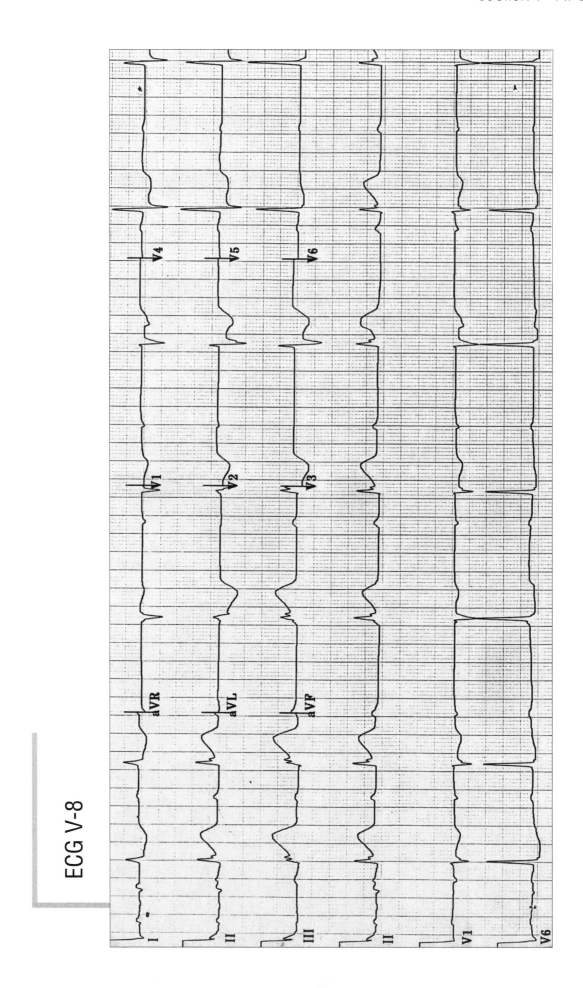

ECG V-8

Diagnoses   ## ECG V-8

1. Acute inferior infarction, with . . .

2. . . . sinus bradycardia with arrhythmia and . . .

3. . . . type I AV block, manifested as a 3:2 Wenckebach, which is followed, as the sinus rate slows, by junctional escape/conducted sinus beat ("escape-capture") sequences

Clinical Data

58-year-old woman

Comments

• A not uncommon mechanism of "bigeminy"—an escape beat followed by a conducted (captured) beat. Here, as usual, beats 4 and 6 are recognized as conducted by the fact that they end cycles shorter than the escape cycles.

• Note that the escape beats, though junctional and appropriately narrow, are—also as usual—slightly different from the conducted sinus beats (in this case taller R in V6, deeper S in V1).

ECG V-9

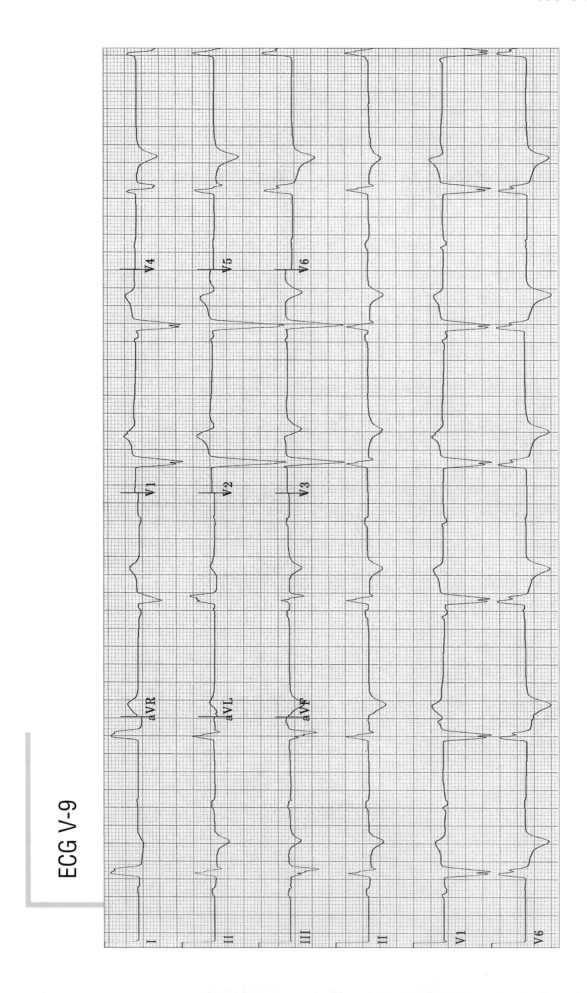

Diagnoses

1. Sinus bradycardia with arrhythmia (rate = 56/min) with . . .

2. . . . complete AV block and . . .

3. . . . idioventricular (or junctional with LBBB) escape rhythm at 39/min

4. Global ischemia suggested by widespread ST-T abnormalities

Clinical Data

82-year-old woman

Comment

It is impossible to be sure whether the escaping pacemaker is junctional or ventricular: the delayed QS nadir in V1 favors ectopic ventricular, while the early peak in V6 favors LBBB.

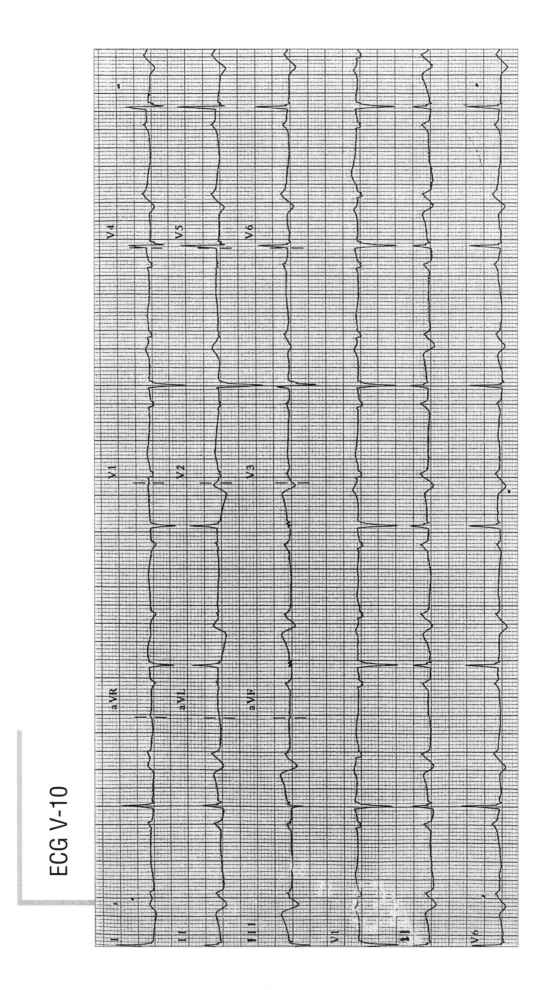

ECG V-10

Diagnoses   **ECG V-10**

1. Sinus rhythm (rate = 78/min) with . . .

2. . . . type I 2:1 AV block (ventricular rate = 39/min)

3. Acute inferior infarction

Clinical Data

81-year-old woman in the critical care unit

Comments

Three things establish the level of the block as AV nodal (type I):

- *inferior* infarction

- prolonged PR interval (0.24 s)

- narrow QRS (absence of bundle-branch block).

In critical care units, type I 2:1 block is 20–30 times more common than type II 2:1 block.

ECG V-11

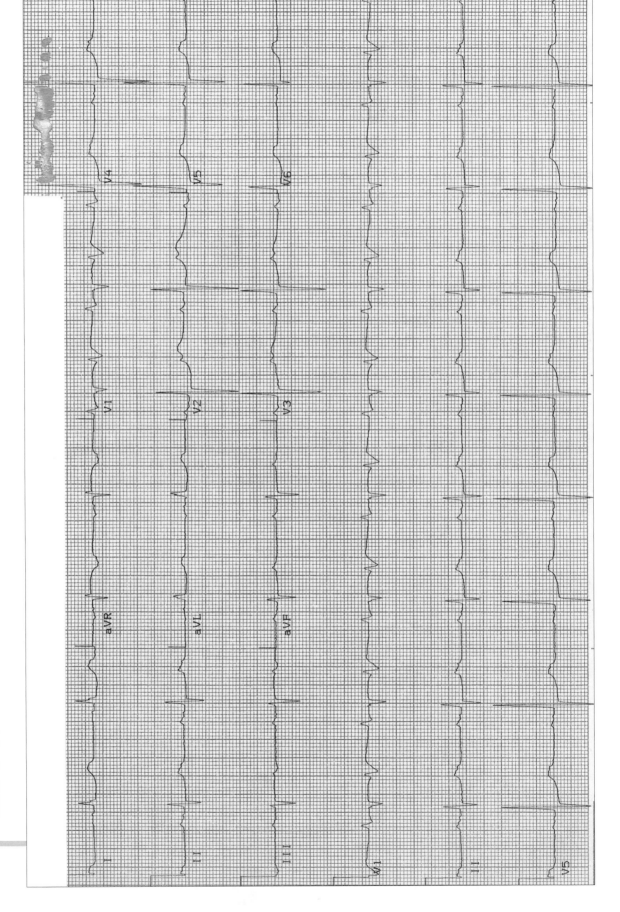

Diagnoses

1. Sinus tachycardia (rate = 106/min) with . . .

2. . . . intra-atrial block (P wave wider than 0.12 s) and biatrial enlargement, and . . .

3. . . . 2:1 type I (AV nodal: prolonged PR, no BBB) AV block

4. Mild left axis deviation (about −30 degrees)

5. Nonspecific, widespread ST depression, probably ischemic

6. Prolonged QT interval; ? prominent U waves, especially V2–3

Clinical Data

93-year-old man

Comment

Though the patient's medications are not known, the ST-T-U pattern, with prominent U waves in V2 and V3, should make you suspect that he was receiving quinidine, with or without digitalis.

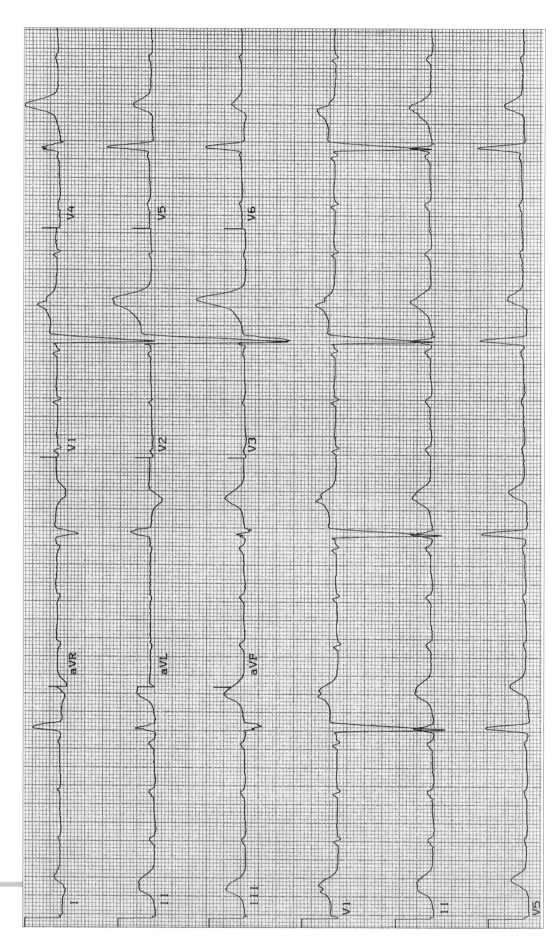

ECG V-12

Diagnoses

ECG V-12

1. Sinus tachycardia (rate = 112/min)

2. Complete (third-degree) AV block

3. Junctional escape rhythm (rate = 28/min)

4. Left bundle-branch block

5. Primary ST-T changes

Clinical Data

69-year-old man

Comments

• Junctional rhythm with BBB is diagnosed because the QRS configuration in lead V1 (slick downstroke to early nadir, 0.05 s) is a strong point in favor of LBBB rather than an ectopic (idioventricular) rhythm.

• The ST-Ts in V4–6 should be downsloping to inverted T waves, but here the T waves are upright, indicating additional (presumably ischemic) disease.

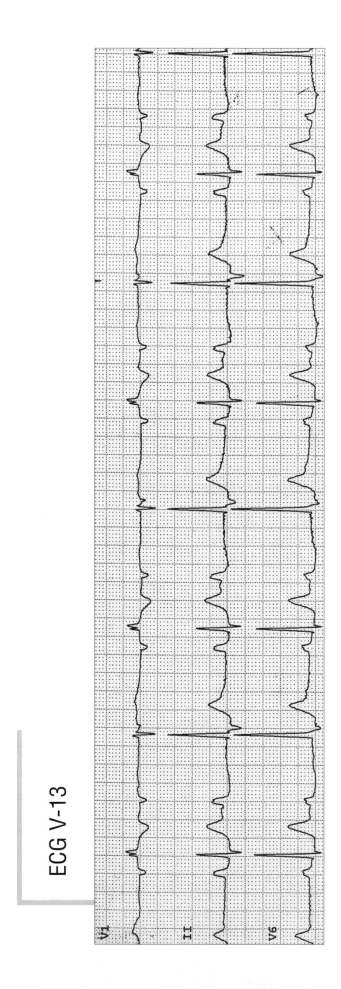

ECG V-13

Diagnoses

1. Sinus rhythm (rate about 75/min) with . . .

2. . . . biatrial enlargement, and . . .

3. . . . 2nd-degree, type I AV block, permitting . . .

4. . . . junctional escape with retrograde conduction to atria

5. Incomplete RBBB and true posterior infarction suspected

Clinical Data

72-year-old woman

Comments

• The prominently positive P waves in lead 2 suggest *right* atrial, while the negative P waves in V1 suggest *left* atrial enlargement—the "P-terminal force" multiples out at 0.16 mm/s, or four times the upper normal limit.

• This is the most common form of escape-capture bigeminy. In this case the atrial cycle (P-P interval) is 80, and therefore the ventricular cycle during 2:1 AV block would be 160. If an escaping pacemaker has a cycle shorter than 160 (the conductible rate)—here it is 130 to 132—the stage is set for escape-capture bigeminy to develop:

    After a beat is conducted, the next atrial impulse is blocked, and before the next impulse can be conducted, the subsidiary pacemaker escapes—that produces the long cycle. The next atrial impulse is blocked (in this case there is retrograde conduction to the atria) and then the *next* impulse is conducted, which creates the shorter cycle and produces the bigeminal effect.

• Note that the QRS of the escape beats, though normally narrow and unmistakably junctional, is different from the sinus QRS—a common finding in junctional escape beats.

• Note the atrial repolarization (Ta or Tᴘ) waves—well seen in all three leads following the blocked P waves.

ECG V-14

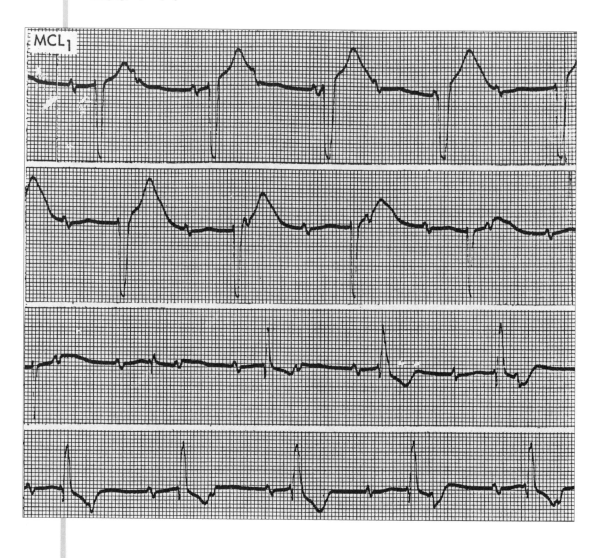

Diagnoses   **ECG V-14**

1. Probable complete AV block (certainly at least high-grade block with complete AV dissociation), with . . .

2. . . . two competing pacemakers having virtually identical rates (47/min): an idioventricular escaping center in the *right* ventricle and a junctional pacer with *right* BBB producing . . .

3. . . . numerous (at least six consecutive) fusion beats

Clinical Data

72-year-old man complaining of lightheadedness

Comments

Junctional beats with RBBB begin to contribute to the QRS with the second beat in the 2nd strip, so that successive beats look more and more normal (note the QRSs getting progressively slimmer and the T waves less tall), until the first beat in the 3rd strip has the contour of a normally conducted beat. In the next few beats there is an increasing contribution from the junctional-with-RBBB beats and less and less from the RV beats until, in the bottom strip, the rhythm is pure junctional with RBBB.

See diagram below. With an ectopic focus on the same side as the bundle-branch block, fusion between the ectopic and descending impulses produces normalization of the QRS complex—because the descending impulses activate the unblocked ventricle while the ectopic focus simultaneously activates the other ventricle.

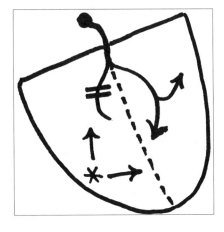

ECG V-15

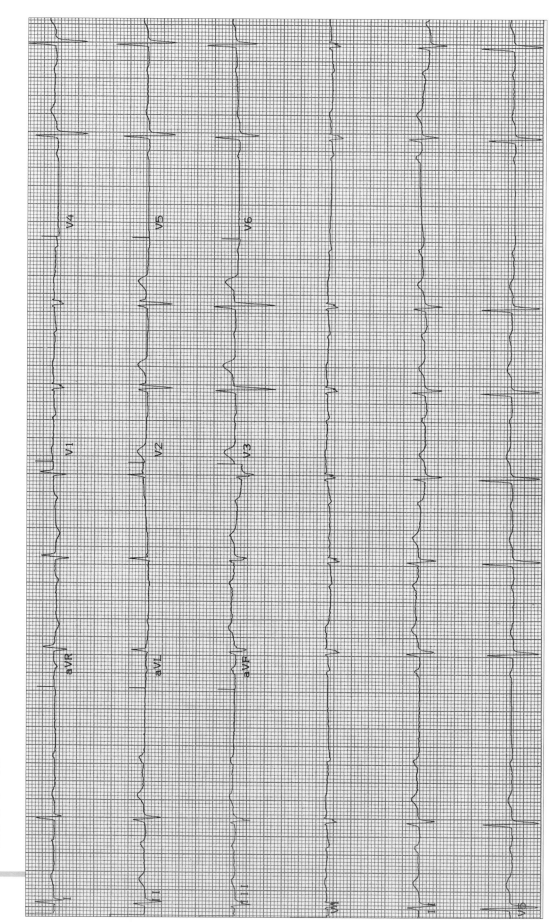

Diagnoses   **ECG V-15**

1. Type I, second-degree AV block, including a 6:5 Wenckenbach period

2. Left axis deviation (-60 degrees), possible left anterior hemiblock

3. Note rSr′ in V2 (? normal variant)

Clinical Data

64-year-old man, aware of irregular heart beat but otherwise asymptomatic

Comments

The axis shift is certainly sufficient to make the diagnosis of LAHB, but lack of increased voltage makes the diagnosis less secure. The prominent S waves through V6 are just an expression of the left axis deviation.

ECG V-16

83-year old man

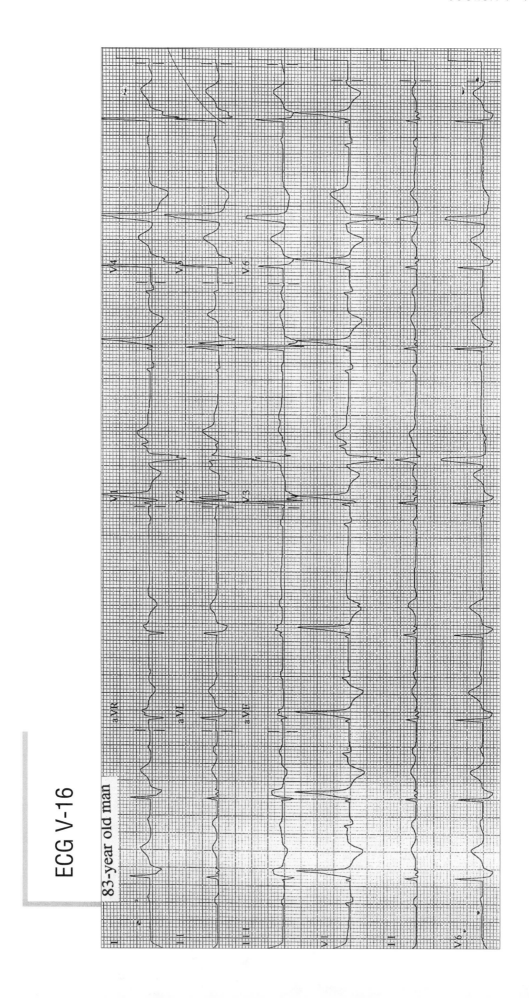

Diagnoses

ECG V-16

1. Sinus rhythm (rate = 70/min) with type I AV block, including one 5:4 Wenckebach period with paradoxical lengthening of the 3rd and 4th PR and the final RR

2. RBBB

3. ? RVH (R' in V1 = 17 mm)

4. Two ventricular premature beats

Clinical Data

83-year-old man

Comments

• In the classic Wenckebach period, the lengthening PR intervals increase by less and less; but in this 5:4 example, the increments are getting bigger—the consecutive PR intervals are 29, 31, 39 and 50, giving consecutive increments of 2, 8 and 11.

• Voltage criteria for RVH in the presence of RBBB are not reliable, but an R' over 10 mm is suspect.

ECG V-17

90-year old woman

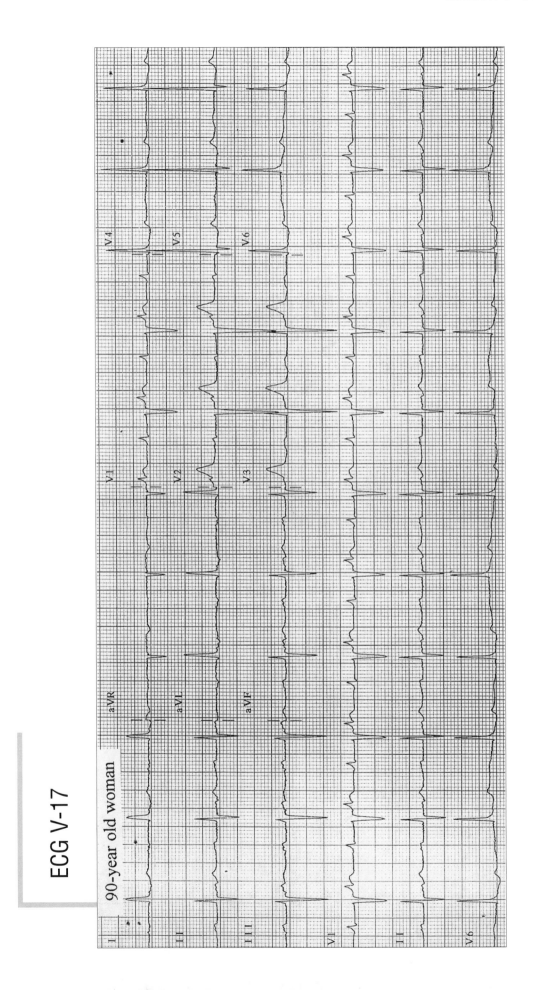

Diagnoses

1. Atrial tachycardia (rate = 135/min), with . . .

2. . . . 2:1 AV block, type I

3. Borderline left axis deviation (−30 degrees)

4. Nonspecific ST-T abnormalities

Clinical Data

90-year-old woman complaining of throbbing in her neck

Comments

• "Throbbing" in the neck is presumably due to the cannon waves resulting from every alternate atrial contraction occurring while the tricuspid valve is still closed.

• The prolonged PR of the conducted beats and absence of BBB indicate AV nodal (type I) block.

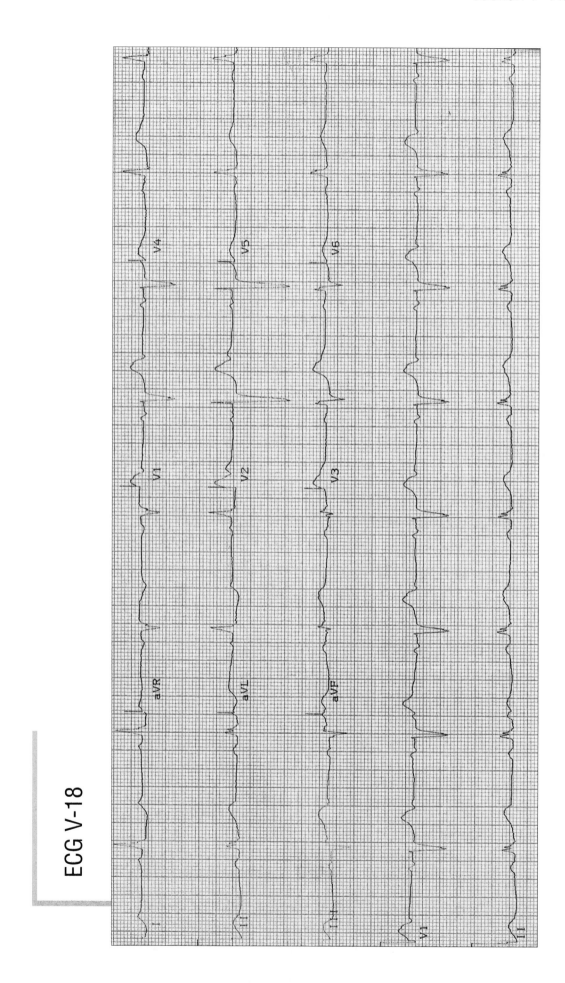

ECG V-18

Diagnoses   **ECG V-18**

1. Sinus rhythm (rate = 96/min) with 2:1 AV block

2. One nonconducted atrial premature beat (just after the second QRS)

3. Acute inferior infarction

4. Atypical LBBB

Clinical Data

66-year-old man complaining of dizzy spells

Comments

• The level of the AV block is uncertain; it could be AV nodal or infranodal. The PR is borderline (0.20–0.22 s), and the QRS interval = 0.12 s. In view of the inferior infarct, it's probably AV nodal, i.e., type I.

• The QRS doesn't look like typical LBBB, but careful measurement shows that the QRS interval is 0.12 s, and clearly the delay is on the left side.

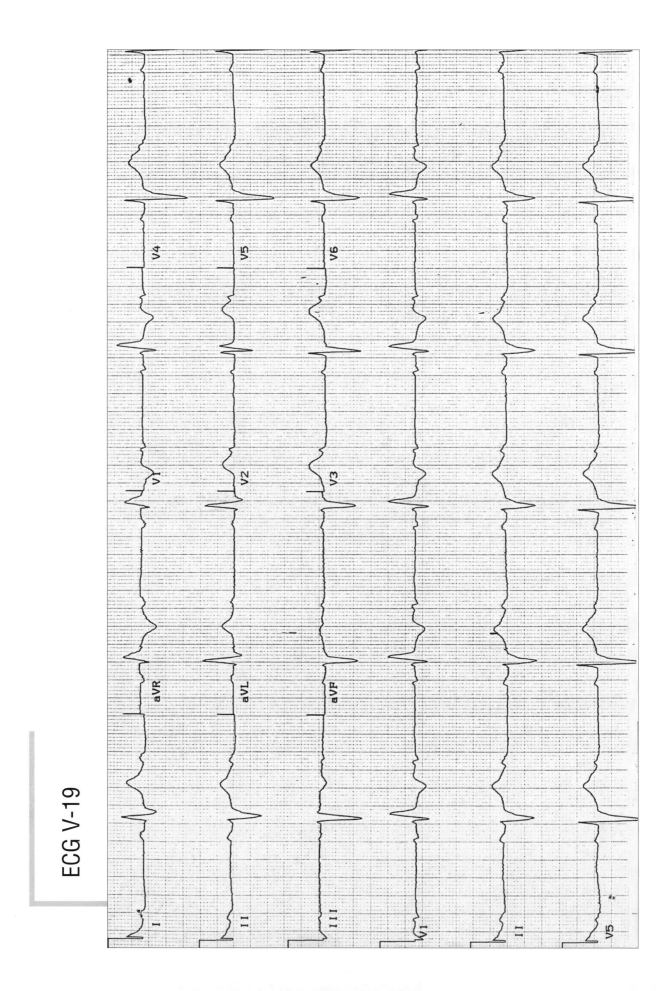

ECG V-19

Diagnoses

ECG V-19

1. Sinus rhythm (rate = 68/min) with . . .

2. 2:1 AV block, ? type

3. Bifascicular block (RBBB + left anterior hemiblock)

Clinical Data

70-year-old man

Comments

• Note that the bifascicular block produces a QRS shape in V6 that is exactly like LV ectopy, i.e., rS with no sign of a q wave.

• Without electrophysiologic studies, the level at which the alternate beats are blocked is uncertain: the slightly prolonged PR (0.22 s) favors AV nodal (type I); the BBB favors infranodal (type II). Statistically, 2:1 type I is much more common than type II.

ECG V-20

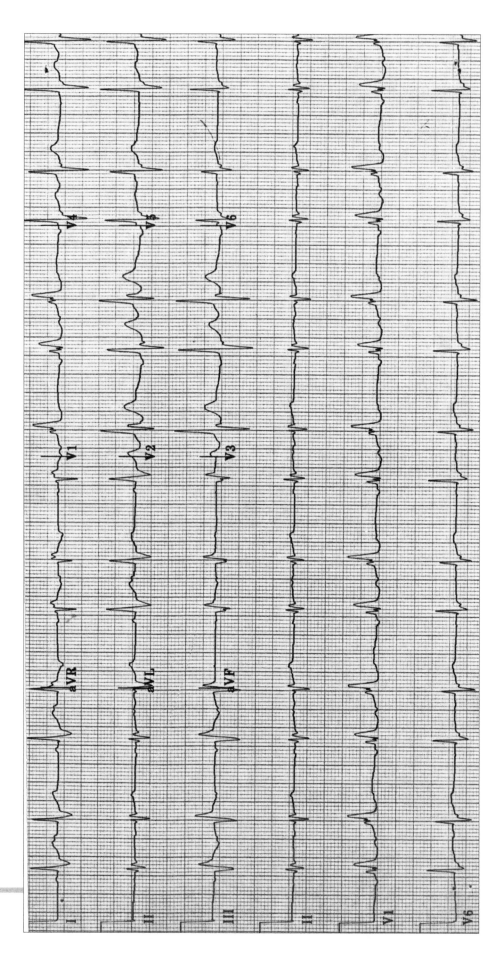

Diagnoses   **ECG V-20**

1. Ectopic atrial rhythm with . . .

2. . . . 3:2 AV Wenckebachs producing bigeminy

3. Inferior infarction of uncertain date, probably recent

4. Right bundle-branch block

Clinical Data

79-year-old man

Comment

Note some unusual features:

• In an AV Wenckebach it is unusual to have the first PR within normal limits, and rare to have both first and second PRs normal—as they are here (0.14 and 0.20 s).

• Unusual wide, splintered notching of the QRS in lead V1

• The slight difference in QRS morphology between the beats of each pair (best seen in the rhythm strips of V1 and V6) is probably secondary to the changed ventricular cycle length (minor aberration— due to slightly increased RBB delay—of beats ending the shorter cycles).

ECG V-21

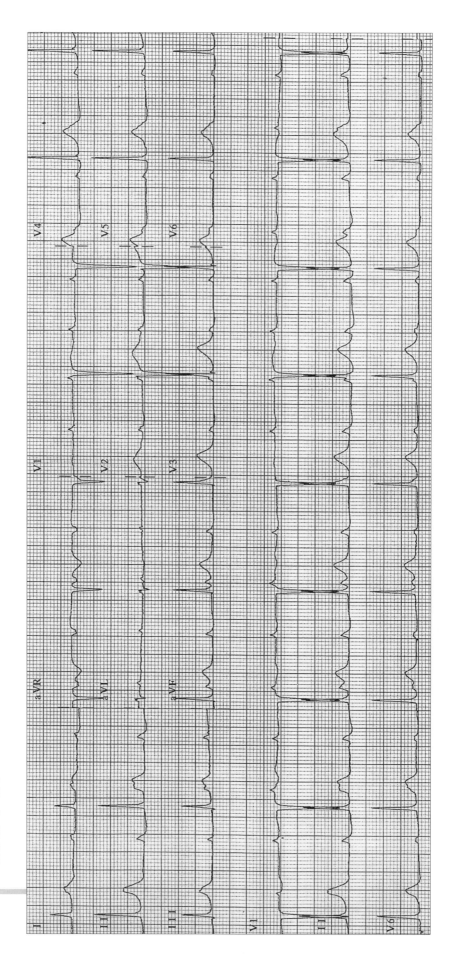

Diagnoses   **ECG V-21**

1. Sinus tachycardia (rate = 106/min)

2. AV block, producing complete AV dissociation

3. Idiojunctional rhythm (rate = 50/min)

4. No QRS-T abnormalities

Clinical Data

22-year-old woman; asymptomatic except aware of intermittent pulsation in neck

Comment

This is probably congenital complete AV block. Most authorities require a ventricular rate under 40, or at least under 45, before labeling the block "complete"; but with congenital block a faster rate is permissible. Pulsations in the neck are presumably due to cannon waves produced when atrial contraction closely follows or coincides with ventricular, as in beats 3, 4, and 5.

ECG V-22

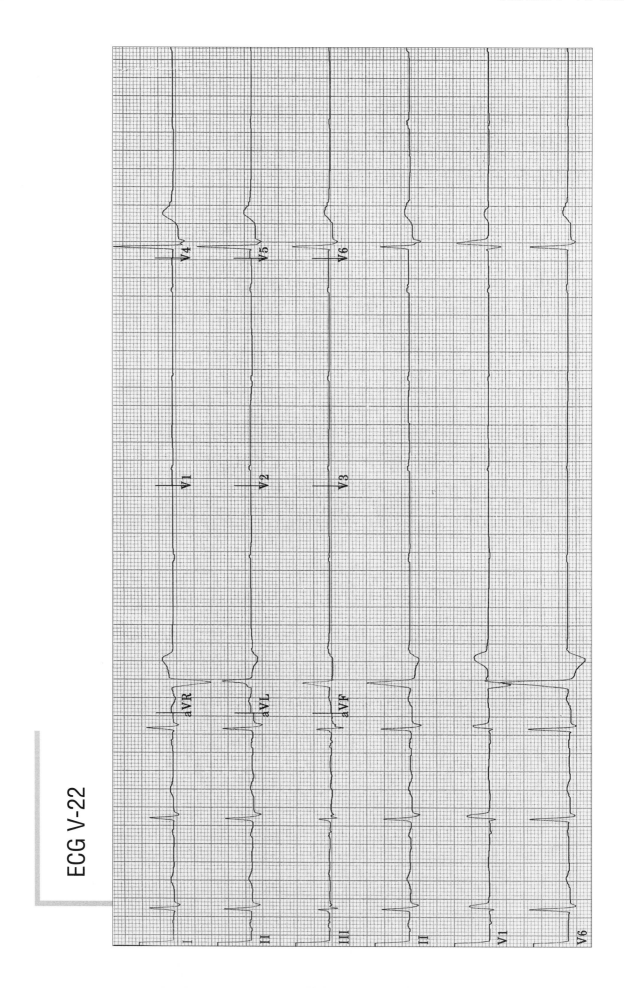

Diagnoses   **ECG V-22**

1. Sinus rhythm (rate = 60/min) with incomplete RBBB interrupted by . . .

2. . . . a ventricular premature beat (VPB) which initiates . . .

3. . . . AV block with ventricular asystole

4. Junctional escape beat with complete RBBB

Clinical Data

73-year-old woman with near-syncope

Comment

• Why does a VPB precipitate AV block and ventricular asystole?

   Answer: Although it is a well-recognized phenomenon, the mechanism is uncertain; but as AV block and asystole can also be precipitated by atrial prematures (even when nonconducted), it is probably a "phase 4" phenomenon, i.e., refractoriness occurring later rather than earlier in the cardiac cycle. This is also sometimes seen in BBB ("paradoxical critical rate" BBB), where LBBB develops at the end of the longer cycle, but not at the end of the shorter (see rhythm strip below).

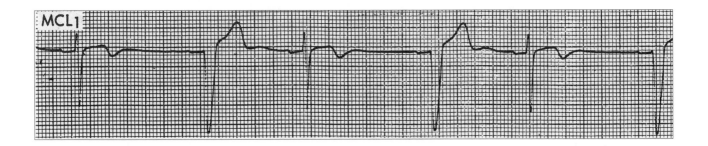

ECG V-23

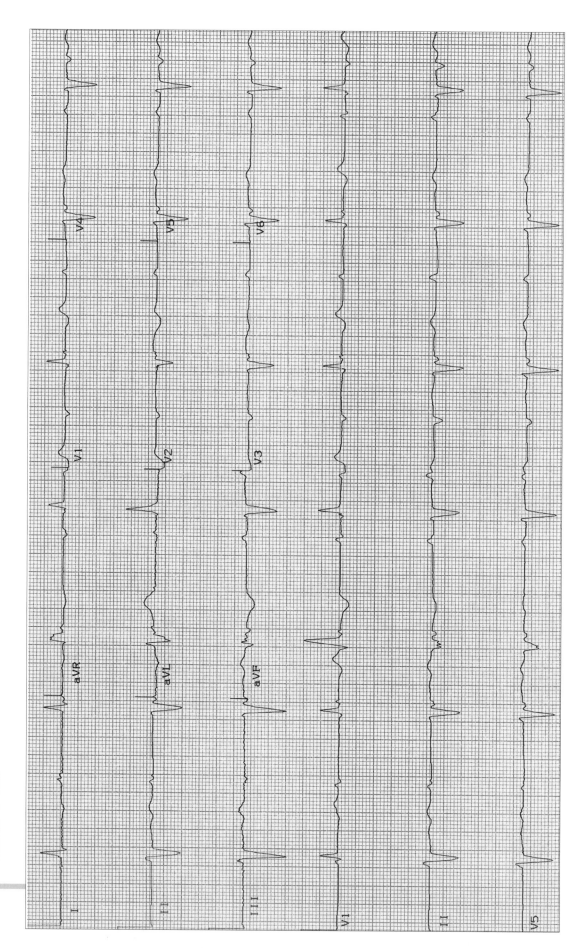

Diagnoses

1. Chaotic (multifocal) atrial rhythm with . . .

2. . . . high-grade AV block and . . .

3. . . . junctional escape rhythm (rate = 38/min) with . . .

4. . . . right bundle-branch block, left anterior hemiblock, and . . .

5. . . . two ventricular capture beats

6. One ventricular premature beat with concealed retrograde conduction depolarizing junctional pacemaker

7. Probable old anteroseptal infarction

Clinical Data

60-year-old woman complaining of lightheaded spells and intermittent "throbbing" in neck

Comments

The first, fourth and fifth cycles are all identical (158) and represent the junctional escape cycle. The third and sixth cycles are shorter (144) and therefore end with captured (conducted) beats. Concealed retrograde conduction discharging the junctional pacemaker is recognized because the next expected junctional beat fails to show up (see X in laddergram below).

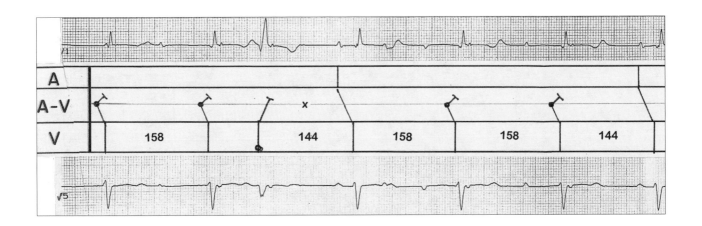

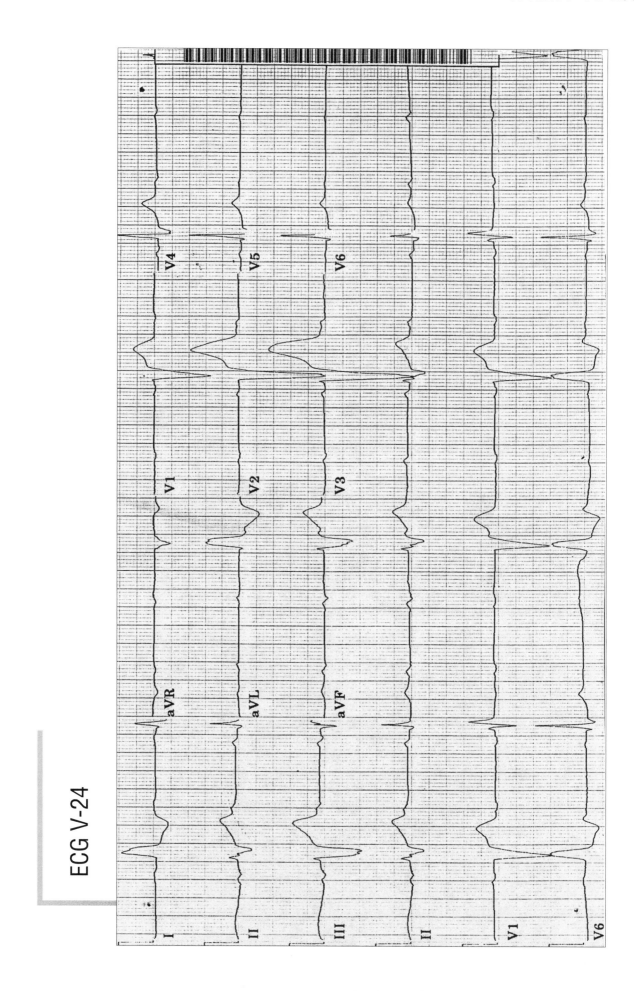

ECG V-24

Diagnoses   **ECG V-24**

1. Sinus rhythm (rate = 78/min) with . . .

2. . . . right bundle-branch block with . . .

3. . . . high-grade AV block, and . . .

4. . . . right ventricular escape at rate 32/min

Clinical Data

82-year-old man

Comments

• The 2nd and 5th beats are ventricular captures (i.e., sinus beats conducted with RBBB interrupting the otherwise dissociated rhythm due to the AV block).

• The escaping beats (3rd, 4th, and 6th) must originate either in the RV myocardium or in the right bundle branch below the level of the block.

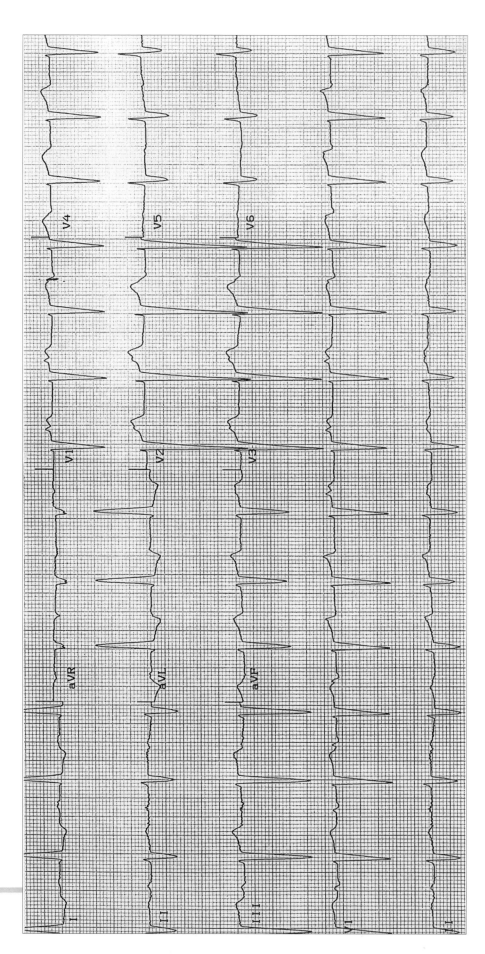

ECG V-25

Diagnoses   **ECG V-25**

1. Sinus arrhythmia (rate about 84/min)

2. Left anterior hemiblock, axis −50 degrees

3. First-degree AV block with varying PR interval (0.28–0.52 s)

4. Left ventricular hypertrophy (?)

Clinical Data

74-year-old woman

Comments

• A classic example of AV nodal block showing the typical reciprocal RP:PR relationship (the stuff of which Wenckebachs are made): as the atrial rate accelerates and the RP shortens, the PR lengthens; and vice versa. For example, in the 2nd cycle the RP is 57, the PR 29; in the 7th cycle the RP is 25, the PR 46.

• The increased QRS voltage in V2 and V3 probably indicates LVH; but note how the hemiblock, by reducing the R-wave height in V5–6, tends to mask LVH.

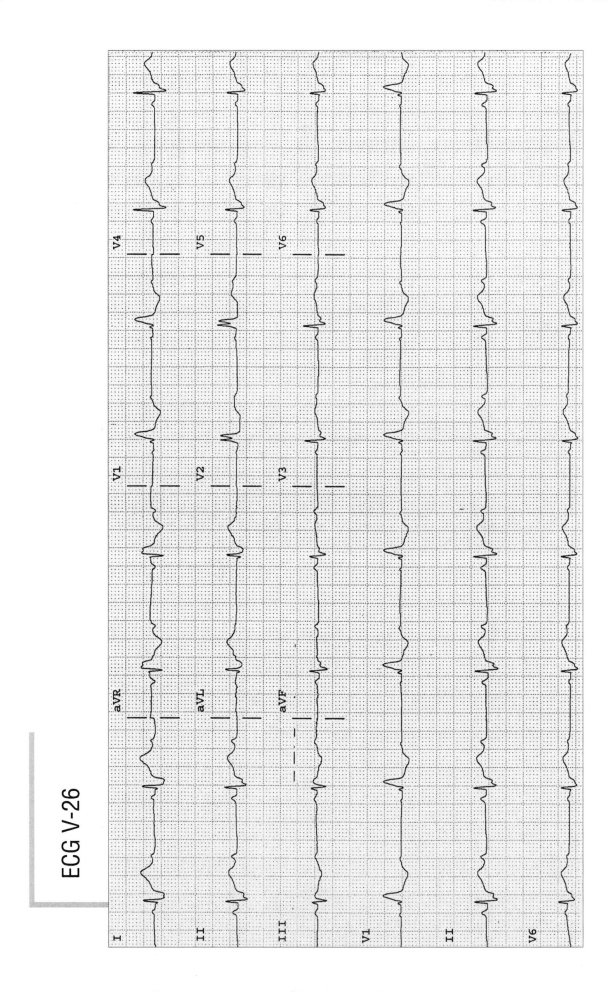

ECG V-26

Diagnoses   **ECG V-26**

1. Sinus rhythm (rate = 94/min) with 2:1 AV block, probably type II

2. Right bundle-branch block

Clinical Data

85-year-old woman

Comments

In 2:1 AV block, the combination of a normal PR with a BBB is more likely type II; but one can only say "probably type II" (with about 70% probability) because a significant minority of type I AV blocks, after dropping a beat, have a normal PR in the returning beat. If such a patient has an unrelated BBB and develops 2:1 AV block, he or she will produce a tracing like this one. In contrast, if a 2:1 block manifests a long PR and narrow QRS, you can be almost 100% certain that you are dealing with AV nodal (type I) block.

ECG V-27

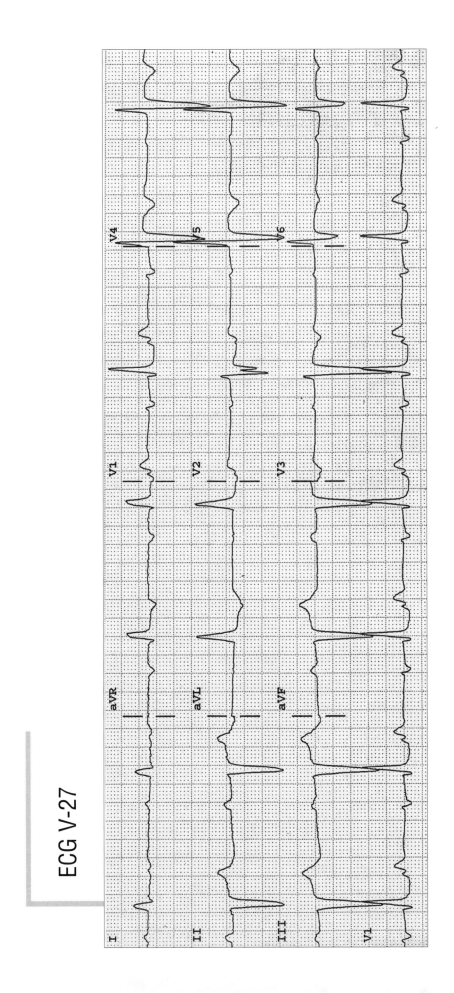

Diagnoses   **ECG V-27**

1. Sinus rhythm (rate = 80/min) with . . .

2. . . . 2:1 AV block, type uncertain

3. Right bundle-branch block with left anterior hemiblock

4. Left atrial enlargement

5. Probable anterior myocardial ischemia

Clinical Data

76-year-old man

Comments

• The level of the AV block is uncertain because the prolonged PR intervals (0.35 s) favor the AV node, whereas the presence of bifascicular, infranodal block suggests that the AV block may be owing to 2:1 block in the surviving posterior fascicle. If the latter is the mechanism, this is a form of trifascicular block.

• The primary ST-T pattern in the V leads probably reflects anterior ischemia or may be the relic of an old anterior infarct.

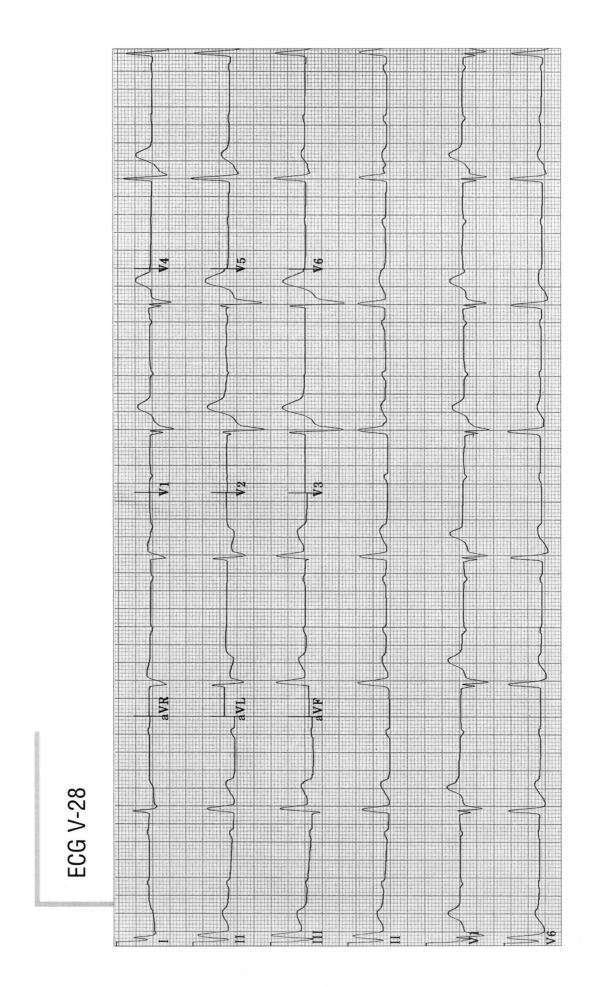

ECG V-28

Diagnoses

1. Sinus tachycardia (rate = 105/min) with . . .

2. . . . complete AV block, and . . .

3. . . . idiojunctional escape rhythm (rate = 42/min) with atypical intraventricular block complicating . . .

4. . . . acute inferior infarction

5. Old anteroseptal infarction is suspect (splintered QS in V1, qrS in V2)

Clinical Data

69-year-old man

Comments

The delayed QS nadir in V1 favors ectopic ventricular, rather than junctional with incomplete LBBB—but perhaps not in the presence of an old anteroseptal infarct. Furthermore, the normal axis would be unusual for an ectopic ventricular rhythm, and the precordial transition from V1 to V6 is characteristic of a conducted rhythm. You can therefore conclude that the mechanism is supraventricular.

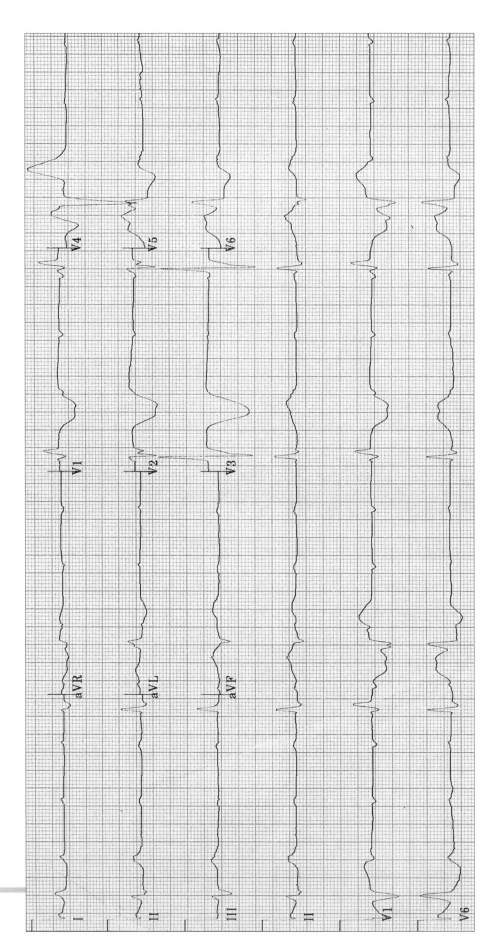

ECG V-29

Diagnoses

1. Sinus rhythm (rate = 92/min) with . . .

2. . . . complete AV block and . . .

3. . . . unusually slow idiojunctional rhythm (rate = 28/min), with . . .

4. . . . right bundle-branch block

5. Three right ventricular premature beats

6. Gross ST-T abnormalities presumably from recent anteroseptal infarction

Clinical Data

90-year-old man complaining of retrosternal pain and dizziness

Comment

Since the idiojunctional cycle and the post-extrasystolic cycles are almost identical, you can conclude that the extrasystoles are conducted retrogradely, and depolarize and re-set the junctional pacemaker (see laddergram below).

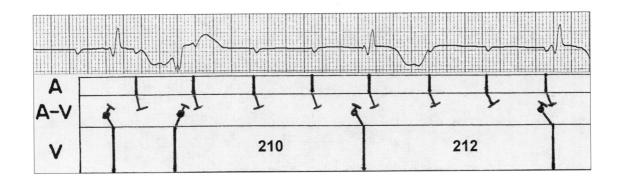

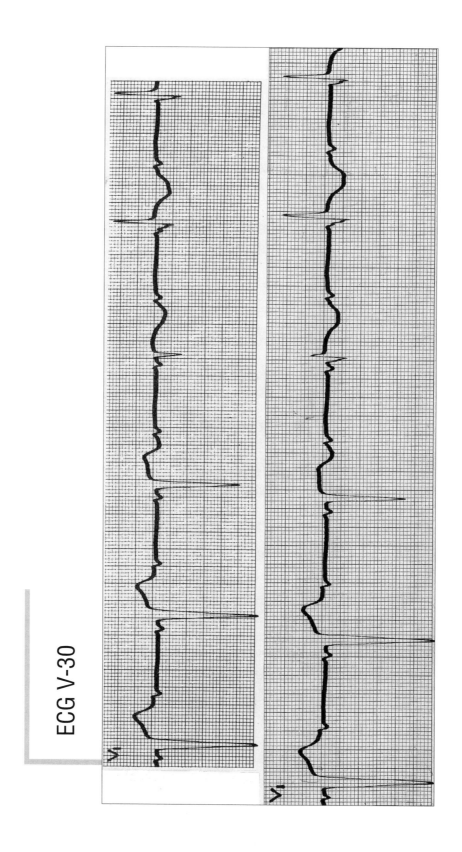

ECG V-30

Diagnoses   ECG V-30

1. Sinus rhythm (rate = 78/min) with . . .

2. . . . 2:1 AV block, probably type II

3. Left bundle-branch block

4. Accelerated idioventricular rhythm (rate = 41/min) producing . . .

5. . . . fusion beats and then AV dissociation

6. Probable acute anteroseptal infarction (judging by the AIVR complexes)

7. Left atrial abnormality (P-terminal force is > 0.04 mm/s)

Clinical Data

82-old-man complaining of weakness and dizziness

Comments

The first two beats in both strips document the underlying rhythm as sinus with 2:1 AV block; because the PR intervals are normal and there is a BBB, you should suspect type II (infranodal) block. In the last two beats we see that an AIVR from the left ventricle has usurped control. The two intervening beats are fusion beats. In the presence of LBBB, the sinus impulse activates the right ventricle first, while the ectopic focus in the LV begins activating the left. When activation in both ventricles begins more or less simultaneously, the fusion QRS is normally narrow and may look completely normal. How about the 4th beat in the upper strip?

Section VI
Sick Sinus, Escape, and Dissociation

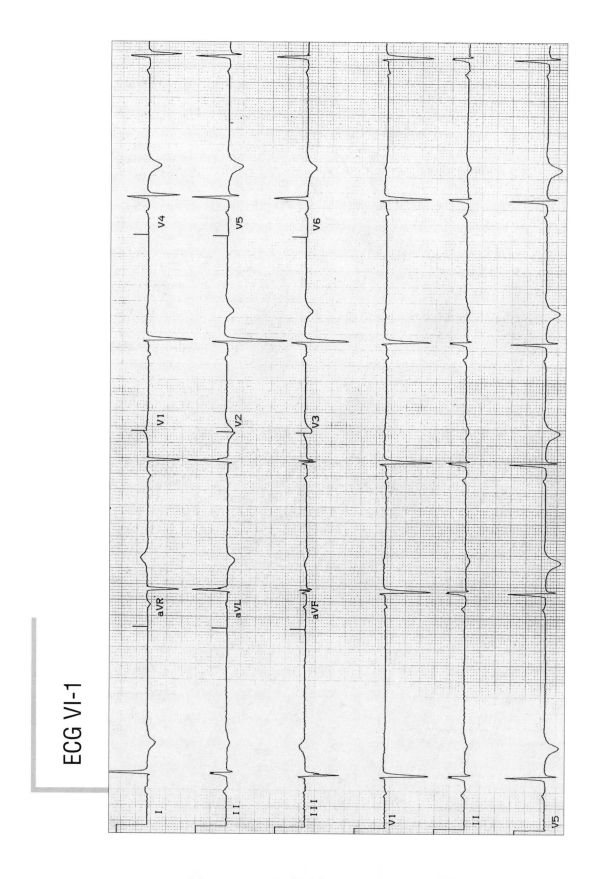

ECG VI-1

Diagnoses   **ECG VI-1**

1. Marked sinus bradycardia with arrhythmia (rate = 32–36/min)

2. First-degree AV block (PR = 0.22–0.24 s)

3. *Probable* left ventricular hypertrophy and "strain" with *probable* superimposed ischemia

Clinical Data

66-year-old woman; taking diltiazem hydrochloride for hypertension; experiencing dizzy spells

Comment

Inversion of the T waves in V2 and V3 where the QRS is predominantly negative, together with the deep T-wave inversion in other leads suggesting more than "strain" alone, add up to the probability of significant, superimposed ischemia.

ECG VI-2

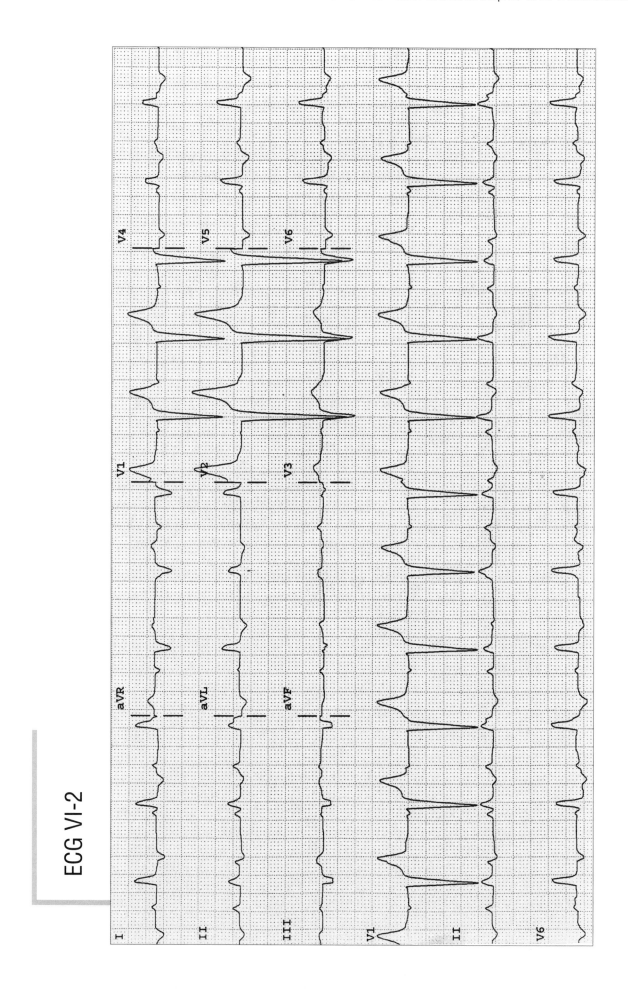

Diagnoses   **ECG VI-2**

1. Accelerated junctional rhythm (rate = 70/min) with . . .

2. . . . left bundle branch block, and . . .

3. . . . *some* degree of AV block, producing . . .

4. . . . complete AV dissociation

5. Sinus tachycardia (rate = 114/min)

Clinical Data

80-year-old woman

Comments

In this rather complex tracing there are good opportunities for diagnostic mistakes:

• Tracings like this are often labeled "complete AV block"—but the ventricular rate is far too fast to allow this diagnosis.

• The ventricular rhythm might be called "idioventricular"—but the morphology in V1 (with slicker downstroke than upstroke) as well as the compatible morphology in the other leads is compelling evidence favoring LBBB.

• "AV dissociation" might be offered as the diagnosis—but AVD is never *the* diagnosis; it is always secondary to some primary condition. Here the dissociation is secondary to an unidentifiable degree of AV block and a collaborating accelerated subsidiary pacemaker.

ECG VI-3

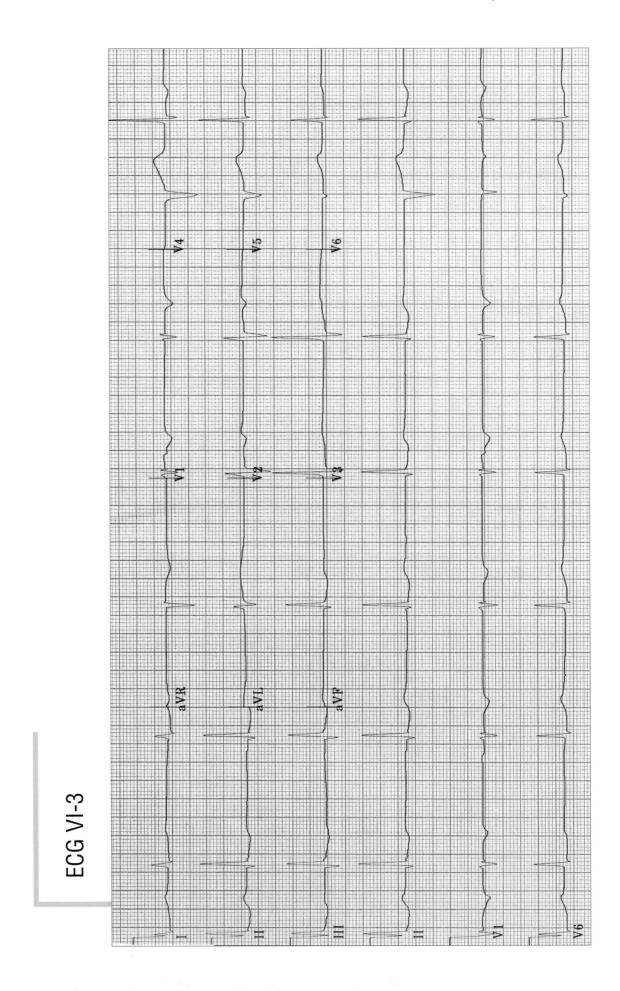

Diagnosis   **ECG VI-3**

1. Sinus bradycardia (rate = 36/min) permitting . . .

2. . . . junctional escape at 42/min, producing . . .

3. . . . incomplete AV dissociation with occasional ventricular capture

4. One ventricular escape beat

5. First-degree AV block (prolonged PR in conducted beats)

6. Nonspecific ST-T abnormalities suggesting ischemia; cannot exclude old inferior infarction

Clinical Data

83-year-old man

Comments

Note on rhythm: The primary rhythmic disturbance here is *sinus bradycardia*; everything else (escape, dissociation, capture) is secondary to the bradycardia.

Analysis of beats (see ECG below): 1 and 7 are ventricular captures; 2 to 5 are junctional escape rhythm; 6 is a ventricular escape.

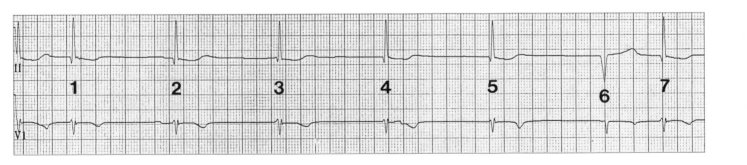

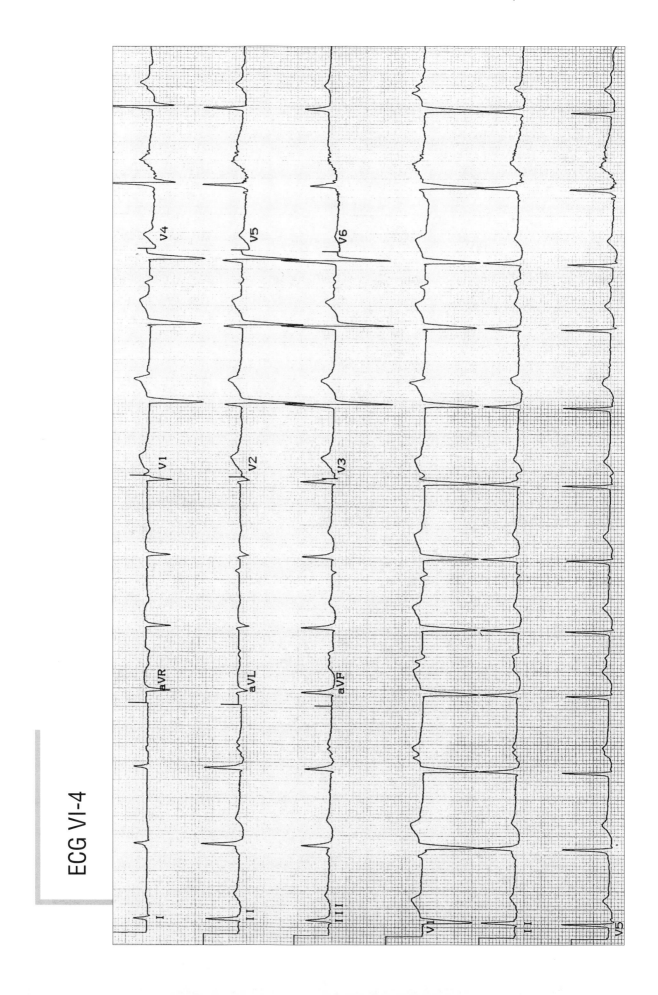

ECG VI-4

Diagnosis   **ECG VI-4**

1. Sinus bradycardia (rate = 57/min) with . . .

2. . . . accelerated junctional rhythm (rate = 70/min) and . . .

3. . . . mild, type I AV block producing . . .

4. . . . AV dissociation with . . .

5. . . . two (maybe three) ventricular captures

6. One atrial premature beat (4th visible P wave) which may or may not be conducted. If conducted, it represents the third ventricular capture.

7. Nonspecific ST-T changes

Clinical Data

76-year-old man with angina; receiving digoxin

Comments

On the rhythm:

- There are three contributors to the dissociation, and all three may be digoxin-related.
- Beats 5 and 10 (and possibly beat 6, the APB) are captures, recognized by shortening of the *ventricular* cycle.
- Type I (AV nodal) block is recognized by the features of the captured beats, namely, long PR, no BBB, and RP/PR reciprocity.

On the ST-T:

- The T waves are upright in all chest leads, but T-V1 is taller than T-V6. This is often, but not always, a useful early sign of trouble (ischemia, LVH, etc).

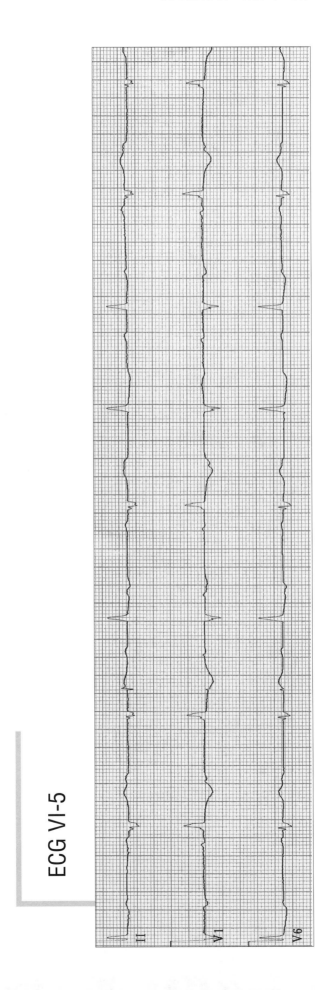

ECG VI-5

Diagnoses   **ECG VI-5**

1. Sinus rhythm (rate = 85/min) with . . .

2. . . . type I AV block, producing . . .

3. . . . AV dissociation with . . .

4. . . . three ventricular captures (4th, 6th, and 7th beats)

5. Idioventricular, or junctional, escape rhythm (rate = 49/min)

Clinical Data

73-year-old man

Comments

• This sort of tracing is sometimes mistaken for complete AV block, despite the irregular ventricular rhythm and the changing QRS complexes.

• The conducted or captured beats (see ECG below, C) are recognized as such simply by the fact that they end shorter ventricular cycles (110–113) than the independent beats (124–128) and have P waves at an appropriate interval in front of them.

• From the first two captured beats we can infer that, if the atrial rate were 55 (cycle length 110) rather than 85, he would be able to conduct 1:1 (every beat) with only "first"-degree block

• Note the reciprocal RP/PR relationship in the three conducted beats, hallmark of AV nodal (type I) block: 70/40, 48/62, 77/36.

• The independent escaping pacemaker has complexes that are not very wide and therefore may be junctional, with the sort of aberration that is commonly seen in junctional beats, i.e., a pacemaking center situated off to one side so that its impulse travels sooner down the ipsilateral BB and produces a pattern of contralateral BB delay.

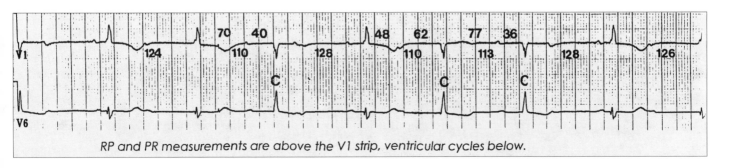

RP and PR measurements are above the V1 strip, ventricular cycles below.

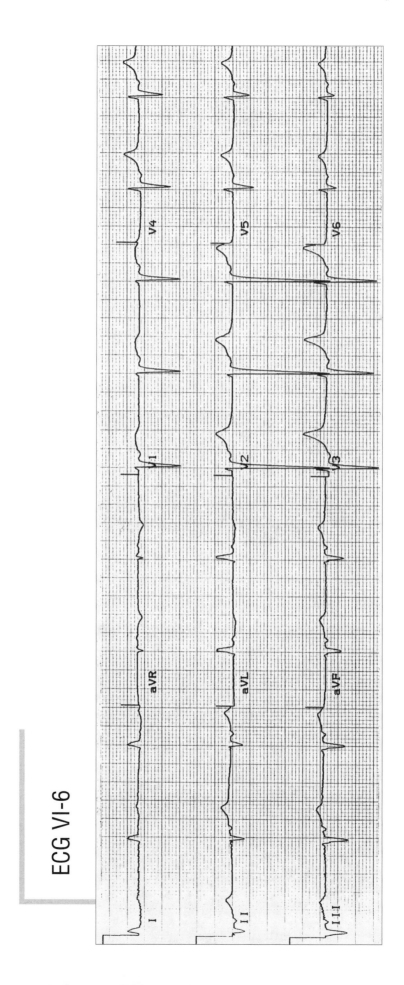

ECG VI-6

Diagnoses   **ECG VI-6**

1. Junctional rhythm (rate = 60/min) with retrograde conduction to atria

2. Left axis deviation (−60 degrees)

3. Poor R wave progression with low voltage in V6

4. Nonspecific ST-T abnormalities

Clinical Data

78-year-old woman with cardiac amyloidosis, end-stage congestive failure; tracing taken the day before death

Comment

The marked left axis, poor R wave progression, and low voltage are obviously nonspecific, but they are common findings in patients with cardiac amyloid.

ECG VI-7

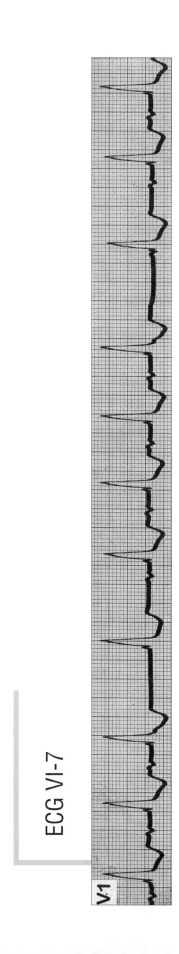

V1

Diagnosis

1. Sinus rhythm (rate = 84/min) with . . .

2. . . . first-degree AV block (PR = 0.24–0.28)

3. Right bundle-branch block

4. Nonconducted atrial premature beats, providing the opportunity for . . .

5. . . . junctional escape at rate 55–60/min

Clinical Data

Unknown

Comments

At first glance, there appear to be rather subtle AV Wenckebach periods; especially since, following each of the junctional escapes, the next two beats show increasing PR intervals. And there is no doubt that, if the sinus rate were a little faster and there were no interruptions by APBs, classic AV Wenckebach periods would develop. But from the rhythm as is, you cannot diagnose more than *first-degree block*.

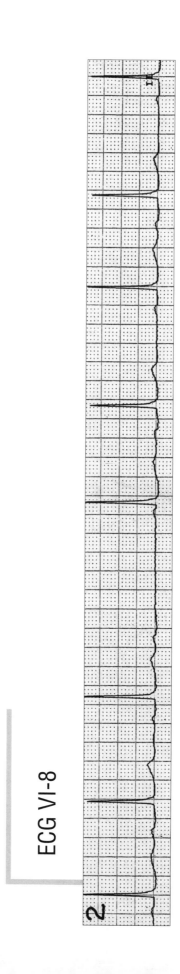

ECG VI-8

Diagnoses   **ECG VI-8**

1. Sinus rhythm with . . .

2. . . . type I SA block (3:2 Wenckebachs out of the sinus node—sinus discharge rate is 86/min) and . . .

3. . . . type I AV block manifested by developing AV Wenckebachs thwarted by the pauses due to the SA block, and one "dropped beat" (after the 4th P wave)

4. The 4th QRS is a junctional escape beat.

Clinical Data

Unknown

Comment

See rhythm strip with laddergram below.

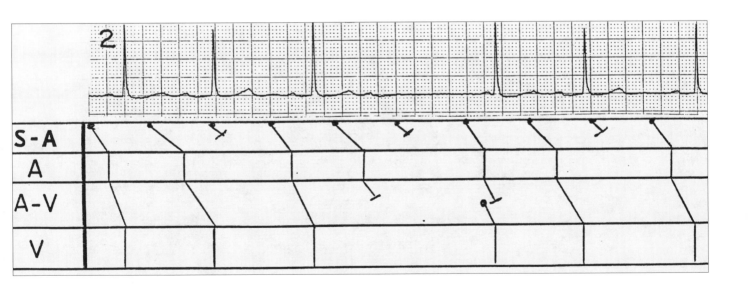

ECG VI-9

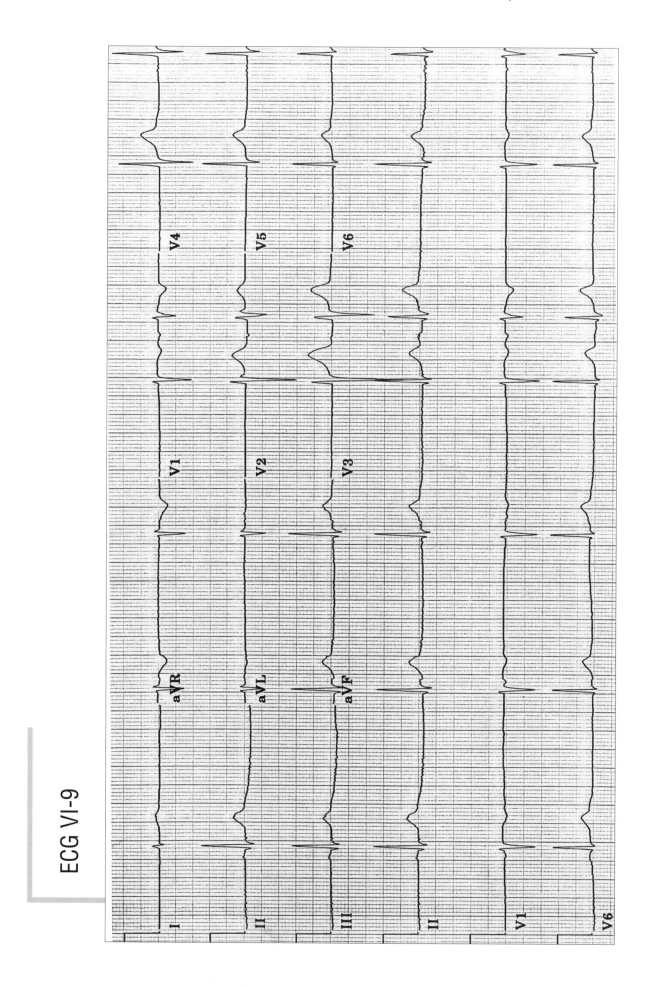

Diagnoses   **ECG VI-9**

1. Sick sinus (sinus bradycardia, rate = 32/min) with resulting . . .

2. . . . junctional escape (rate = 36/min), producing . . .

3. . . . AV dissociation with . . .

4. . . . two ventricular capture beats (5th and last beats), the first showing . . .

5. . . . prolonged PR (0.23 s) and minor RBB delay

Clinical Data

53-year-old Marfanoid man with right-sided chest pain; rhythm spontaneously reverted to normal sinus

Comments

• This sort of tracing is often misconstrued as some sort of AV block (of which there is *no* evidence), when it is actually a sick sinus from which everything else (escape, dissociation, capture) follows.

• The two earliest signs of delayed conduction in the right bundle branch are shrinkage of the S wave and slurring of the terminal upstroke in V1, both of which are well seen here. In confirmation, there is also a corresponding widening of the terminal S wave in leads 2 and V6.

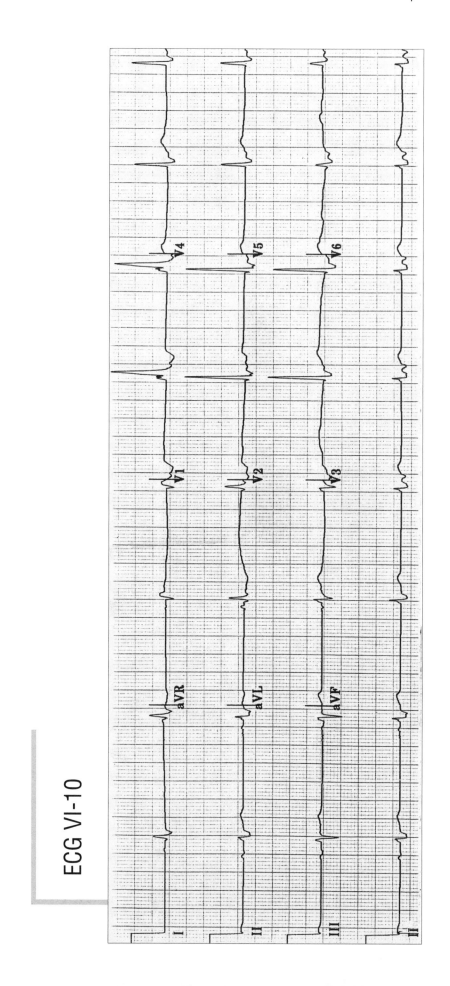

ECG VI-10

Diagnoses   **ECG VI-10**

1. Sinus bradycardia (rate = 42/min)

2. Junctional escape (at 45/min accelerating to 56/min)

3. Right bundle-branch block

4. Left axis deviation of initial forces (−30 degrees)

Clinical Data

86-year-old man

Comments

• The escaping junctional pacemaker at first (for two beats) produces AV dissociation; then retrograde conduction to the atria (atrial capture) supervenes and persists through the rest of the strip.

• The acceleration of the junctional pacemaker is a good example of a common phenomenon ("warm-up"), often seen at the start of an automatic rhythm as the ectopic pacemaker reaches its stride.

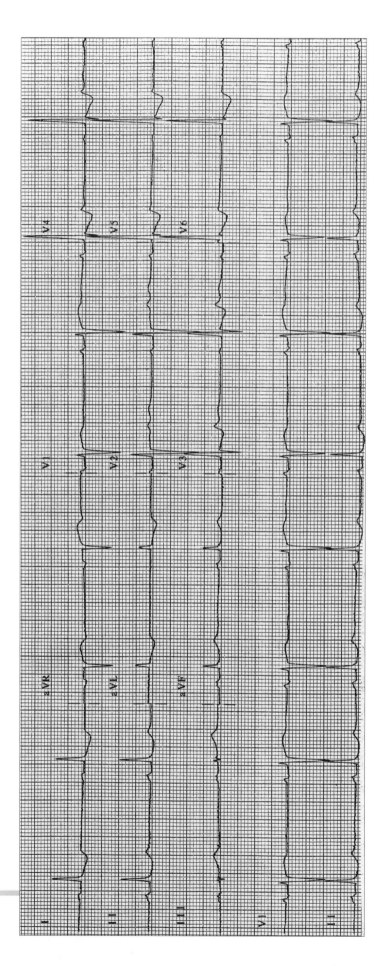

ECG VI-11

Diagnoses   ## ECG VI-11

1. Sinus rhythm (intrinsic rate = 70/min) with . . .

2. . . . 3:2 S-A Wenckebachs, and . . .

3. . . . borderline first-degree AV block (PR = 0.22 S)

4. Nonspecific ST-T abnormalities, indicating probable LV ischemia

Clinical Data

71-year-old retired nurse complaining of irregular pulse

Comments

With paired supraventricular beats, the two likely possibilities are atrial extrasystolic bigeminy and 3:2 Wenckebachs, either sinus or AV. In this patient:

• The long coupling (P-P) interval makes atrial extrasystolic bigeminy very unlikely.

• There is no recognizable, consistent change in the earlier P wave—which you would expect if the early beats were atrial extrasystoles.

Therefore 3:2 exit Wenckebach conduction out of the sinus is the probable diagnosis (see laddergram below).

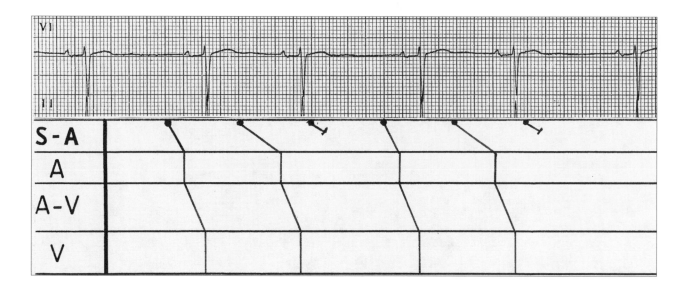

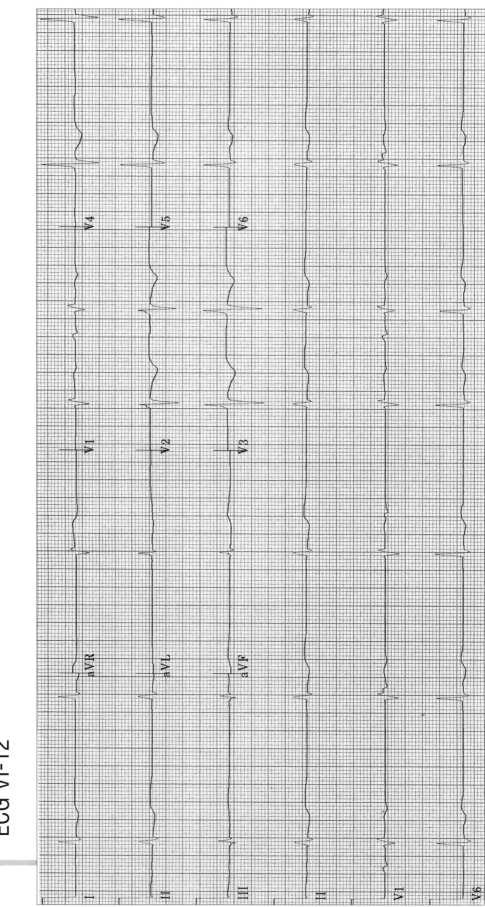

ECG VI-12

Diagnoses

ECG VI-12

1. Sick sinus (marked sinus bradycardia, rate = 30/min), permitting . . .

2. . . . junctional escape (rate = 36/min) producing AV dissociation with . . .

3. . . . one ventricular capture beat

4. First-degree AV block (long PR of capture beat)

5. Widespread ST-T negativity (diffuse ischemia ?)

6. Incomplete RBBB (rSr′ in V1, QRS interval 0.10 s)

Clinical Data

77-year-old man, 2 months after coronary artery bypass graft

Comments

Note that the *primary* arrhythmic diagnosis is sinus bradycardia—everything else (escape, dissociation, capture) is *secondary* to the bradycardia.

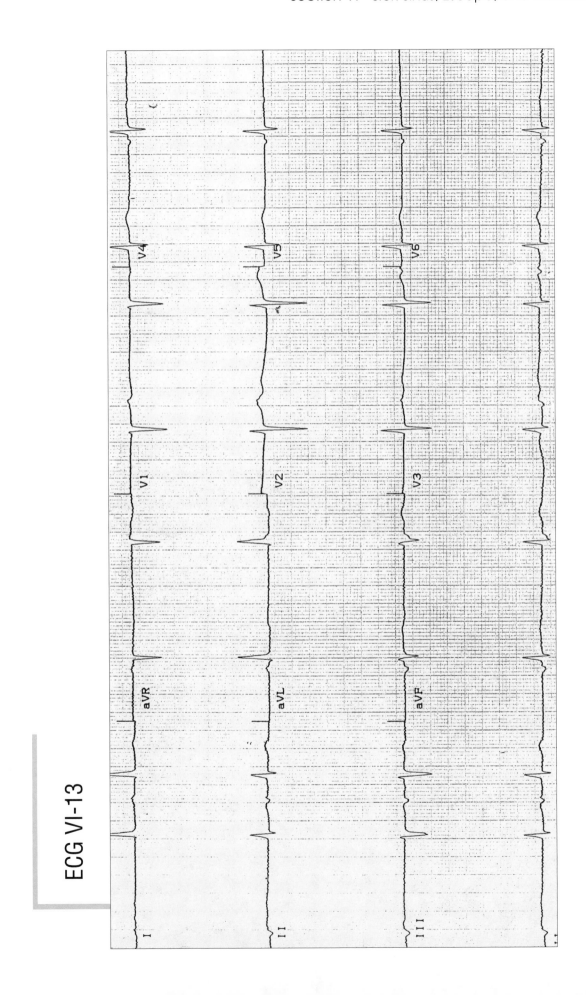

ECG VI-13

Diagnoses   **ECG VI-13**

1. Sick sinus (iatrogenic), with resulting . . .

2. . . . junctional escape by two dissociated pacemakers, the upper controlling the atria (at 39/min), the lower the ventricles (at 46/min)

3. Two ventricular captures by the upper pacemaker (see ECG below, *C*)

4. Minor AV block (prolonged PR intervals in captured beats)

5. Nonspecific ST-T abnormalities

Clinical Data

77-year-old woman on verapamil

Comments

• Computer diagnosis was "undetermined rhythm"; physician interpretation was "complete heart block."

• The upper pacemaker, with its inverted P waves, *could* be ectopic atrial, but escape at a rate of 39/min is more likely to be junctional.

• This form of dissociation is likely to be confused with reciprocal beating, but is distinguished from it by the *regularity* of the atrial rhythm; in **reciprocal rhythm,** the P-P intervals vary because they result from varying retrograde conduction.

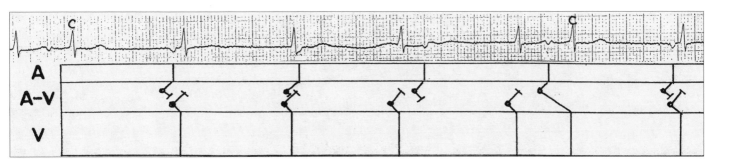

ECG VI-14

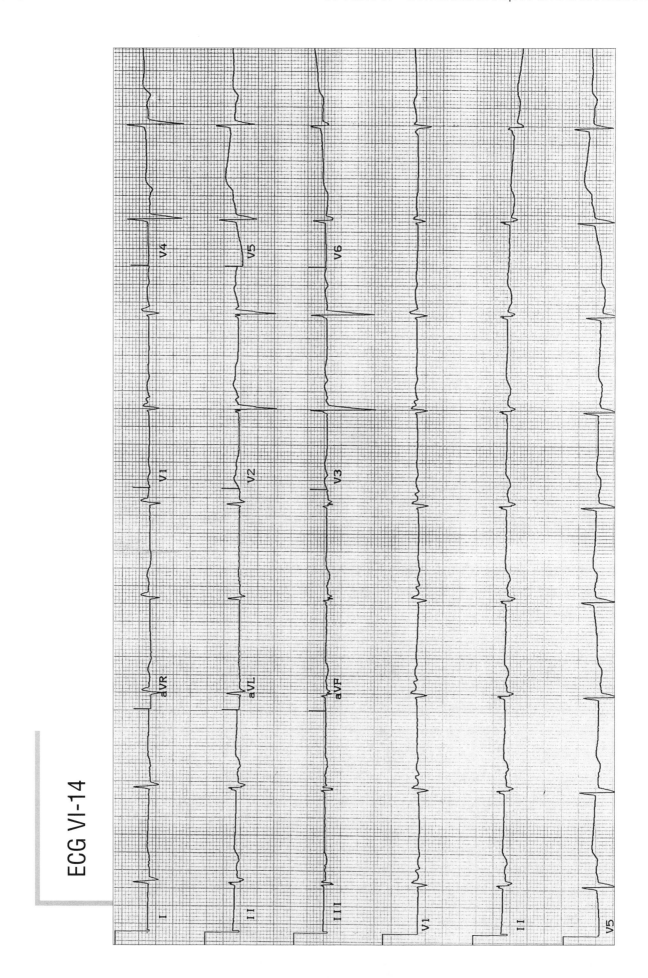

Diagnoses

ECG VI-14

1. Sinus bradycardia (rate = 57/min) permitting . . .

2. . . . junctional escape at 56/min producing isorhythmic AV dissociation

3. Low voltage in limb leads with "indeterminate" axis

4. Incomplete RBBB pattern

5. ST-T-U abnormalities are nonspecific, but hypokalemia should be ruled out.

Clinical Data

77-year-old woman complaining of weakness, throbbing in neck, and shortness of breath

Comments

• The two slow pacemakers are beating independently in a run of isorhythmic AV dissociation; toward the end of the strip, the sinus accelerates slightly and the P wave begins to emerge in front of the QRS (best seen in the V1 rhythm strip).

• The throbbing in her neck is presumably due to cannon waves when the right atrium contracts against the closed or closing tricuspid valve, i.e., when the dissociated P wave closely follows or coincides with the QRS.

ECG VI-15

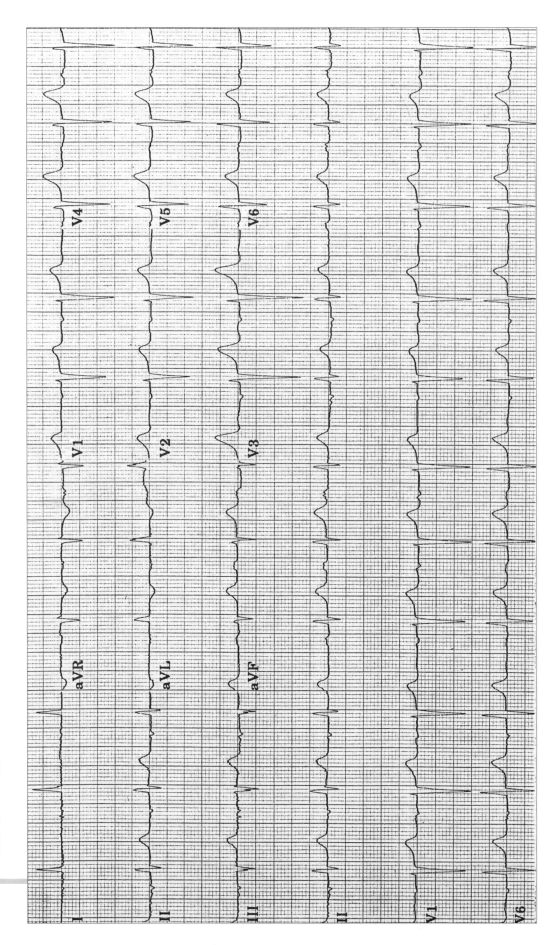

Diagnosis   **ECG VI-15**

1. Shifting atrial pacemaker with . . .

2. . . . first-degree AV block (PR = 0.23–0.33 s)

3. Mild left axis deviation (−15°) with abnormal QRS-T angle (105°)

4. T waves flat in lead 1 with . . .

5. . . . suspiciously horizontal STs in several leads

Clinical Data

56-year-old man with angina of effort

Comments

Note the tendency to RP/PR reciprocity, indicating that at a sinus rate of about 75/min he would have Wenckebach periods ("type 1, second-degree AV block"). The mood for progressive PR lengthening in successive beats is well seen in beats 4, 5, and 6 (at which point the developing Wenckebach is aborted by the atrial—? sinus—pause and pacemaker shift), and again in the last three beats.

ECG VI-16

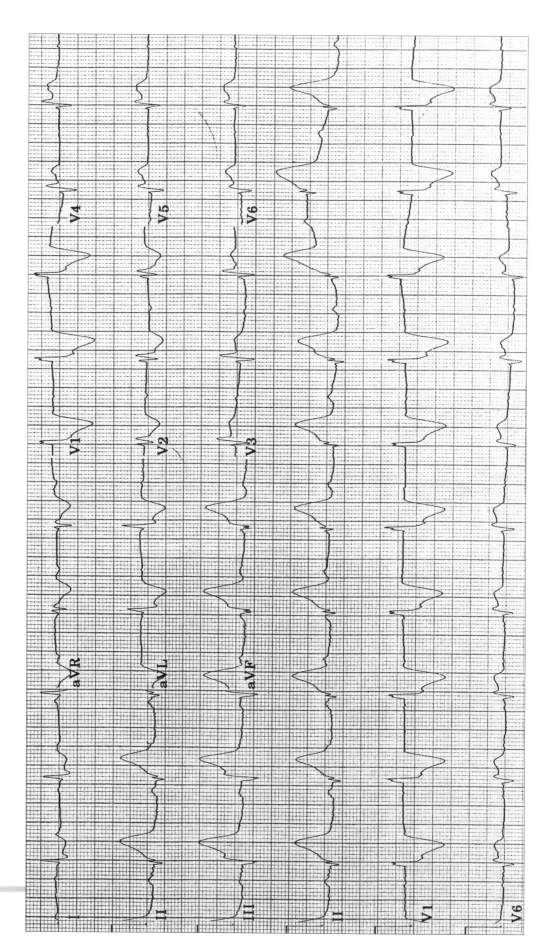

Diagnosis   **ECG VI-16**

1. Acute infero-postero-lateral infarction complicated by . . .

2. . . . sinus tachycardia (rate = 129/min) with . . .

3. . . . some (unspecified) degree of AV block, and . . .

4. . . . accelerated junctional rhythm (rate = 67/min) causing . . .

5. . . . complete AV dissociation

Clinical Data

51-year-old man

Comment

• The prominent early R in V1 with gross ST depression indicates posterior involvement in addition to the obvious inferolateral.

• The "degree" of AV block cannot be assessed because, although there is no conduction and the dissociation is therefore complete, the ventricular rate is too fast to permit the diagnosis of complete block. A convenient, though clumsy, term for this indefinable situation is **block/acceleration dissociation.**

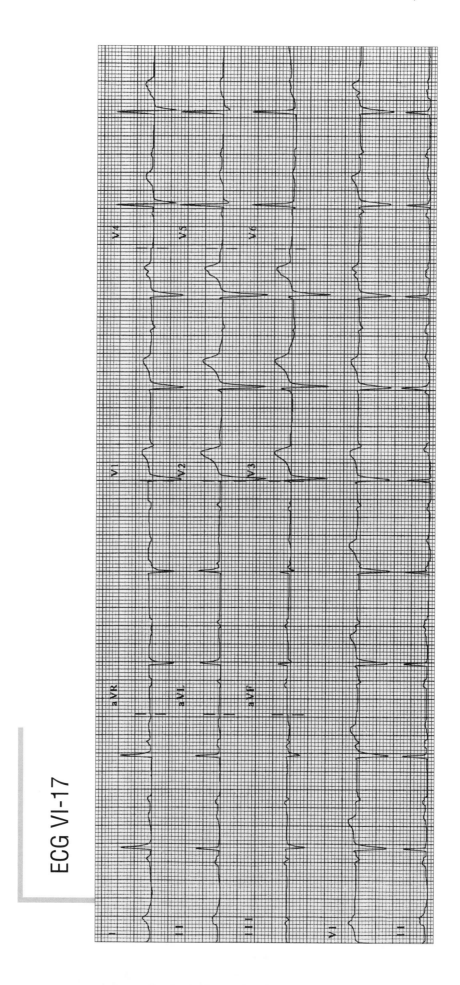

ECG VI-17

Diagnoses   **ECG VI-17**

1. AV dissociation partly due to AV block, partly to accelerated pacemakers (sinus rate = 91/min, junctional rate = 59/min)

2. Nonspecific ST-T abnormalities

Clinical Data

72-year-old man

Comments

The presence of AV block is obvious because no matter where the P waves land, there is no AV conduction (the junctional rhythm is absolutely regular with no shortening of any cycles). The dissociation is therefore complete, but the ventricular rate is too fast to permit the diagnosis of complete AV block. The most descriptive name for this combination of features is block/acceleration dissociation.

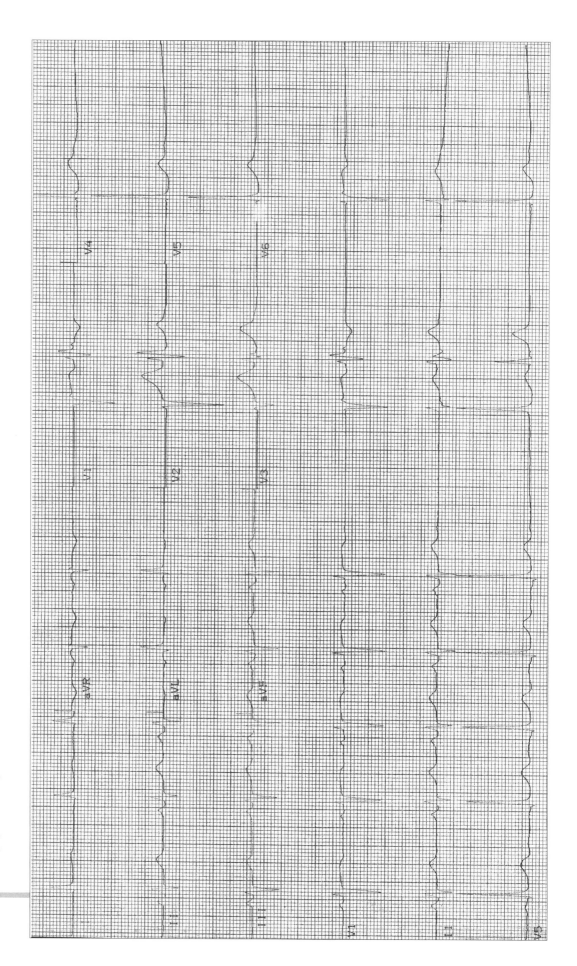

ECG VI-18

Diagnoses   **ECG VI-18**

1. Sick sinus, evidenced by prolonged sinus pause

2. Junctional escape (rate = 32/min)

3. Probable junctional premature beat with incomplete RBBB aberration and retrograde conduction to atria

4. Left axis deviation (−30 degrees)

5. Nonspecific T-wave abnormalities (QRS-T angle = 100 degrees)

6. LVH suggested by 20-mm QRS voltage in V5–6

Clinical Data

85-year-old woman

Comments

Notice that the QRSs of the junctional escape beats are slightly different from the QRSs of the conducted sinus beats—a common finding and presumably due to an **eccentric location** of the escaping focus.

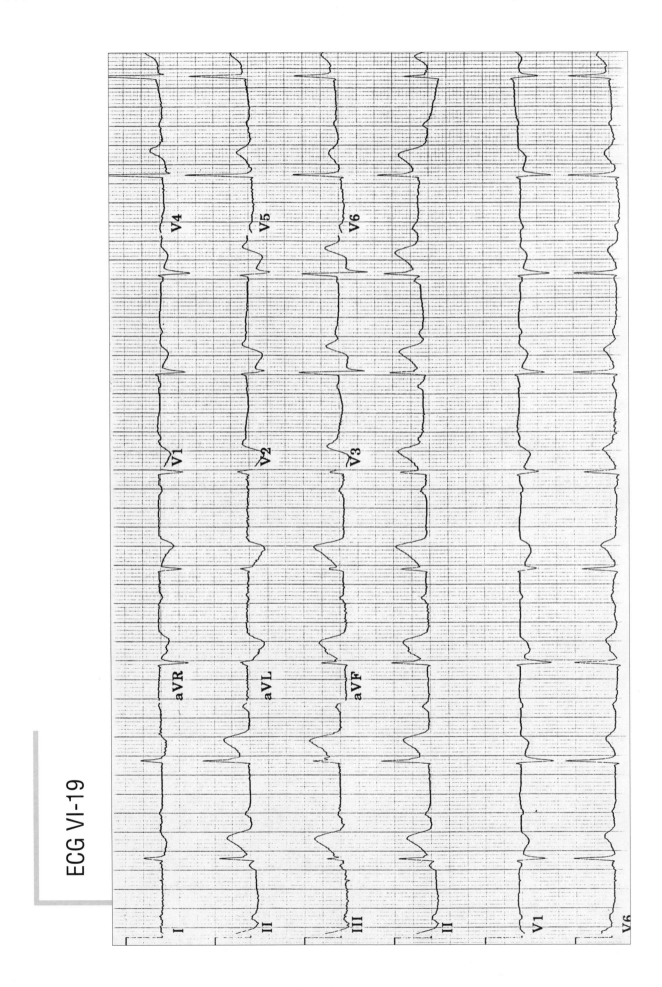

ECG VI-19

Diagnoses   ECG VI-19

1. Acute inferior infarction with probable posterolateral extension, complicated by . . .

2. . . . sinus tachycardia (rate = 106/min) with . . .

3. . . . a mild degree of AV nodal (type I) block, and . . .

4. . . . junctional rhythm (rate = 57/min), producing . . .

5. . . . incomplete AV dissociation with one, perhaps two, ventricular captures

Clinical Data

65-year-old man

Comments

• "Type I block" because:

   that's the usual level of block with *inferior* infarctions
   there's no BBB
   the first captured beat (see ECG below, *C*) has a prolonged PR.

• The captured beats are recognized not only by the fact that the first one ends a measurably shorter ventricular cycle, but also because this corresponds with a distinct change in the QRS contour (best seen in V1).

This is an example of the sort of tracing that is almost always misread as complete or advanced AV block when, in fact, it represents minor block—indeed, it is the equivalent of only "first-degree" AV block at an atrial rate of 60/min. (You can deduce from the captured beat that if the sinus rate were a normal 60/min instead of the uncomfortably rapid 106/min, the patient would enjoy 1:1 AV conduction with only a somewhat prolonged PR interval.)

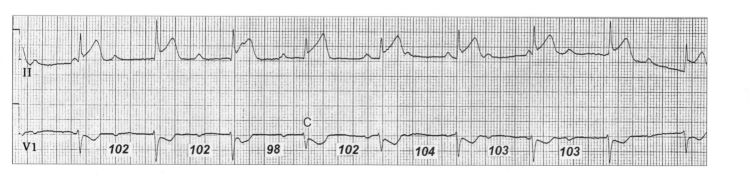

ECG VI-20

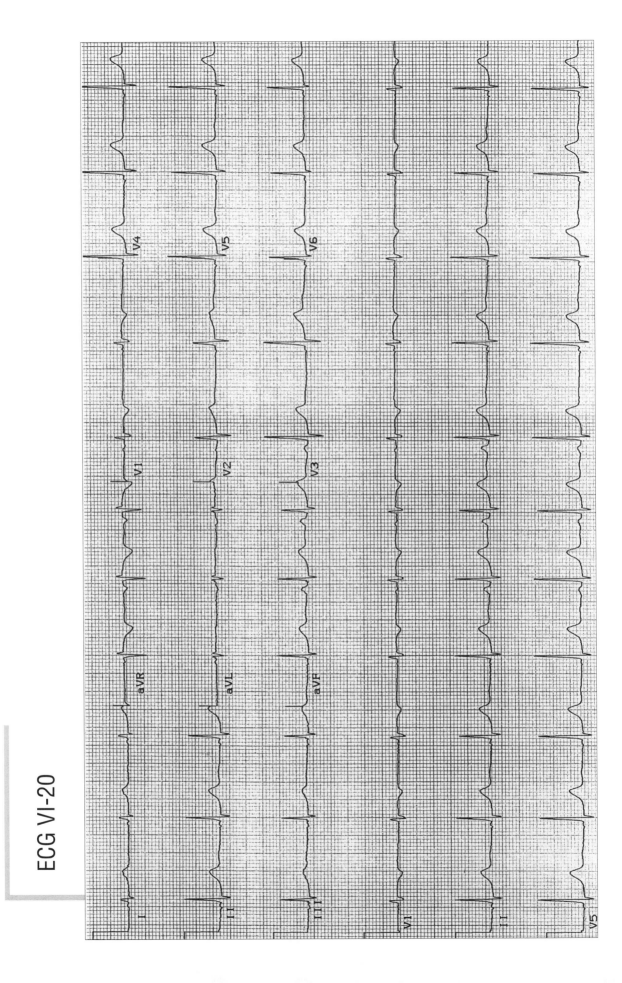

Diagnoses

1. Shifting (or wandering) pacemaker and sinus arrhythmia

2. Otherwise a probably normal variant

Clinical Data

Asymptomatic 49-year-old woman

Comments

• The first four and last four beats are presumably low atrial or junctional; the middle three are sinus. For the ectopic rhythm to take over, the sinus has to slow down, producing an underlying sinus arrhythmia. This is common with a shifting pacemaker.

• The dominant R in V1 and V2 is probably a normal variant.

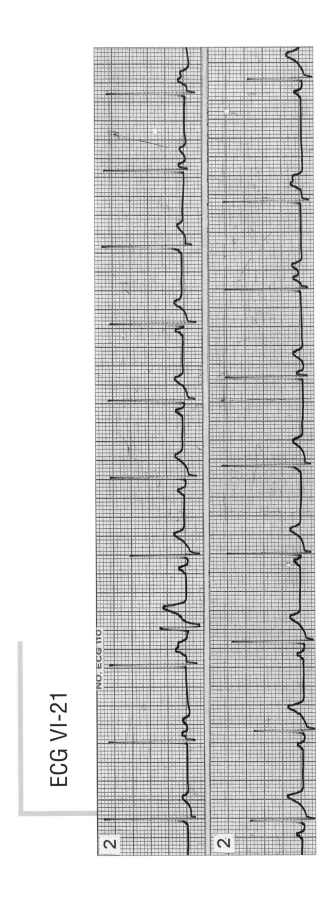

ECG VI-21

Diagnoses   **ECG VI-21**

1. AV dissociation between . . .

2. . . . accelerated junctional rhythm (rate = 74/min) and . . .

3. . . . sinus rhythm (rate = 61/min) with . . .

4. . . . one capture beat in top strip showing . . .

5. . . . ventricular aberration and . . .

6. . . . concealed conduction into the junction at the end of bottom strip (capturing junction but not ventricles)

Clinical Data

8-year-old child with rheumatic fever

Comments

• A quick way of spotting which beats are junctional and which are conducted sinus is the height of the R wave: the junctional beats are taller than the sinus beats. Thus the fifth beat in the top strip and the first two beats and last beat in the bottom strip are conducted sinus beats—as is the fourth beat in the top strip, which is a captured beat with aberration because of its prematurity.

• Toward the end of the bottom strip there is another attempted ventricular capture (see below); this time, however, the impulse fails to reach the ventricles but "captures" and resets the junction. Since this conduction as far as the junction can be recognized only from the failure of the next expected junctional beat to appear, it qualifies as **concealed conduction.**

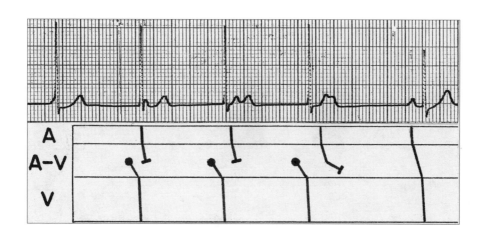

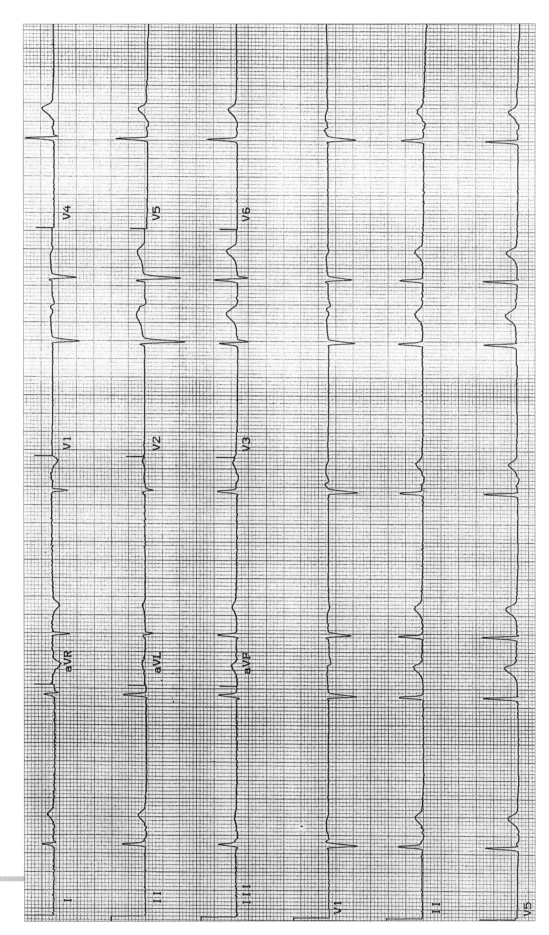

ECG VI-22

Diagnoses   ECG VI-22

1. Sinus bradycardia (rate = 31/min) with . . .

2. . . . junctional escape rhythm at 36/min, producing . . .

3. . . . AV dissociation, with . . .

4. . . . two ventricular capture beats, with . . .

5. . . . first-degree AV block (PR = 0.32 s)

Clinical Data

Elderly woman after cardioversion of atrial fibrillation

Comment

This is the context that gave the "sick sinus" its name—Lown in Boston first applied the term when, after cardioverting a patient with atrial fibrillation, what resulted was a profound sinus bradycardia.

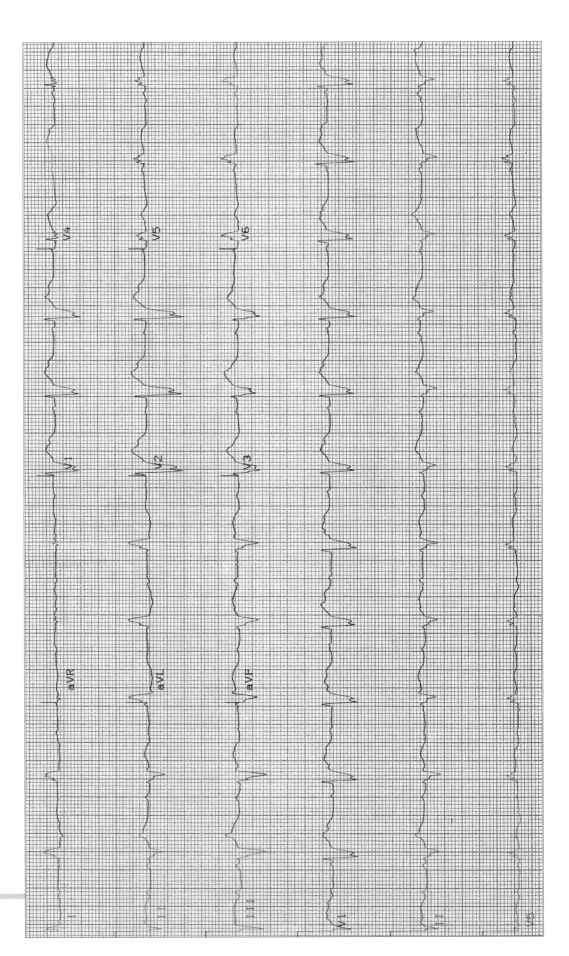

ECG VI-23

Diagnoses   **ECG VI-23**

1. Irregular atrial tachycardia, rate about 175/min

2. Some degree of AV block with . . .

3. . . . accelerated junctional rhythm (rate = 70/min), producing . . .

4. . . . block/acceleration dissociation

5. LBBB with left axis deviation

6. Probable acute inferolateral infarction

Clinical Data

77-year-old woman with chest pain

Comments

• Although the P′ waves are not very prominent, they are quite well seen in almost all leads.

• The ventricular rhythm is absolutely regular, so there are no conducted beats and the dissociation is complete (but the ventricular rate is much too fast to permit the diagnosis of complete AV *block*).

• The ventricular rhythm is junctional rather than ventricular because the QRS morphology in V1 (slick downstroke to early nadir) is typical of LBBB rather than ventricular ectopy.

• Although you cannot be absolutely sure of the acute infarction, the loss of upward ST concavity (2, 3, and aVF), with primary T-wave changes (V4–V6) and hint of ST elevation in these leads, is certainly enough to keep the patient under observation until the situation is resolved.

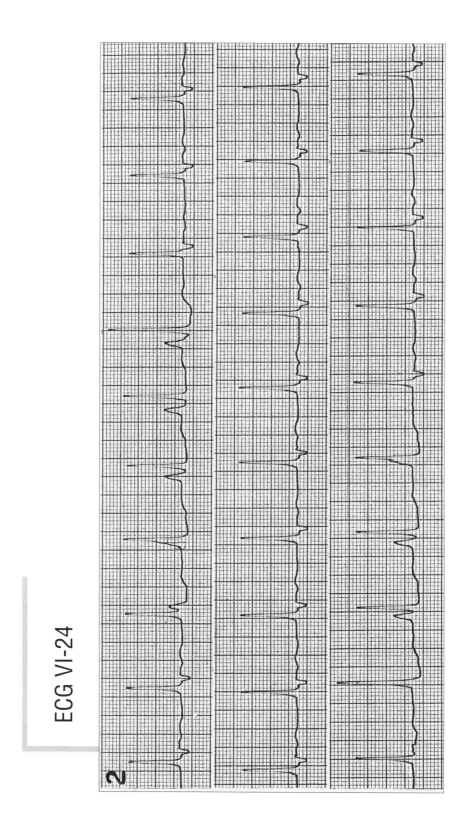

ECG VI-24

Diagnoses   **ECG VI-24**

1. Sinus arrhythmia (rate = 75–80/min) whose longer cycles permit . . .

2. . . . a junctional rhythm to escape at 73/min with . . .

3. . . . retrograde conduction to the atria

4. AV dissociation for 3–4 beats when the sinus wakes up

5. One atrial fusion beat (just after first QRS in bottom strip)

6. Probable right atrial enlargement (? P-pulmonale)

7. Nonspecific ST-T abnormalities

Clinical Data

46-year-old woman with emphysema

Comments

Clearly the basic rhythm is junctional with retrograde conduction to the atria. The sinus tries to assert itself every now and then, but fails miserably.

• The top strip begins with two junctional beats. The sinus awakens too late to take control, but in time to thwart retrograde conduction and produce three dissociated beats. The next two (6th and 7th) beats may or may not be successfully conducted sinus beats (the PR is 0.15–0.16 s).

• But then the sinus pauses long enough for the junction to take over again, and its control is undisputed through the middle strip.

• Right after the first beat in the bottom strip (see below), there is a deformed P wave replacing the retrograde—presumably representing fusion (partial dissociation) between sinus and retrograde impulses. After four dissociated beats, the sinus again pauses, and the junction resumes control.

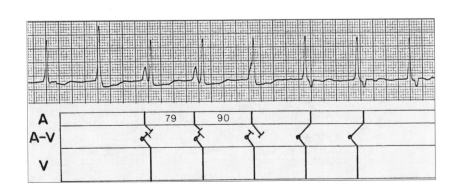

Section VII

Myocardial Ischemia and Infarction

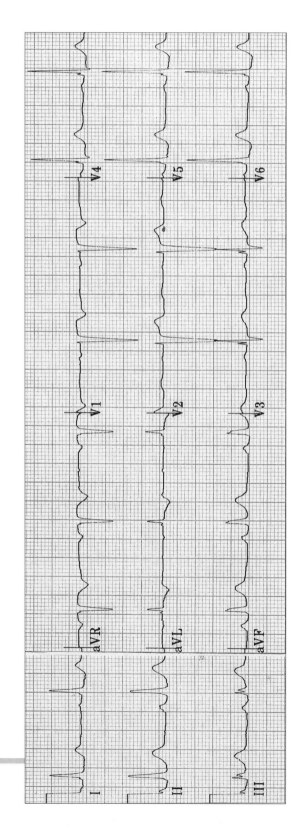

ECG VII-1

Diagnoses   **ECG VII-1**

1. Sinus rhythm (rate = 62/min)

2. Early acute inferior infarction

Clinical Data

69-year-old woman

Comments

This is a good example of:

- The sort of early, inferior infarction that can easily be missed in the ECG

- The sometimes great value of lead aVL in early diagnosis of inferior infarction.

There is very slight ST elevation in leads 3 and aVF, and the T waves in those leads perhaps look disproportionately large. But the inescapable clue is the ST-T pattern in lead aVL, with less conspicuous reciprocal changes in other leads (1, V4–V6). An hour later (see ECG below) the diagnosis was in full bloom.

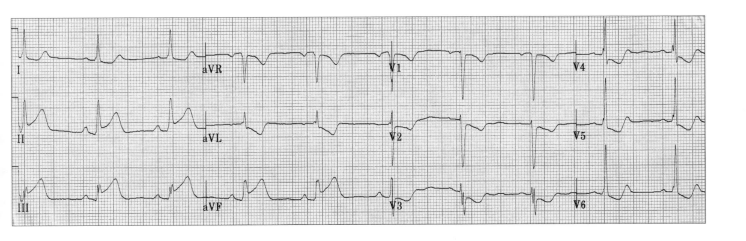

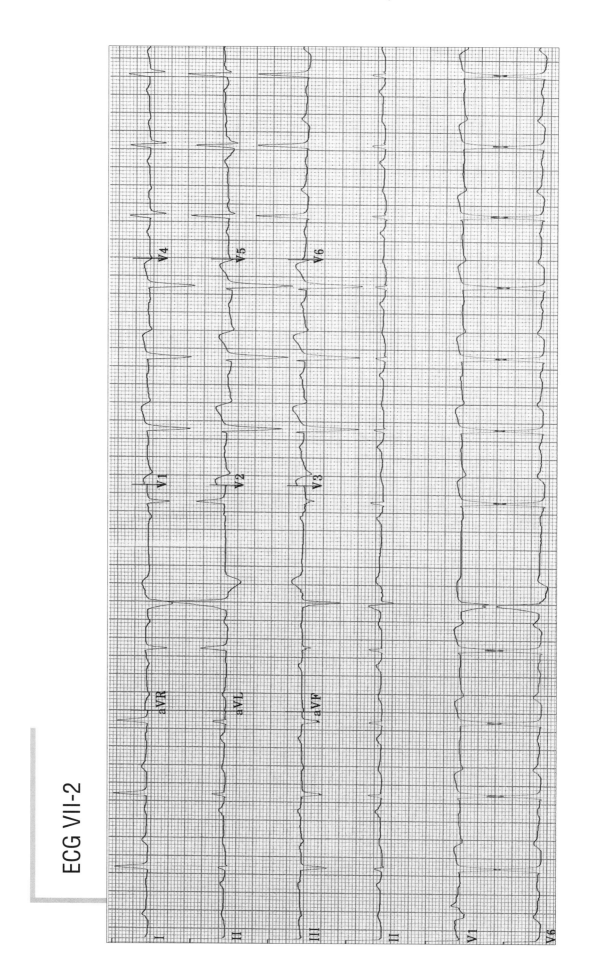

ECG VII-2

Diagnoses   ECG VII-2

1. Sinus rhythm (rate = 74/min)

2. One RV premature beat

3. Anteroseptal myocardial ischemia

4. Diffuse ST-T abnormalities

Clinical Data

69-year-old man

Comments

• Note the typical shape of the RV ectopic beat in V1 with slower downstroke than upstroke, requiring > 0.06 s (here 0.09 s) to reach the QS nadir.

• The ST-T pattern in V2–3 has been dubbed "**Wellens' warning**" because it often indicates a critical, proximal LAD lesion, suggesting an imminent, massive anterior infarct (based on a widely overlooked article by Wellens and colleagues; see Am Heart J 103:730, 1962).

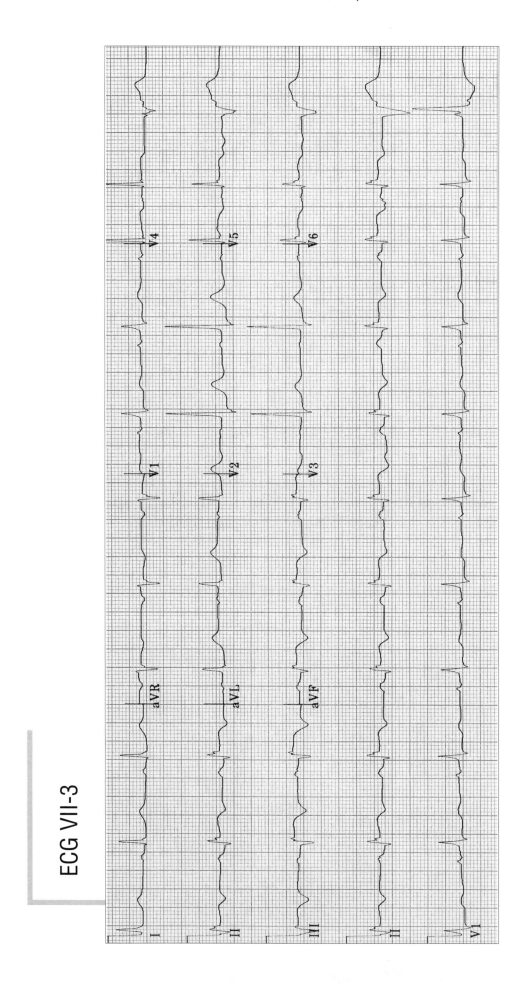

ECG VII-3

Diagnoses   **ECG VII-3**

1. Sinus rhythm (rate = 64/min)

2. Acute infero-postero-lateral infarction

3. One atrial premature beat

4. One ventricular premature beat with retrograde conduction to atria

Clinical Data

76-year-old woman

Comment

The atrial activation seen just following the VPB might be thought to be the returning sinus P wave; but the deflection appears to be mainly negative in leads 2 and V4–6 and positive in V1, and this polarity is typical for a retrograde P.

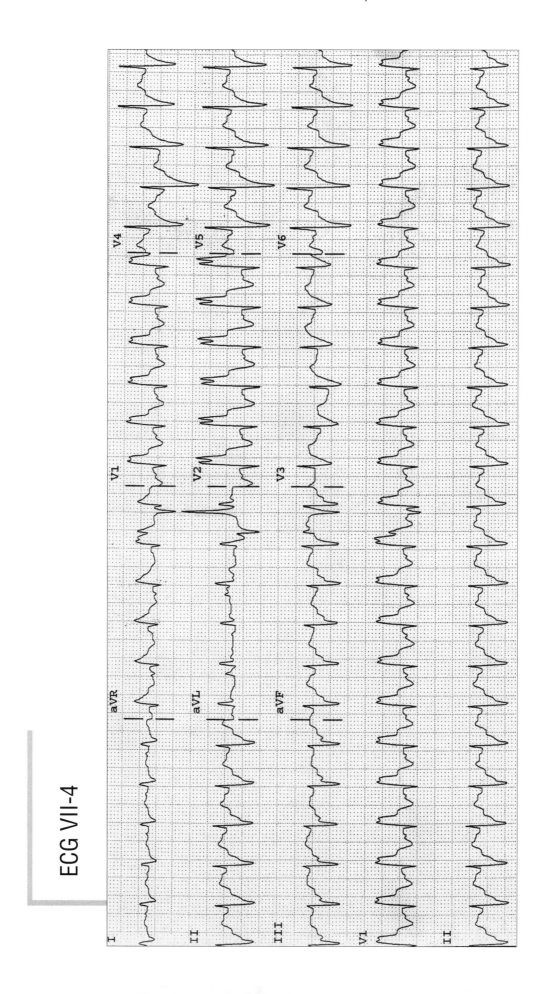

ECG VII-4

Diagnoses   **ECG VII-4**

1. Acute anteroseptal infarction

2. Sinus tachycardia (rate = 136/min)

3. Bifascicular block (RBBB + LAHB)

Clinical Data

75-year-old man; died due to computer misdiagnosis

Comments

• This case exemplifies the folly of relying on the computer's interpretation: Because the patient had an elevated BUN and the computer diagnosed "old" infarction, the patient was not admitted to CCU and was not seen by a cardiologist for 4 hours.

• At this rate of 136/min you cannot exclude the possibility of atrial flutter with 2:1 AV conduction.

ECG VII-5

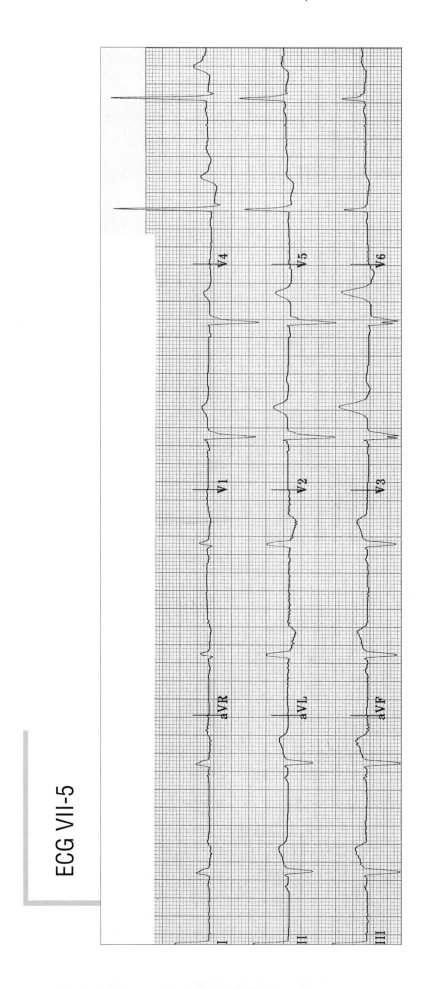

Diagnoses   **ECG VII-5**

1. Sinus bradycardia (rate = 48/min) with . . .

2. . . . left anterior hemiblock (QRS axis = −65 degrees)

3. ? Possible/probable LVH

4. Acute inferior infarction

Clinical Data

77-year-old man with three-vessel disease

Comments

The high voltage in lead V4 suggests LVH; combined with the hemiblock, you may at first wonder if the ST-T pattern in leads 2, 3, and aVF is not secondary to these two abnormalities. But the STs in the inferior leads lack the expected concavity upward of a typical "secondary" change. Additionally, the contours of the ST-T in V2 and V3 are highly suspicious of an acute reciprocal pattern.

Thus, the diagnosis of acute inferior infarction is made with reasonable confidence.

(The computer diagnosed *anterior* infarction of uncertain age, presumably because of the "poor R-wave progression.")

ECG VII-6

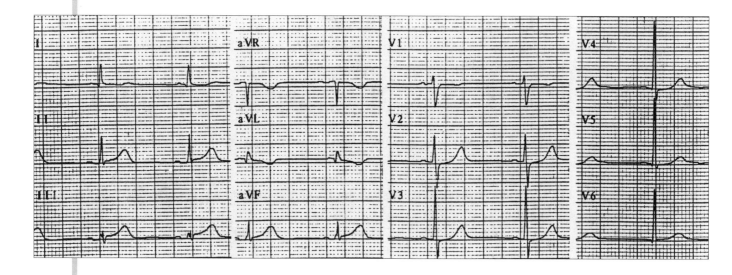

Diagnoses   **ECG VII-6**

1. Sinus rhythm (rate = 62/min) with . . .

2. . . . early acute inferior infarction

Clinical Data

70-year-old man

Comments

This is another good example of an acute infarction that could easily be missed. There is a little elevation of the ST take-off in the inferior leads, but no more than is sometimes seen normally, and the upward concavity of the ST is preserved. Perhaps the T waves are disproportionately large relative to their QRSs, but it is the suspicious-looking ST-T negativity in aVL and the unequivocally abnormal repolarization in lead 1 that fill the bill as *reciprocal changes* and confirm the probable diagnosis. (Compare with ECG VII-1.)

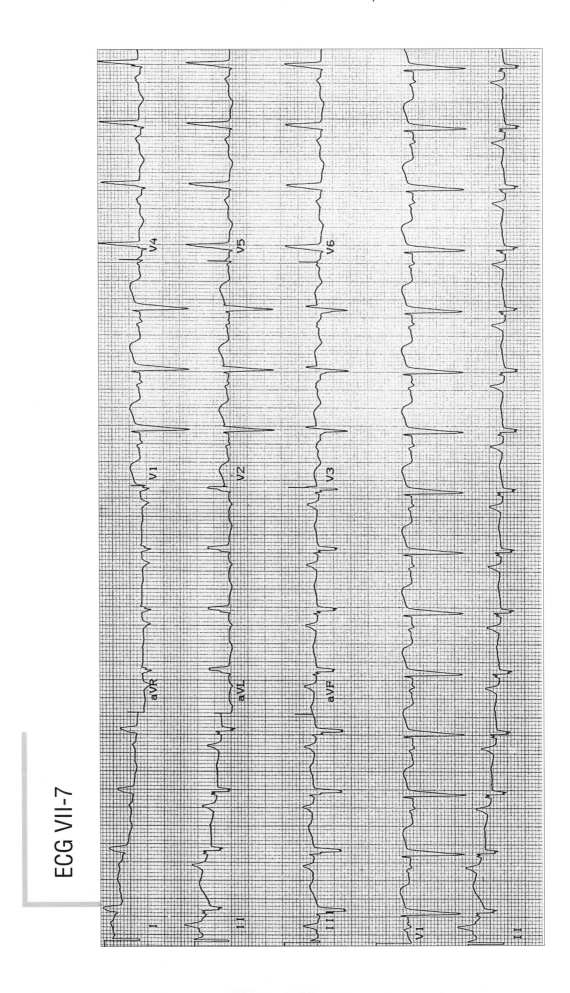

ECG VII-7

Diagnoses   **ECG VII-7**

1. Sinus rhythm (rate = 90/min) with P-pulmonale (P waves 3–4 mm tall in 2, 3, and aVF; P-wave axis +75°)

2. Left axis deviation (axis −45°), possible left anterior hemiblock

3. Anteroseptal infarction of uncertain date, probably recent

Clinical Data

Unknown

Comments

• Despite the ST elevation, without knowledge of the clinical history you cannot assume that the infarction is acute; for example, this could be an old anteroseptal infarct with residual aneurysm.

• The QRS axis is only about −45°, and the increased voltage one would expect with LAHB is absent; so *that* diagnosis is tentative.

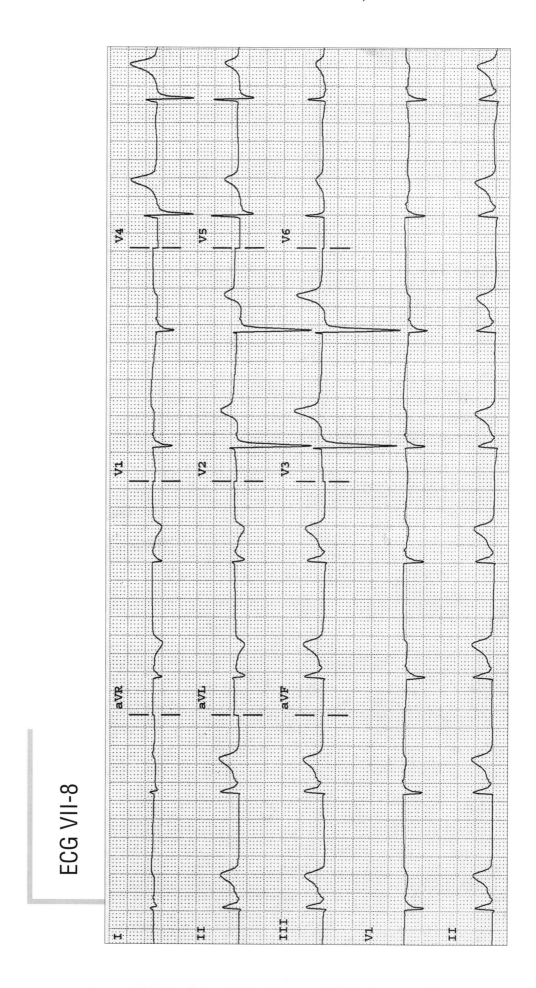

ECG VII-8

Diagnoses

1. Acute inferior infarction

2. Sick sinus (secondary to the infarction) with resulting . . .

3. . . . junctional bradycardia (rate = 47/min) with . . .

4. . . . retrograde conduction to atria

Clinical Data

96-year-old man

Comment

The retrograde P waves just following the QRS are particularly well seen in V1—where they are, as usual, at least partly upright.

ECG VII-9

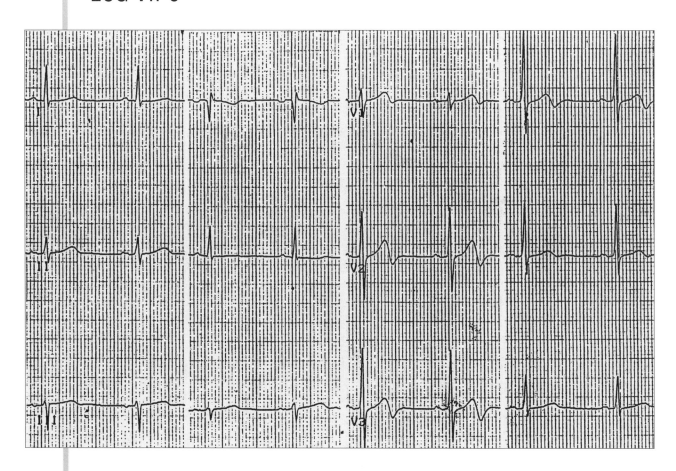

Diagnoses   ## ECG VII-9

1. Normal sinus rhythm (rate = 60/min)

2. Anteroseptal ischemia

Clinical Data

47-year-old man with atypical chest pain, referred for cardiac catheterization

Comment

This ST-T pattern in V1–4 is a typical "**Wellens' warning**"—an alert to look for a critical, proximal LAD lesion (see ECG VII-2). Such a lesion was found at catheterization, and angioplasty was successful.

ECG VII-10

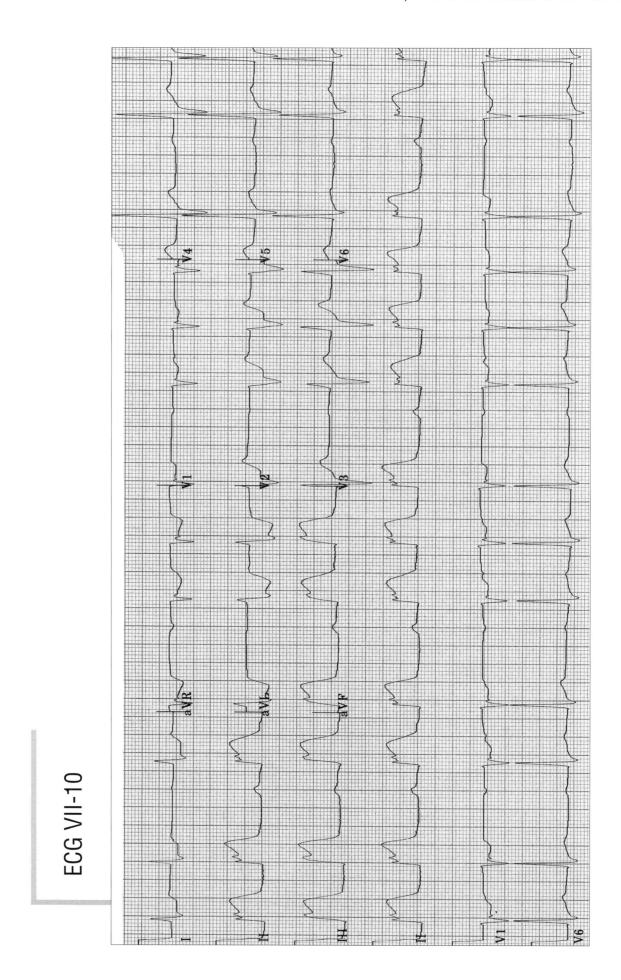

Diagnoses   **ECG VII-10**

1. Sinus tachycardia (rate = 100/min) with . . .

2. . . . 3:2, 4:3, and 5:4 AV Wenckebach periods complicating . . .

3. . . . acute inferior myocardial infarction

Clinical Data

64-year-old man

Comment

Note the "**group beating**" that immediately suggests Wenckebach-type conduction, which is then confirmed by observing and measuring PR and RR intervals.

ECG VII-11

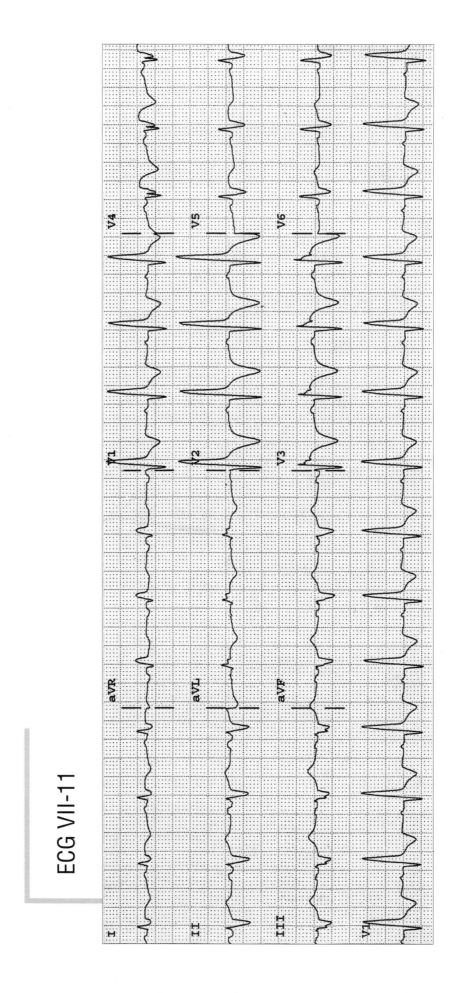

Diagnoses   **ECG VII-11**

1. Sinus rhythm (rate = 84/min)

2. Acute, extensive anterior infarction

3. Right bundle-branch block

4. Left axis deviation (initial 0.06 s about −70 degrees)

Clinical Data

36-year-old man

Comment

There is certainly *enough leftward axis* (−70) of the first half of the QRS to diagnose left anterior hemiblock, but be hesitant to pronounce hemiblock without a significant increase in QRS voltage.

ECG VII-12

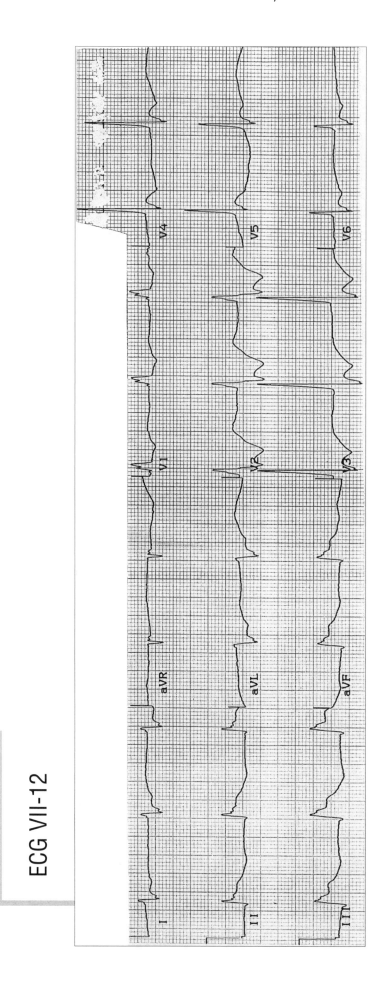

Diagnoses   **ECG VII-12**

1. Acute inferoposterior infarction

2. Right bundle-branch block

3. Accelerated junctional rhythm (rate = 63/min)

Clinical Data

A fatal infarct in a 79-year-old woman

Comments

• "Posterior" as well as inferior infarction is diagnosed because the *initial* R waves are prominent in V1 and V2, and ST-T depression is present as well.

• Complete absence of any evidence of atrial activity may be due to sinus arrest secondary to the infarct; or retrograde P waves from the junctional pacemaker may be buried in each QRS complex.

ECG VII-13

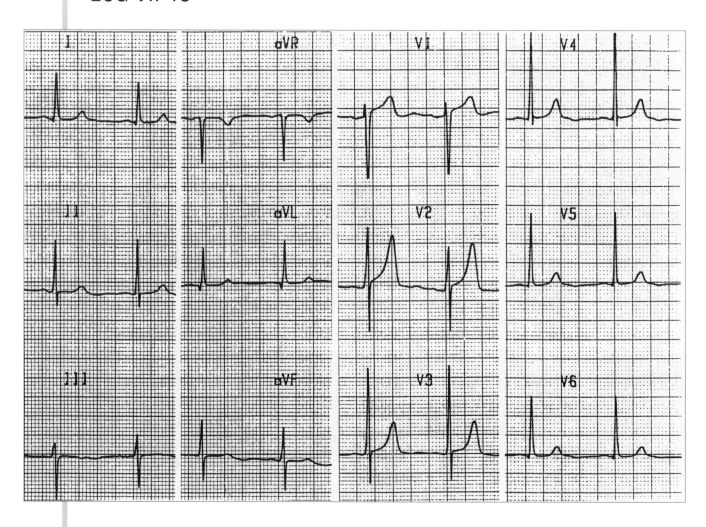

Diagnoses   **ECG VII-13**

1. Left ventricular hypertrophy

2. Probable myocardial ischemia

Clinical Data

56-year-old diabetic man with mild angina of effort, BP 182/102

Comments

• From the ECG, one suspects LVH from the **QRS voltage** (total > 175 mm, here = 218).

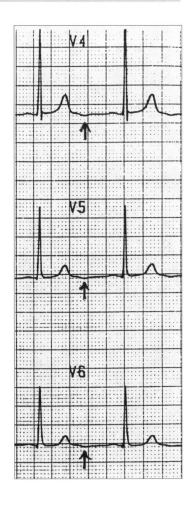

• An eye-catching feature is the **TV1-taller-than-TV6 pattern,** which is not always abnormal but should be regarded as an "alert" to look for further evidence of trouble.

• Here, the unequivocal clincher is the **U-wave inversion** (see ECG at right, *arrows*) in V4–6 (probably also in lead 2).

Both the precordial T-wave imbalance and the U-wave negativity are common findings in early LVH and probably imply significant myocardial ischemia.

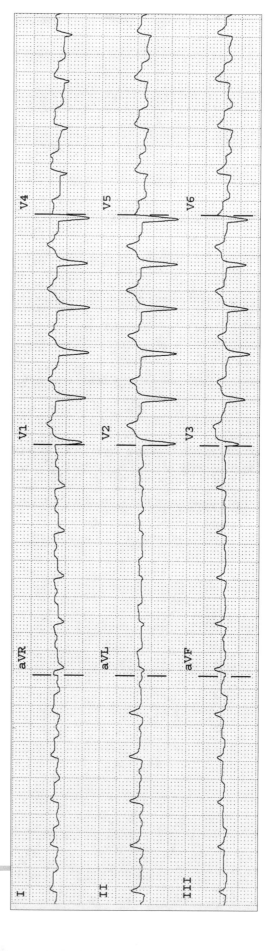

ECG VII-14

Diagnoses

1. Sinus tachycardia (rate = 120/min)

2. Acute global infarction

3. Incomplete LBBB

4. Low voltage

Clinical Data

38-year-old diabetic man with severe three-vessel disease who died in the cath lab

Comment

Indicative changes (ST elevation) in anterior, lateral, and inferior leads equate to "global" infarction—perhaps due to occlusion of a long LAD wrapping around the apex and supplying part of the inferior wall as well.

ECG VII-15

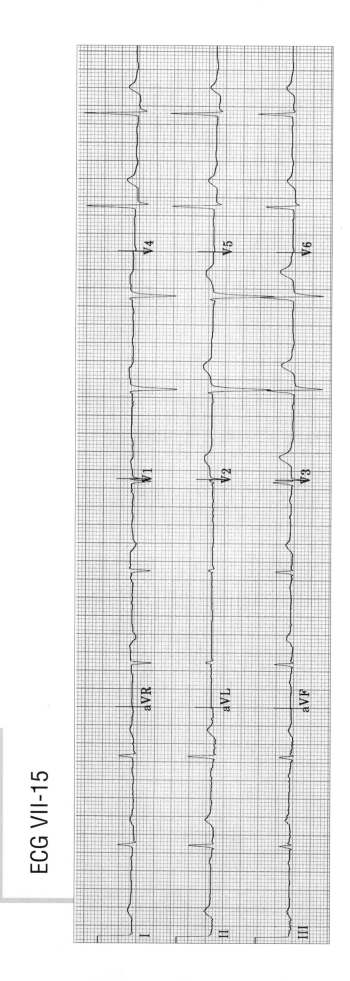

Diagnoses   **ECG VII-15**

1. Borderline sinus bradycardia (rate = 59/min)

2. Myocardial ischemia

Clinical Data

75-year-old man with angina

Comment

The clues to ischemia here are:

- *Horizontal* ST segments in many leads, with and without slight depression

- ST-T angulation

- Inverted U waves in V3–6.

ECG VII-16

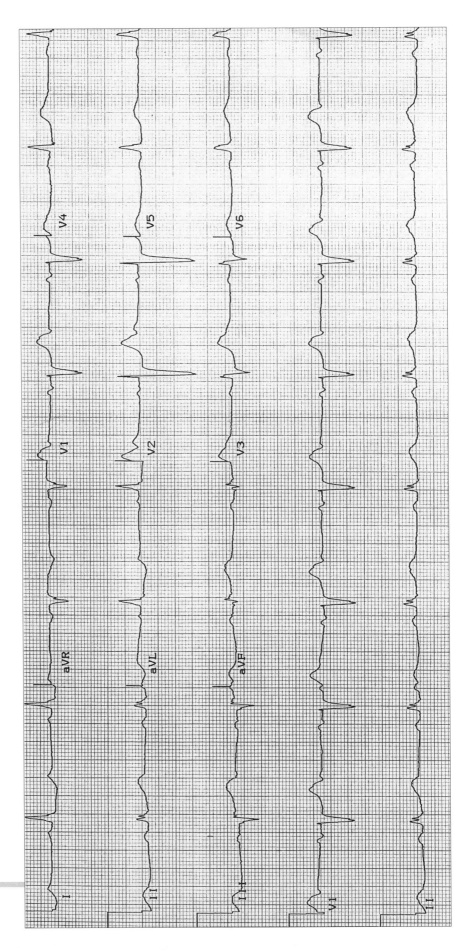

Diagnoses   **ECG VII-16**

1. Sinus rhythm (rate = 96/min) with 2:1 AV block

2. One nonconducted atrial premature beat (just after the second QRS)

3. Acute inferior infarction

4. Atypical LBBB

Clinical Data

66-year-old man complaining of dizzy spells

Comments

• The level of the AV block is uncertain; it could be AV nodal or infranodal. The PR is borderline (0.20–0.22 s), and the QRS interval is 0.12 s. In view of the inferior infarct, it's probably AV nodal, i.e., type I.

• The QRS doesn't look like typical LBBB, but carefully measured the QRS interval is 0.12 s, and clearly the delay is on the left side.

ECG VII-17

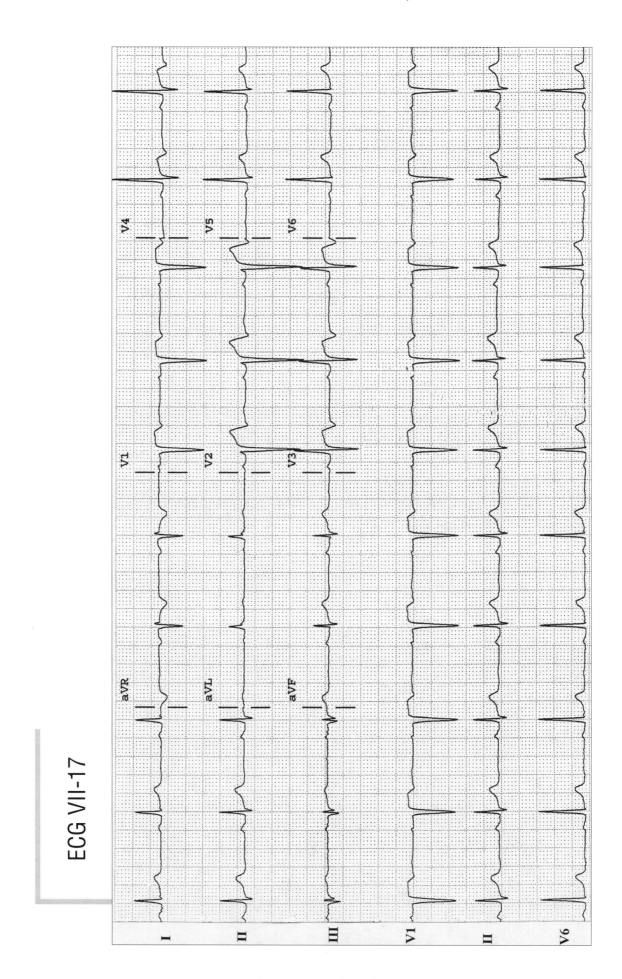

Diagnoses   **ECG VII-17**

1. Sinus rhythm (rate = 60/min)

2. Compatible with anteroseptal ischemia

Clinical Data

43-year-old man

Comments

This is a classic example of "Wellens' warning"—a pattern not to be taken lightly. He and his colleagues in Holland described the pattern in anteroseptal leads well seen here. It is strongly suggestive of an obstructive, proximal lesion in the LAD requiring aggressive investigation to ward off an impending anterior infarct. (Compare to ECGs VII-2 and VII-9.)

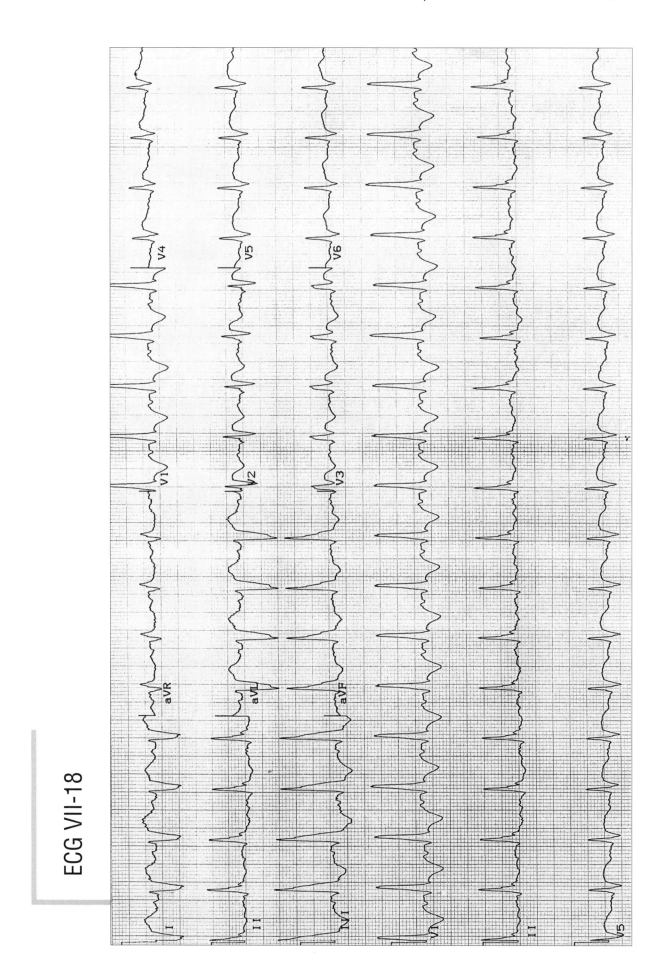

ECG VII-18

Diagnoses   **ECG VII-18**

1. Sinus tachycardia (rate = 108/min)

2. Bifascicular block (RBBB + left posterior hemiblock)

3. Extensive anterior infarction

4. Possible RVH (R waves in V1 of 13–14 mm)

Clinical Data

73-year-old woman with severe retrosternal pain and shortness of breath

Comments

None

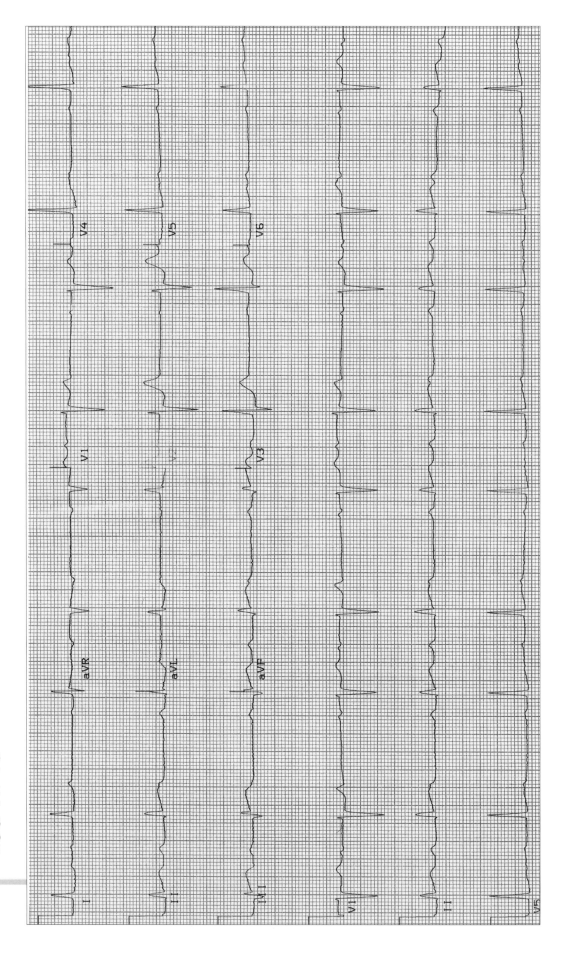

ECG VII-19

Diagnoses   **ECG VII-19**

1. Sinus rhythm (rate = 80/min) with . . .

2. . . . type I, second-degree AV block (in the form of 3:2 Wenckebach periods) reducing the ventricular rate to 52/min

3. Acute inferior infarction

Clinical Data

72-year-old woman with severe chest pain, sweating profusely and short of breath

Comments

None

ECG VII-20

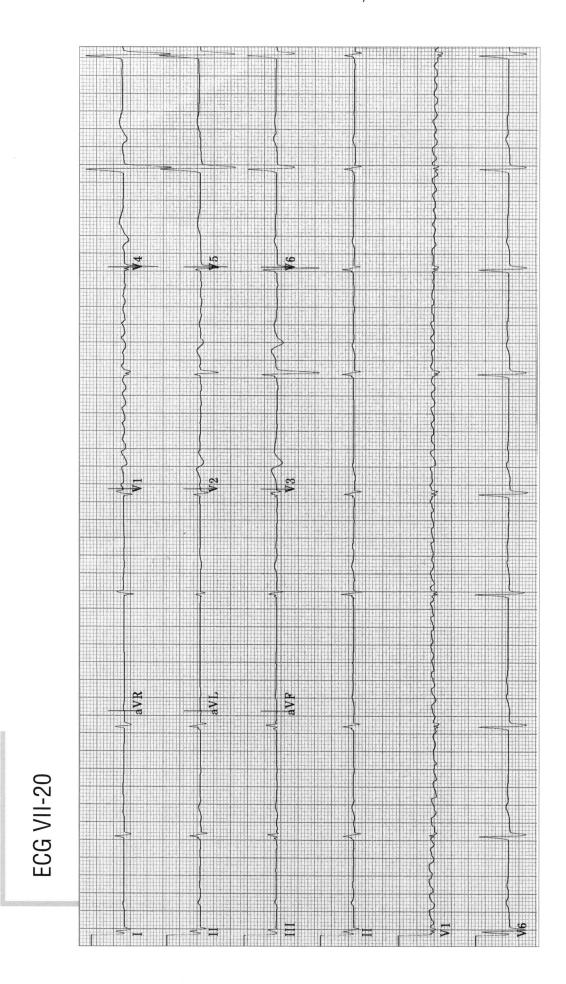

Diagnoses   **ECG VII-20**

1. Atrial fibrillation with slow ventricular response (about 48/min)

2. Anteroseptal ischemia

3. Low voltage in limb leads

Clinical Data

84-year-old man diagnosed with unstable angina

Comment

Although the main reason for including this record is the excellent sample of "Wellens' warning" (see also ECGs VII-2, VII-9, and VII-17), it is worth drawing attention to the miniscule QRS complexes in V1, a lead that is generally accepted as one of the best leads for monitoring QRS morphology.

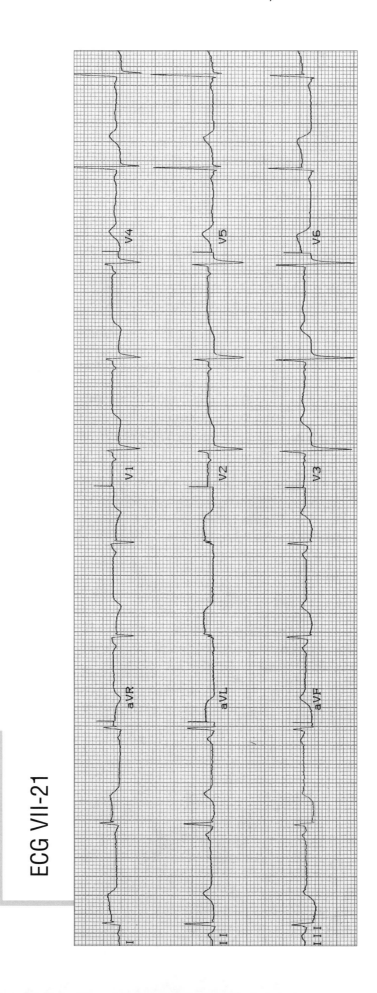

ECG VII-21

Diagnoses   **ECG VII-21**

1. Sinus rhythm (rate = 60/min)

2. Acute lateral infarction

Clinical Data

52-year-old man with clinical picture of myocardial infarction

Comment

Indicative changes (ST elevations) are confined to leads 1, aVL, and V6, making the diagnosis of *lateral* infarction.

ECG VII-22

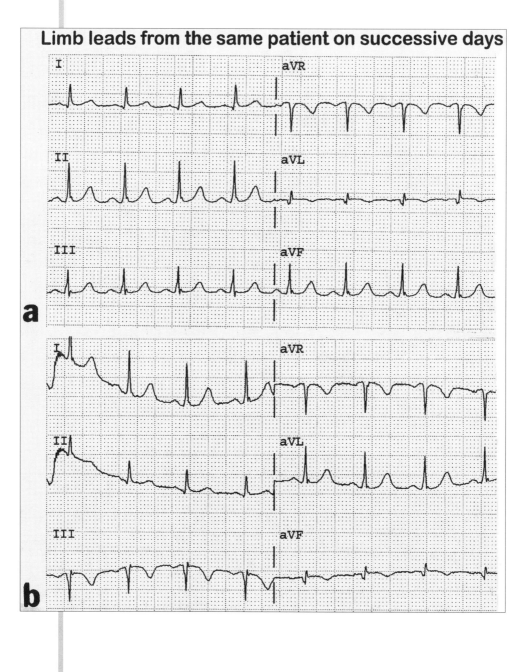

Limb leads from the same patient on successive days

Diagnoses   **ECG VII-22**

1. *a* = Normal limb leads

2. *b* = Switched left arm and left leg electrodes (producing pseudo-infarction pattern in leads 3 and aVF)

Clinical Data

44-year-old asymptomatic man

Comment

Reversing the left arm and left leg electrodes switches leads 1 and 2, and leads aVL and aVF, and records lead 3 upside down. The resulting Q and T pattern in 3 and aVF simulates an inferior infarction.

Check your connections!

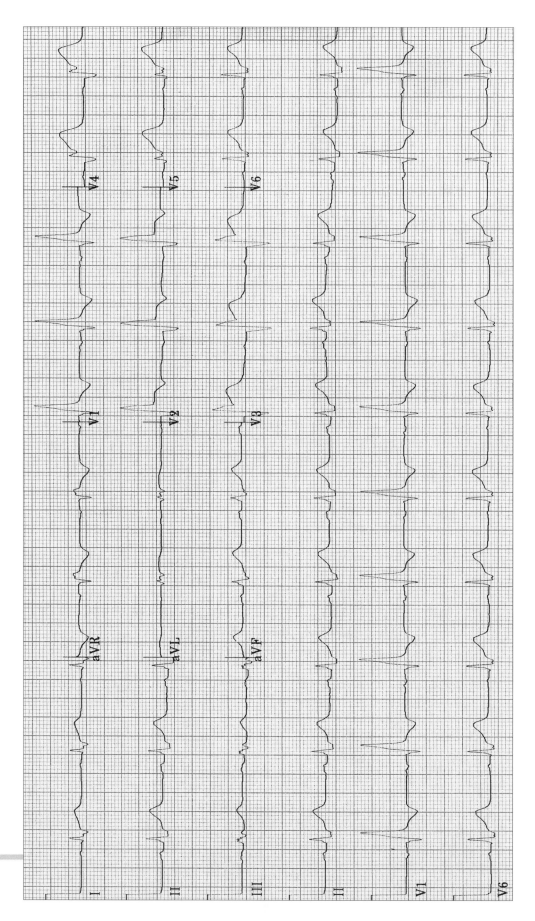

ECG VII-23

Diagnoses   **ECG VII-23**

1. Normal sinus rhythm (rate = 66/min) with borderline PR interval (0.20 s)

2. Acute extensive anterior (anterolateral) infarction

3. Right bundle-branch block

Clinical Data

69-year-old man

Comments

None

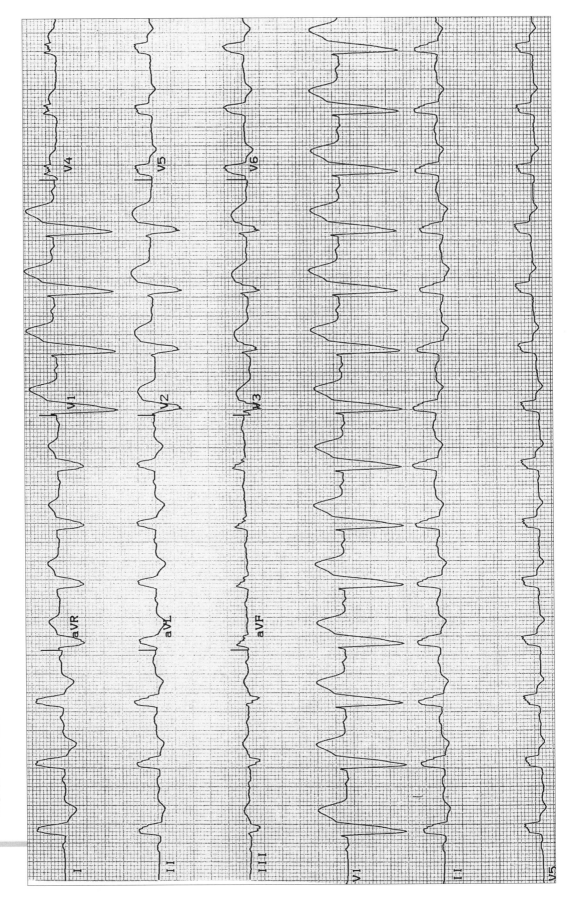

ECG VII-24

Diagnoses   **ECG VII-24**

1. Borderline intra-atrial block (P-wave width 0.12 s)

2. Left bundle-branch block

3. Acute anterolateral infarction

Clinical Data

76-year-old man with severe chest pain

Comments

It is sometimes taught that infarction cannot be recognized in the presence of LBBB (probably because development of QRS changes are relatively uncommon). However, if attention is paid to the ST-T, the diagnosis is often easy—as in this case where the ST elevation with convexity upward in V2–5 indicates acute injury.

Section VIII

12-Lead Miscellany

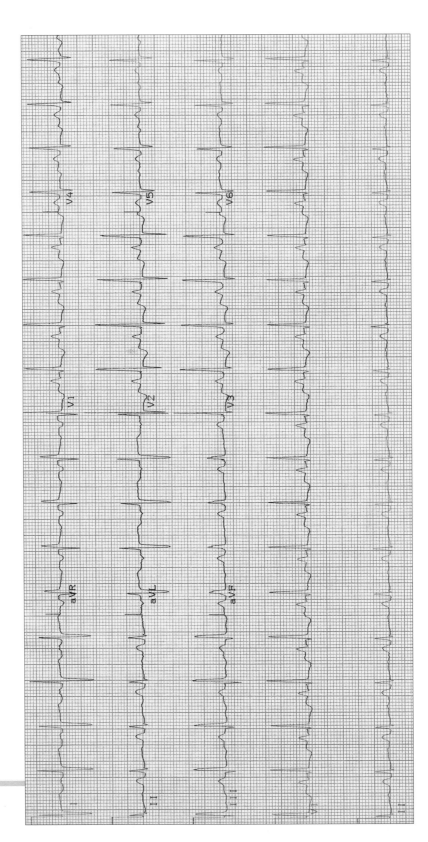

ECG VIII-1

Diagnoses   **ECG VIII-1**

1. Sinus tachycardia (rate = 107/min)

2. Right atrial hypertrophy (P-pulmonale)

3. Right ventricular hypertrophy

4. Right axis deviation (axis about +120°)

Clinical Data

33-year-old man weighing 300+ lbs; hypoventilation, recurrent pneumonia, and pulmonary emboli

Comment

The right atrial and ventricular hypertrophy and right axis deviation are all secondary to the pulmonary hypertension and chronic cor pulmonale, which resulted from his clinical disasters.

ECG VIII-2

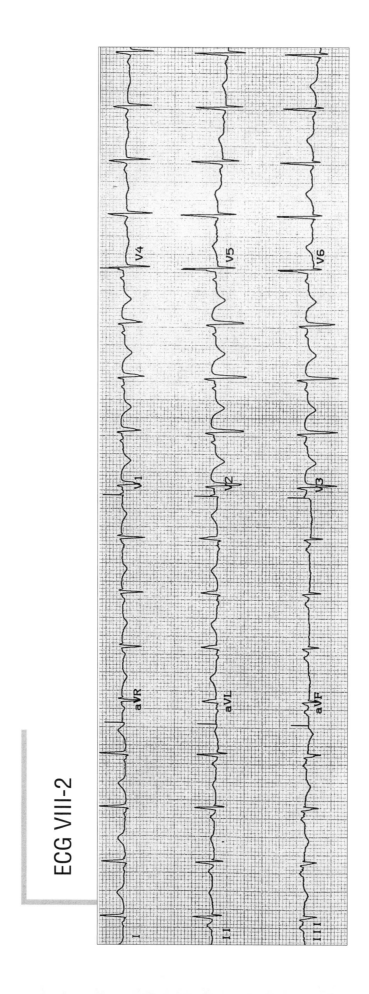

Diagnoses   **ECG VIII-2**

1. Sinus tachycardia (rate = 101/min)

2. Borderline short PR interval (0.12 s)

3. Acute cor pulmonale

Clinical Data

45-year-old woman with pulmonary embolism

Comment

Significant T-wave inversion simultaneously in inferior (here in lead 3) and anteroseptal leads (here in leads V1–3) should make you think of pulmonary embolism.

ECG VIII-3

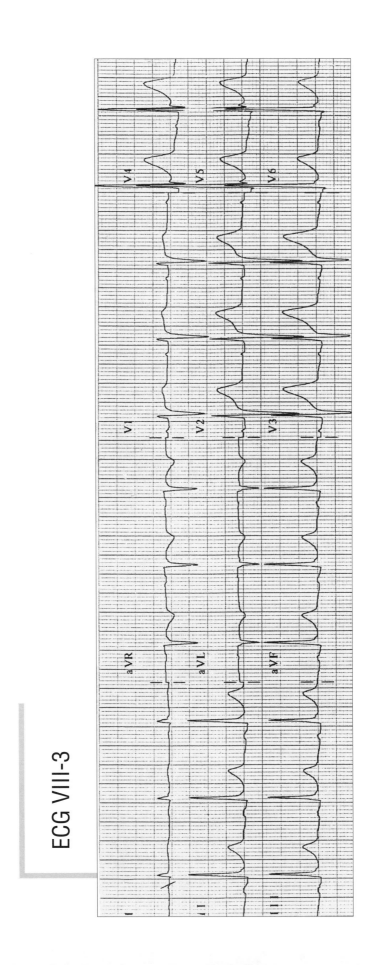

Diagnoses   **ECG VIII-3**

1. Sinus rhythm (rate = 75/min)

2. "Early repolarization"

3. Normal tracing

Clinical Data

45-year-old man

Comments

• "Early repolarization," which Spodick has again pointed out is "an underinvestigated misnomer" (Clin Cardiol 20:913, 1997), has to be differentiated from pericarditis (see table below).

• Typical of "early repolarization" in this tracing are: (a) the barb at the J point which, with the associated ST-T, creates the image of a fishhook (especially in V5), and (b) the level of the J point in V5–6, which is less than 25% the height of the T wave.

Early Repolarization	**Pericarditis**
Mostly males	Both sexes
Taller T waves	Less tall T waves
"Fishhook" at J point	No "fishhook"
In V6, ST < 25% of T	In V6, ST > 25% of T
Bradycardia often	Tachycardia usually

ECG VIII-4

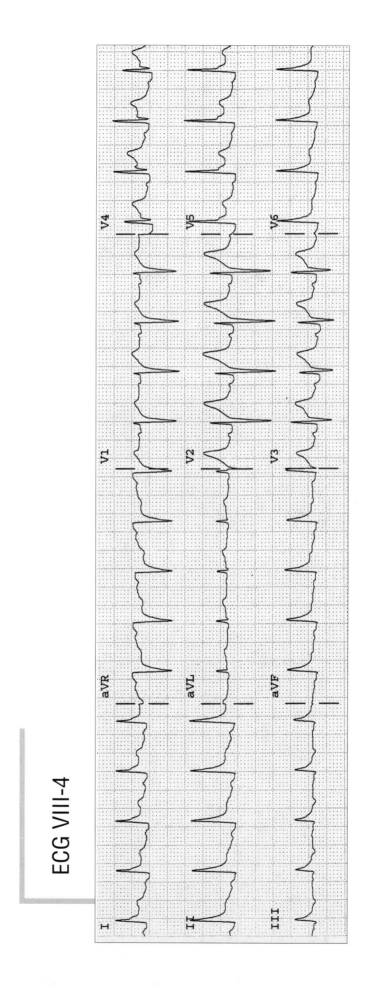

Diagnoses

ECG VIII-4

1. Sinus tachycardia (rate = 110/min)

2. Acute pericarditis

Clinical Data

60-year-old man with staphylococcal joint infection, bacteremia, and purulent pericarditis (360 cc of pus on tap)

Comment

Note especially in V6 that, unlike the benign "early repolarization" pattern, the J-point level almost equals the height of the T wave. (In early repolarization, the J-point level is usually less than 25% of the T-wave height; see ECG VIII-3.)

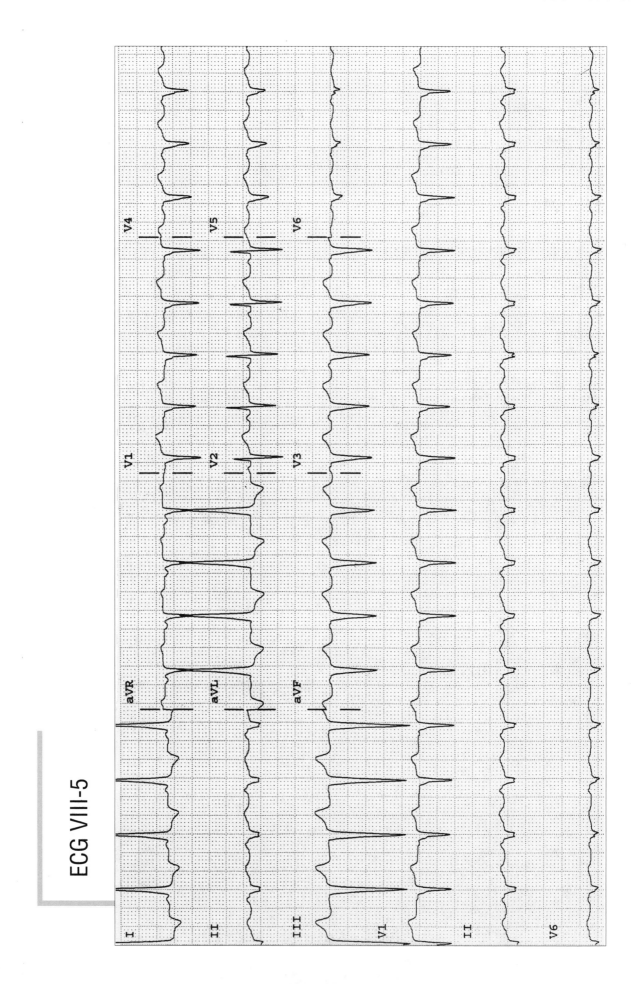

ECG VIII-5

Diagnoses   **ECG VIII-5**

1. Sinus tachycardia (rate = 104/min)

2. Left axis deviation (axis −40 degrees)

3. Wolff-Parkinson-White syndrome

Clinical Data

41-year-old woman

Comments

This is a beautiful example of the way in which lead V2 can be left out in the cold—looking as though it did not belong to the precordial series—because of the way we stagger the electrodes across the chest.

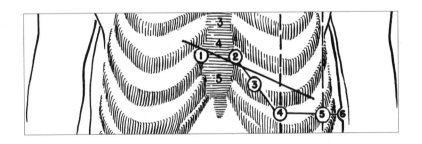

ECG VIII-6

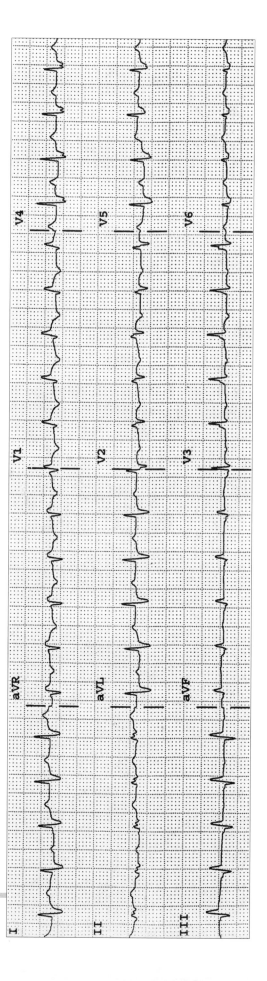

Diagnoses

ECG VIII-6

1. Sinus tachycardia (rate = 126/min)

2. Acute cor pulmonale

Clinical Data

64-year-old woman in sickle cell "crisis." Hematocrit dropped from 30 to 8, but because she was a Jehovah's Witness she refused transfusion. Diffuse pulmonary hemorrhages developed, and she died.

Comments

The simultaneous suspicion of inferior (Q in lead 3) and anteroseptal infarcts—not to mention the classic S1Q3 pattern—should immediately make you think of acute cor pulmonale (usually, of course, due to pulmonary embolism, but here owing to the uncontrolled pulmonary hemorrhages). A good, but apparently little known, clue to acute cor pulmonale is the suspicion of ischemia, injury, or infarction *simultaneously in inferior and anteroseptal leads.*

ECG VIII-7

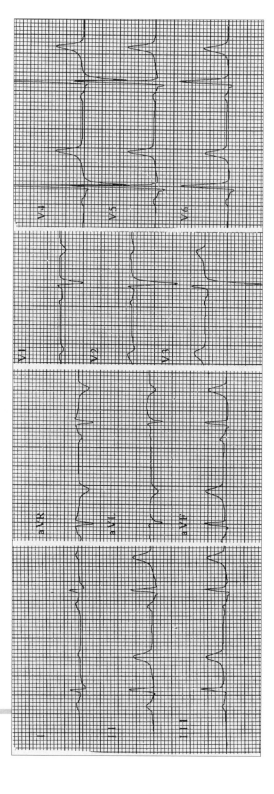

Diagnoses

ECG VIII-7

1. Sinus bradycardia (rate = 56/min)

2. Hyperkalemia

3. Hypocalcemia

Clinical Data

23-year-old man undergoing dialysis for chronic renal disease; potassium 5.8 meq/L and calcium 7.6 meq/L

Comment

The tracing is rather typical of this combination of electrolyte disorders—the narrow-based, peaked T waves (high potassium effect) at the end of an elongated ST segment (low calcium effect) are characteristic.

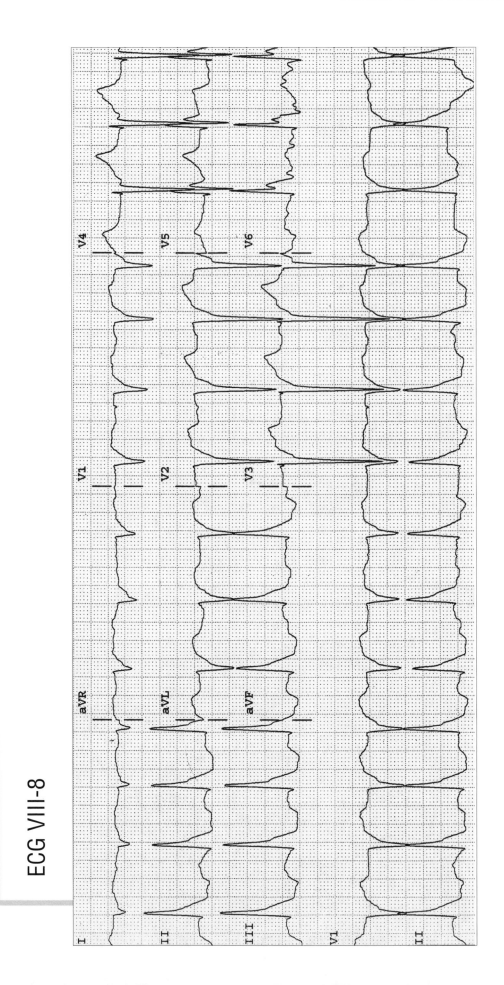

ECG VIII-8

Diagnoses   **ECG VIII-8**

1. Atrial fibrillation with moderate ventricular response at about 80/min

2. Right axis deviation

3. Hypothermia

Clinical Data

61-year-old man found unconscious with BP 60/40 and temperature 84 degrees

Comment

Note the **Osborn waves** "buttressing" the QRSs.

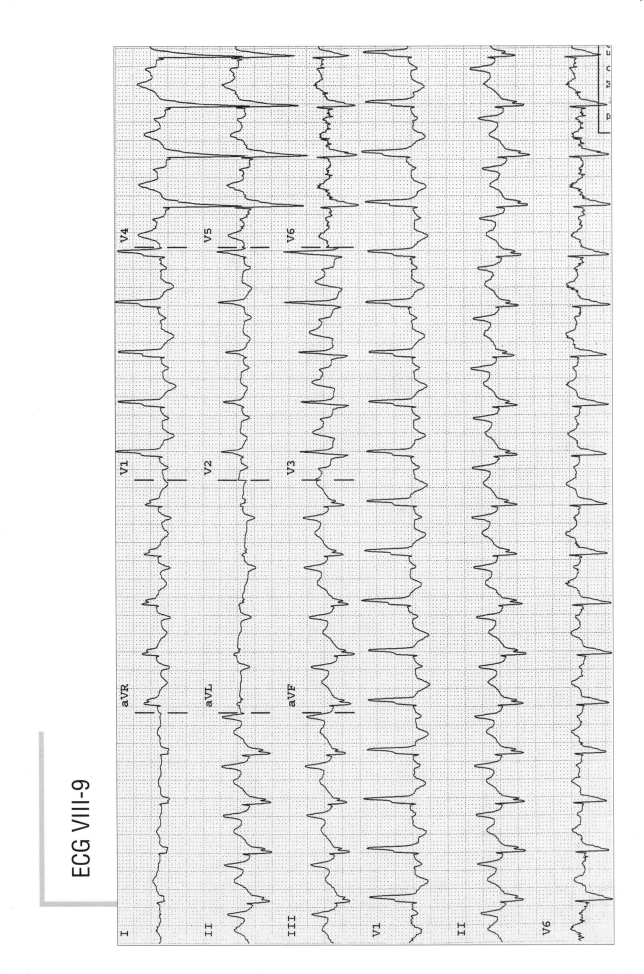

ECG VIII-9

Diagnoses   **ECG VIII-9**

1. Sinus tachycardia (rate = 110/min)

2. Right bundle-branch block

3. Bizarre frontal plane QRS axis ($-120°$)

4. Chronic cor pulmonale with exaggerated P-pulmonale

5. Cannot exclude left atrial enlargement

6. Old anterior infarction

Clinical Data

67-year-old woman with severe emphysema

Comments

• Note that the P-wave axis is almost $+90°$, and the height of the P waves in leads 2, 3, and aVF is 5–7 mm, i.e., an exaggerated P-pulmonale.

• Note also the bizarre axis and the rS complex in V6 which, with a wide QRS, are usually good clues to ventricular ectopy.

• The abnormally large P-terminal force in V1, though almost always due to *left* atrial enlargement, *can* result from an enlarged *right* atrial appendage extending leftward.

ECG VIII-10

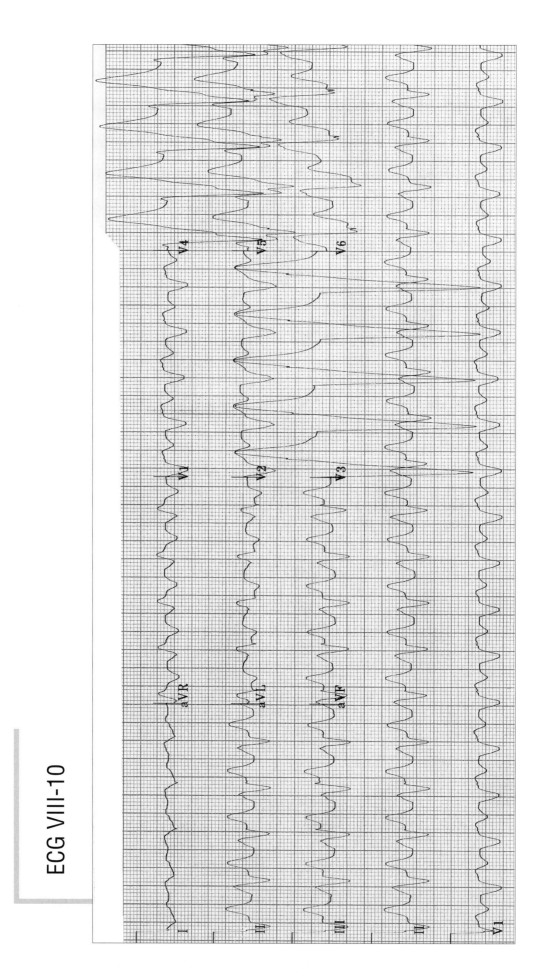

Diagnoses   **ECG VIII-10**

1. Tachycardia (rate = 117/min), mechanism uncertain

2. Hyperkalemia

Clinical Data

79-year-old woman in end-stage renal failure with pulmonary edema and potassium level of 6.2 meq/L

Comment

• Note the wide (QRS interval = 0.20 s), grotesque QRS shapes and the almost straight line from the S wave to the apex of the T in V3–5.

• The mechanism of the tachycardia is necessarily uncertain; if the atria are potassium-paralyzed it could be sino-ventricular (i.e., sinus in control, with impulse conducted to ventricles via internodal pathways and no atrial activation).

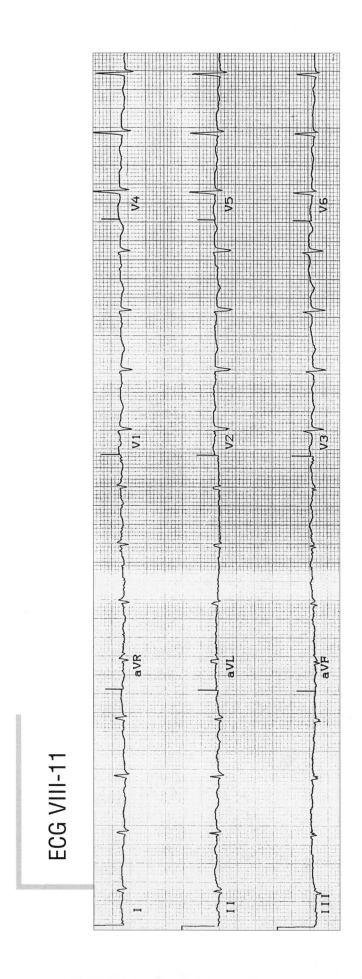

ECG VIII-11

Diagnoses   ### ECG VIII-11

1. Sinus rhythm (rate = 97/min)

2. Hypothyroidism

Clinical Data

45-year-old man with myxedema

Comment

Although nonspecific, low voltage with T wave flattening to mild inversion in the absence of associated ST abnormalities is characteristic of hypothyroidism.

ECG VIII-12

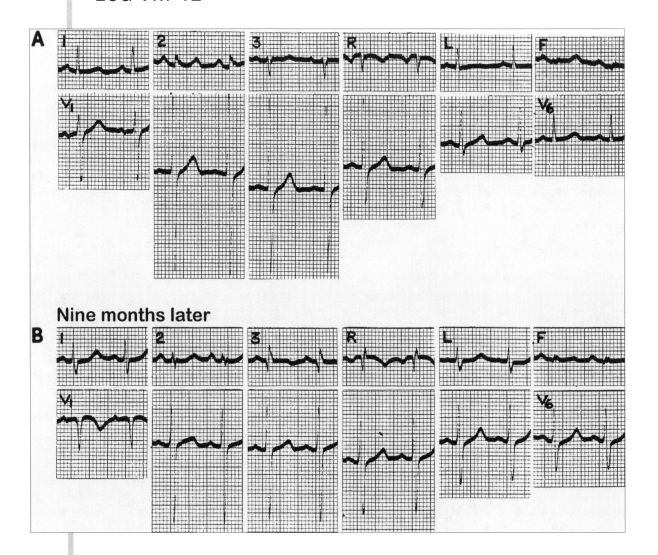

Nine months later

Diagnoses   **ECG VIII-12**

1. *A* = Within normal limits, except for unusually high total QRS voltage in V2–3

2. *B* = Mild sinus tachycardia; acute cor pulmonale from pulmonary embolism

Clinical Data

53-year-old man

Comments

The embolus was fatal. Features suggesting or compatible with pulmonary embolism are:

- S1/Q3 pattern

- Development of S waves in almost all leads

- *Simultaneous* new T-wave inversion in leads 3 and V1—the most important clue, and a rather subtle manifestation of the clue stressed in ECG VIII-6.

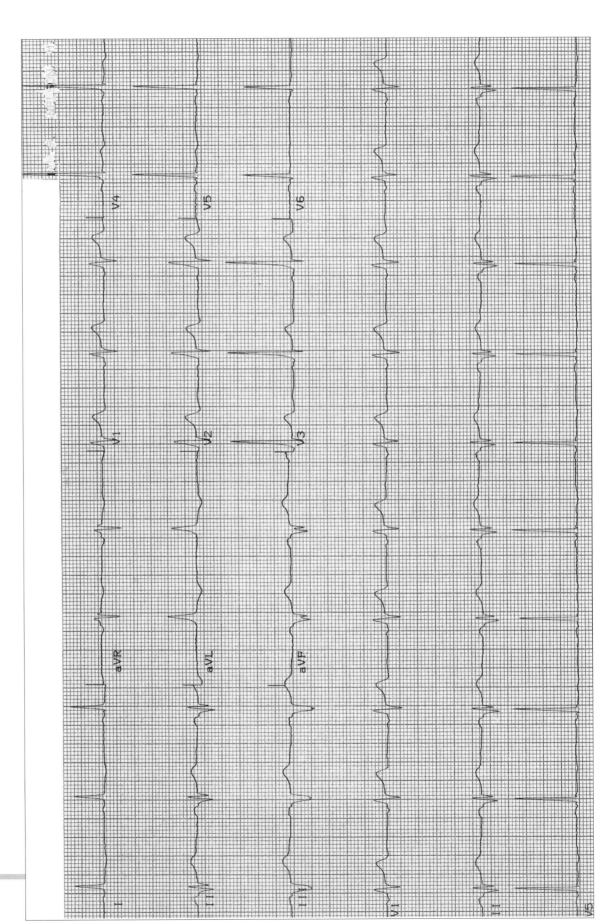

Diagnoses   **ECG VIII-13**

1. Sinus rhythm (rate = 63/min)

2. Preexcitation (WPW type)

Clinical Data

68-year-old man, asymptomatic

Comment

This tracing was diagnosed by the hospital panel reader as "inferoposterior infarction of uncertain date." The three things a WPW is most likely to be mistaken for are:

- Myocardial infarction (negative delta waves = wide Q waves)

- Ventricular hypertrophy (increased QRS voltage)

- Bundle-branch block (wide QRS complexes).

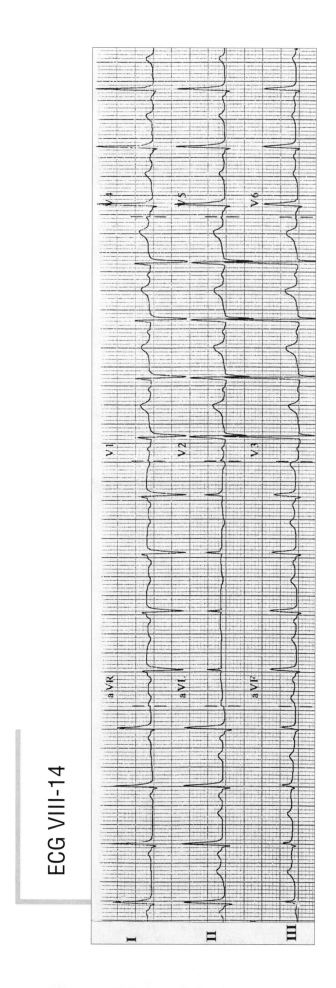

ECG VIII-14

Diagnoses   **ECG VIII-14**

1. Sinus rhythm/tachycardia (rate = 99/min)

2. Hypocalcemia (calcium 7 meq/L)

3. Nonspecific T-wave abnormalities (flat in 1, TV1 > TV6)

Clinical Data

49-year-old woman on dialysis for end-stage renal failure

Comment

Think of hypocalcemia when:

- The ST segment is prolonged, lengthening the QT interval.

- The T wave, while remaining relatively normal, rubs shoulders with the next P wave.

ECG VIII-15

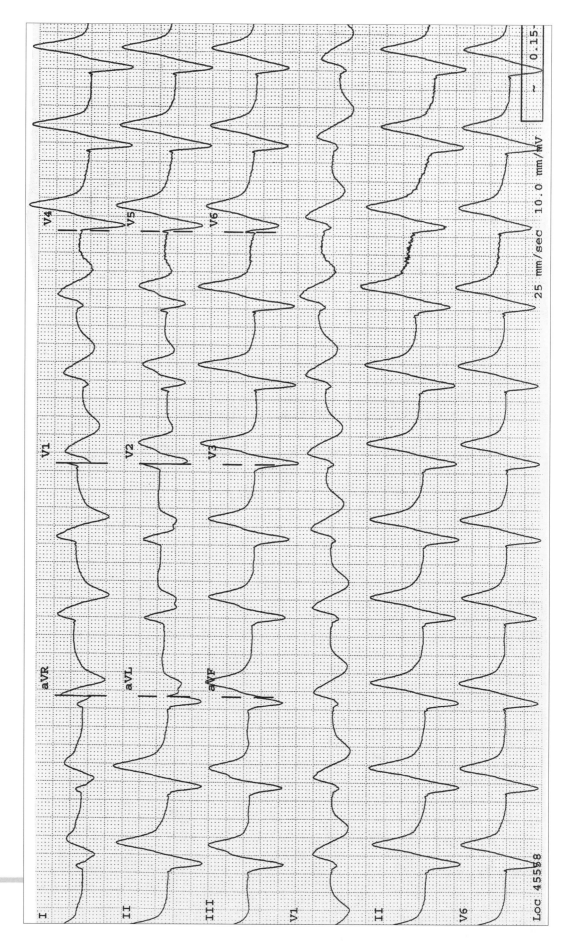

Diagnoses   **ECG VIII-15**

1. Rhythm uncertain, rate 70/min

2. Hyperkalemia (potassium 8.5 meq/L)

Clinical Data

68-year-old woman in chronic renal failure

Comments

This is the typical "**Z-fold pattern**" of severe hyperpotassemia. Note the absence of P waves and the wide QRSs with, in many leads, a *virtual straight line from the nadir of the S wave to the apex of the T wave.*

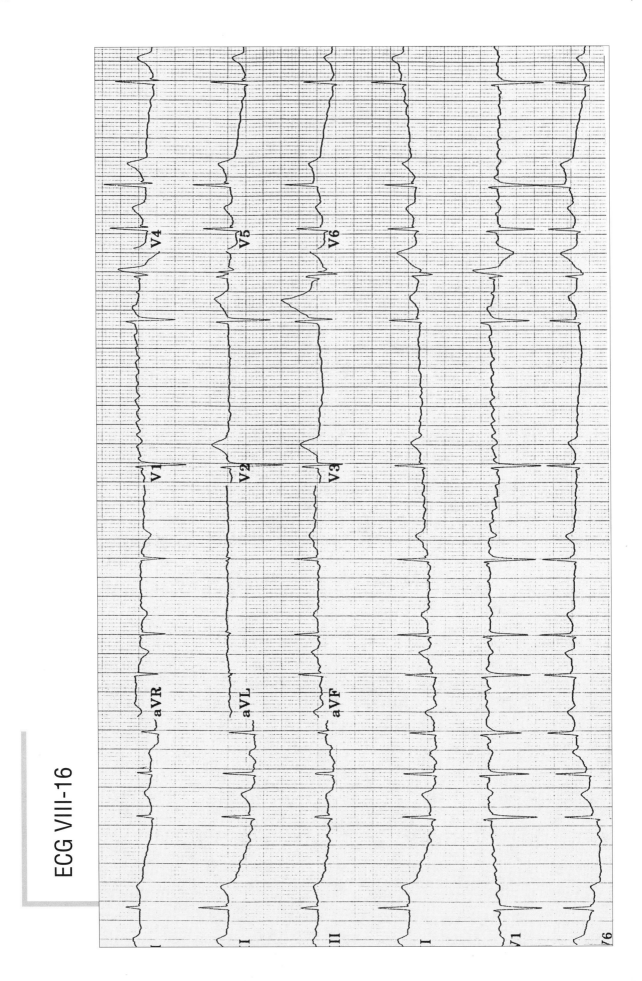

ECG VIII-16

Diagnoses

ECG VIII-16

1. Atrial fibrillation with moderate ventricular response (rate about 75/min)

2. One beat conducted with RBBB aberration

3. Acute pericarditis

Clinical Data

38-year-old man with pericardial rub; cocaine user, arrested for robbery, complaining of chest pain aggravated by his apprehension!

Comments

• The aberrant beat is a classic example of the **Ashman phenomenon,** i.e., aberration of a beat ending a long-short cycle sequence during atrial fibrillation. The long cycle, by lengthening the refractory period of the ventricular conduction system, sets the stage for aberration to appear when a relatively early beat follows. The rsR′ morphology in V1 is typical of RBBB aberration, but the computer is usually (as here) unable to distinguish aberration from ectopy.

• Note the varied ventricular cycles, representing rates from 40 to 150/min. This marked irregularity is due to the unpredictably varying numbers of the fibrillatory impulses that get as far as the junction, but no further (concealed conduction).

ECG VIII-17

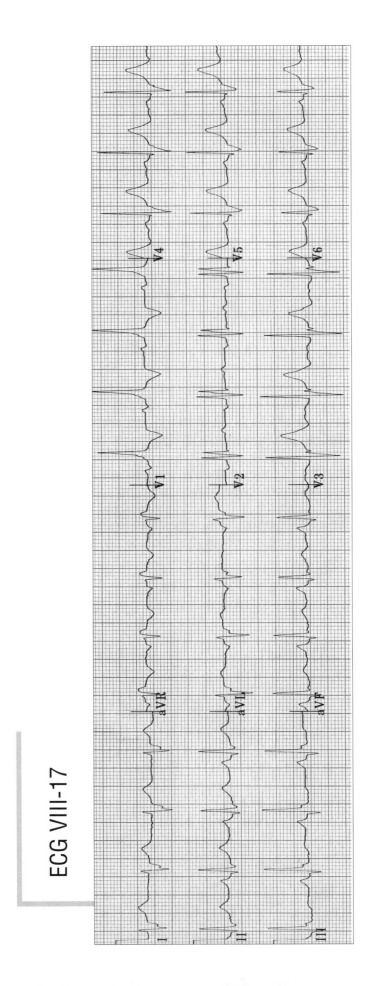

Diagnoses ECG VIII-17

1. Sinus rhythm (rate = 90/min)

2. P-pulmonale (P-wave axis +90 degrees)

3. Right bundle-branch block, with . . .

4. . . . *possible* left posterior hemiblock (axis of initial 0.04 s is +110 degrees), or . . .

5. . . . right ventricular hypertrophy (RV1 = 14 mm)

Clinical Data

72-year-old woman

Comments

It is tempting to diagnose bifascicular block (RBBB + LPHB). However, since one of the criteria for diagnosing LPHB is "no evidence of RVH," and since the P-pulmonale and the R wave voltage in V1 suggest an underlying RVH, you cannot diagnose LPHB. (In the limb leads, RVH and LPHB may produce identical patterns, and therefore you cannot make the assumption of LPHB in the presence of known or suspected RVH.)

ECG VIII-18

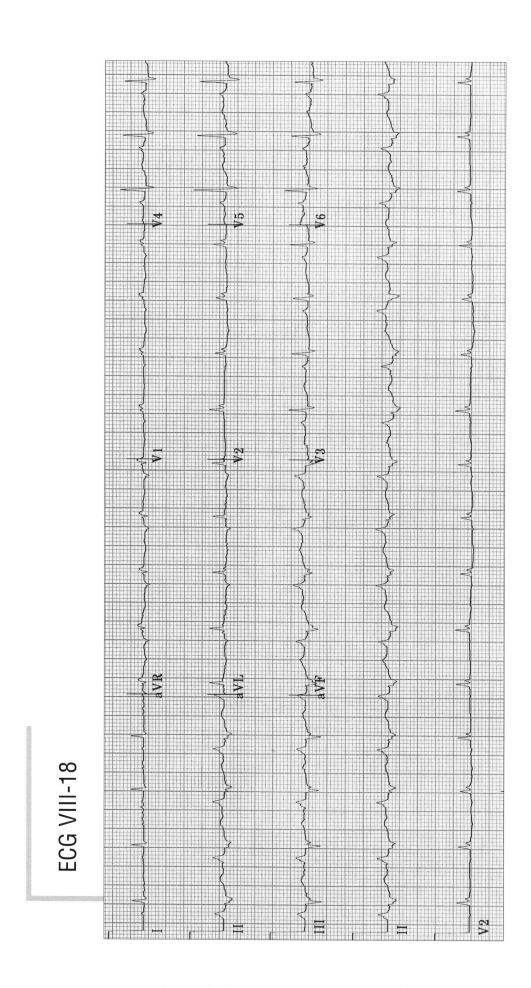

Diagnoses   **ECG VIII-18**

1. Sinus tachycardia (rate = 102/min)

2. Chronic cor pulmonale (CCP)

Clinical Data

70-year-old man with chronic asthma and hypothyroidism

Comments

• The features *suggestive of* CCP are P-pulmonale (P axis about +80 degrees) and low QRS voltage.

• The features *consistent with* the diagnosis are the positive QRSs in V1–2 and the marked left axis deviation (about −70 degrees) which is found in a significant minority of CCPs.

With this background diagnosis of CCP, there is no way the additional diagnosis of hypothyroidism can be made from the ECG.

ECG VIII-19

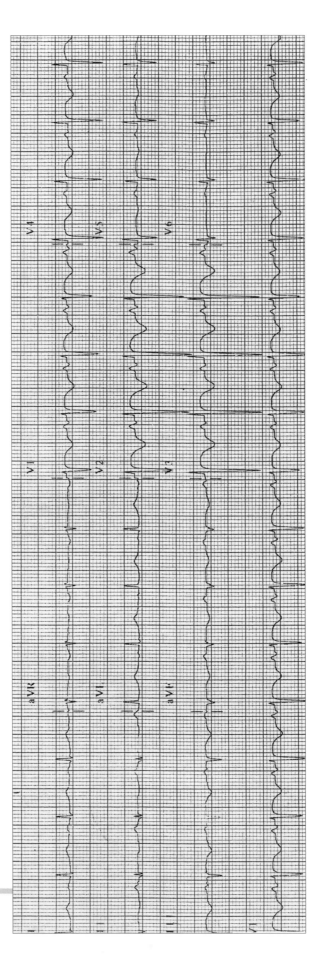

Diagnoses

ECG VIII-19

1. Sinus rhythm (rate = 93/min)

2. Acute cor pulmonale

Clinical Data

84-year-old man

Comment

This is another classic example of the ECG of pulmonary embolism—an often missed diagnosis. Note the *simultaneous, abnormal* T-wave inversion in the inferior leads (3 and aVF) and the anteroseptal leads.

ECG VIII-20

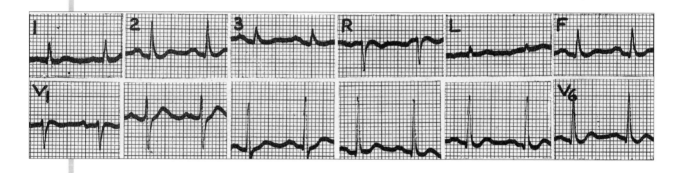

Diagnoses   ## ECG VIII-20

1. Sinus rhythm/tachycardia (rate = 100/min)

2. Hypercalcemia

Clinical Data

57-year-old man with bronchogenic carcinoma and calcium of 13 meq/L

Comments

The changes are subtle, but definite. Look especially at lead V2: loss of the ST segment results in a steeper upstroke than downstroke of the T wave, so that the *apex* of the T is reached early (shortened QaT interval). The QT interval remains normal.

ECG VIII-21

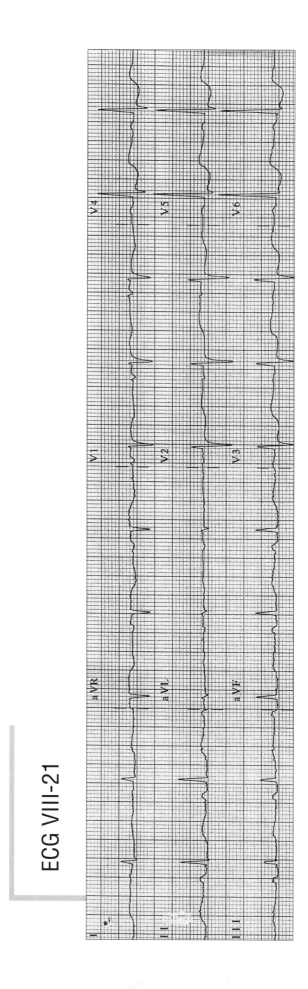

Diagnoses   **ECG VIII-21**

1. Sinus rhythm (rate = 68/min)

2. Hypokalemia (2.9 meq/L)

Clinical Data

62-year-old woman with potassium depletion from diuretics and vomiting

Comments

Note the typical down-up, "roller-coaster" effect in leads V3–6; and the broad T-U amalgam in 2 and aVF making it *look like* a long QT.

ECG VIII-22

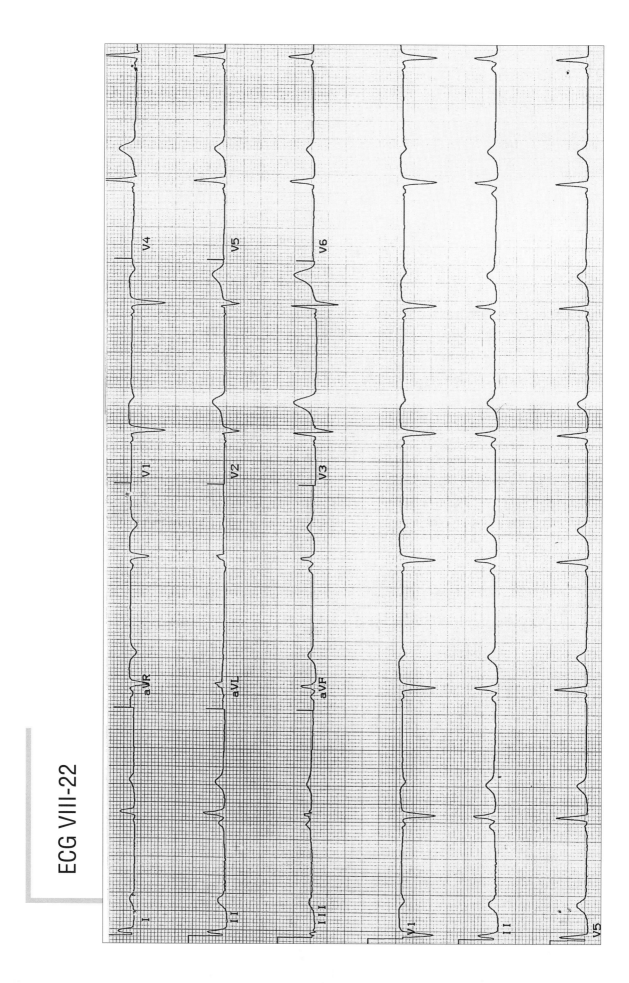

Diagnoses   **ECG VIII-22**

1. Sinus bradycardia (rate = 43/min)

2. Short PR interval (0.11 s)

3. WPW syndrome

Clinical Data

88-year-old man

Comments

An interesting tracing for discussion. The computer interpretation was "isochronic AV dissociation," but it is most unlikely that the sinus and the junction would both have the same independent rate of 43 and maintain precisely the same P to QRS relationship throughout the strip. There are two other possibilities.

• Short PR with incomplete (what Sodi-Pallares would call "first degree") LBBB, i.e., minimal widening of the QRS with loss of evidence of septal activation (loss of q waves in V5–6, etc., and of r waves in V1)

• Preexcitation, which is favored by the short PR and also readily explains the loss of initial septal activation

Conduction via an accessory pathway, therefore, is the most likely explanation for the constant, close PR relationship.

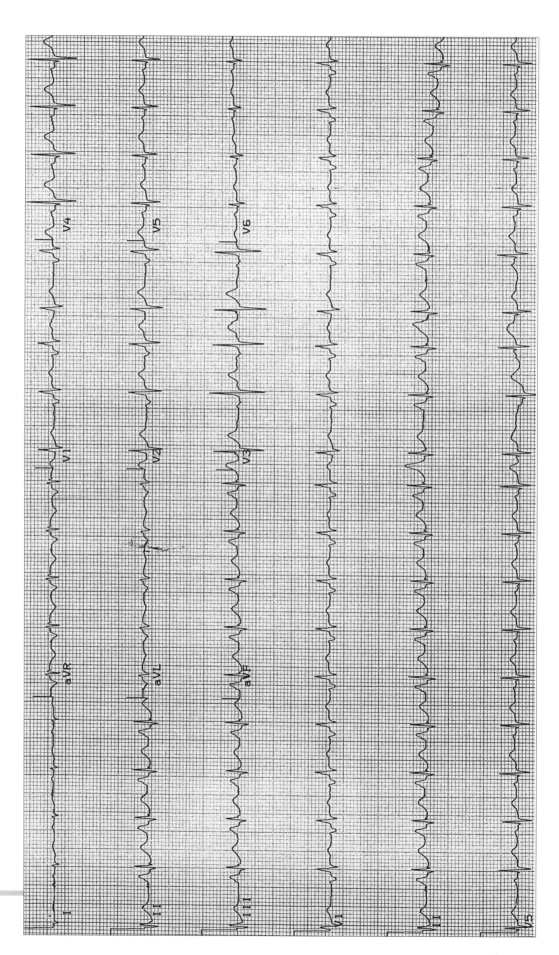

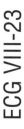

Diagnoses   **ECG VIII-23**

1. Sinus tachycardia (rate = 115/min)

2. Two atrial premature beats

3. Chronic cor pulmonale

4. ? Left atrial abnormality/enlargement (prominent P-terminal force in V1)

Clinical Data

65-year-old man with emphysema

Comments

This tracing shows many of the classic features of chronic cor pulmonale due to emphysema:

- P-pulmonale (prominent P waves in inferior leads, with P-wave axis about +80 degrees)
- Vertical QRS axis with relatively low voltage in limb leads
- Prominent RV1 (RVH)
- Significant S waves through V6
- Strikingly low QRS amplitude in V6.

ECG VIII-24

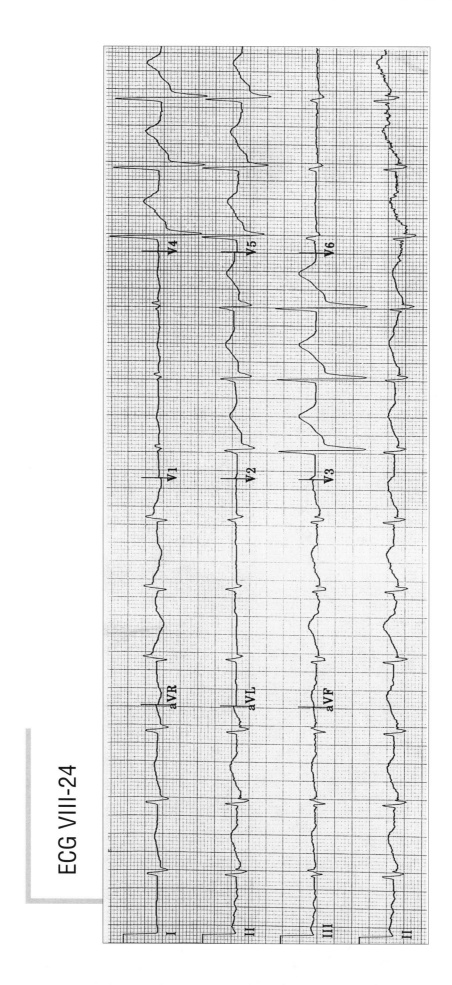

Diagnoses   **ECG VIII-24**

1. Sinus rhythm (rate = 77/min)

2. Hypokalemia

Clinical Data

78-year-old man with carcinoma of prostate, subarachnoid hemorrhage, and potassium of 2.8 meq/L

Comments

• Another case in which V1 would be a poor choice for QRS monitoring (compare with ECGs III-34 and VII-20)

• The large U waves, surprisingly prominent at this potassium level, are presumably exaggerated by the intracranial disturbance.

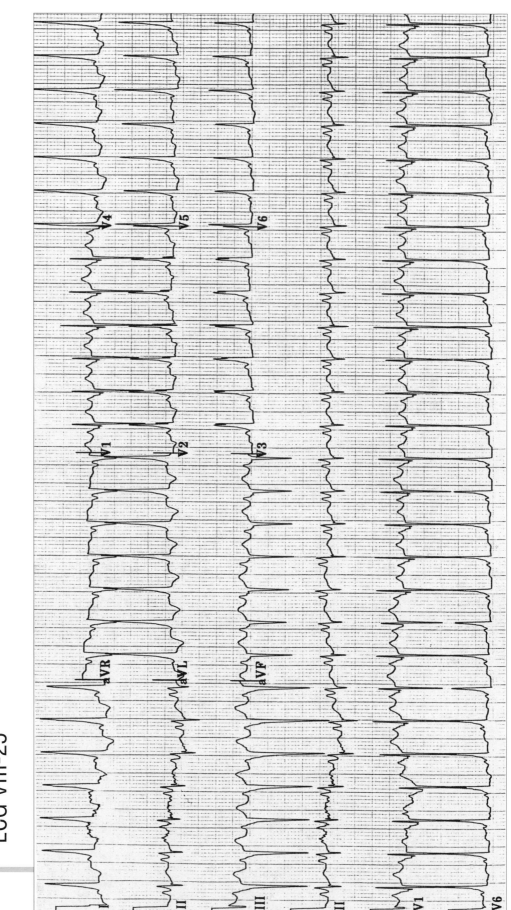

ECG VIII-25

Diagnoses

ECG VIII-25

1. Sinus tachycardia (rate = 163/min)

2. WPW syndrome

Clinical Data

3-week-old baby boy

Comment

The short PR is evident in most leads; the delta wave is best seen in the left-sided V leads. Note how the delta wave becomes a wide little Q wave in V1.

(The computer interpretation was: "Wide QRS tachycardia . . . nonspecific intraventricular block.")

ECG VIII-26

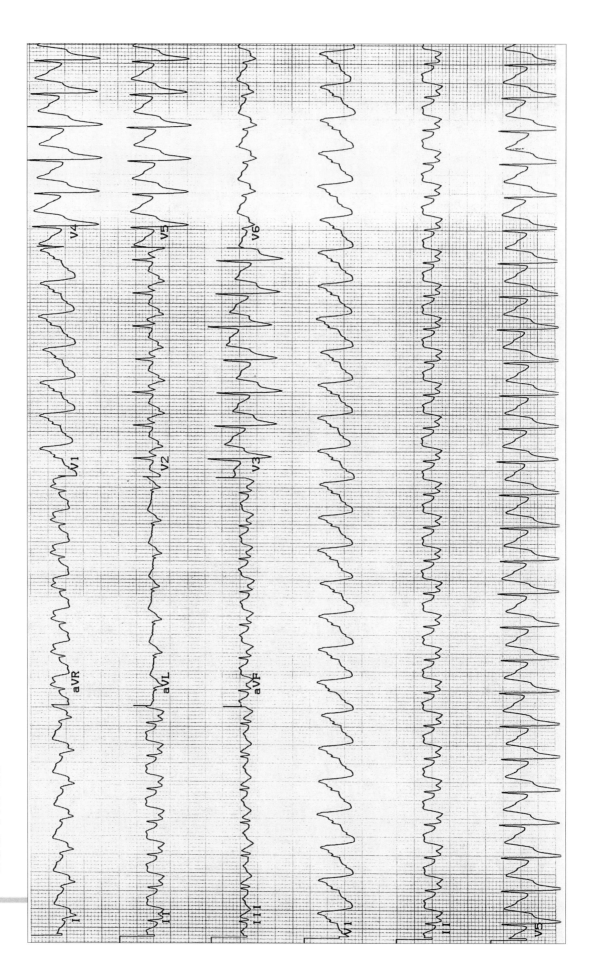

Diagnoses

ECG VIII-26

1. Hyperkalemia (potassium = 9 meq/L)

2. Sinus tachycardia (166/min)

Clinical Data

2-day-old baby girl, dying of renal failure

Comment

Note the almost vertical upstroke of T waves in V3–V5, one of the patterns typical of severe hyperkalemia.

ECG VIII-27

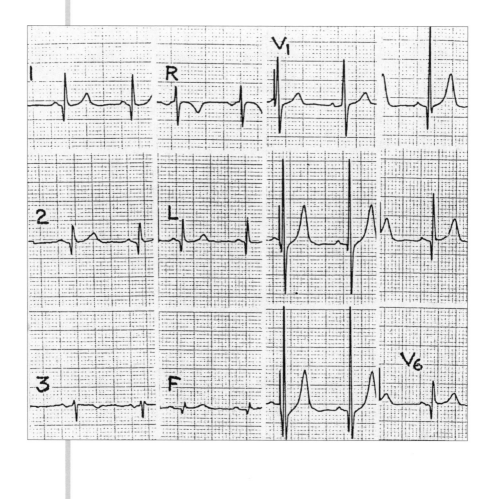

Diagnoses   **ECG VIII-27**

1. Sinus rhythm (rate = 76/min)

2. Septal hypertrophy (hypertrophic cardiomyopathy)

Clinical Data

Unknown

Comment

The dominant R wave in V1 requires differentiation among RVH, true posterior infarction, septal hyper-trophy, WPW, and normal variant. The association of large but narrow Q waves (in leads where Q waves represent septal activation) confirms septal hypertrophy as the diagnosis.

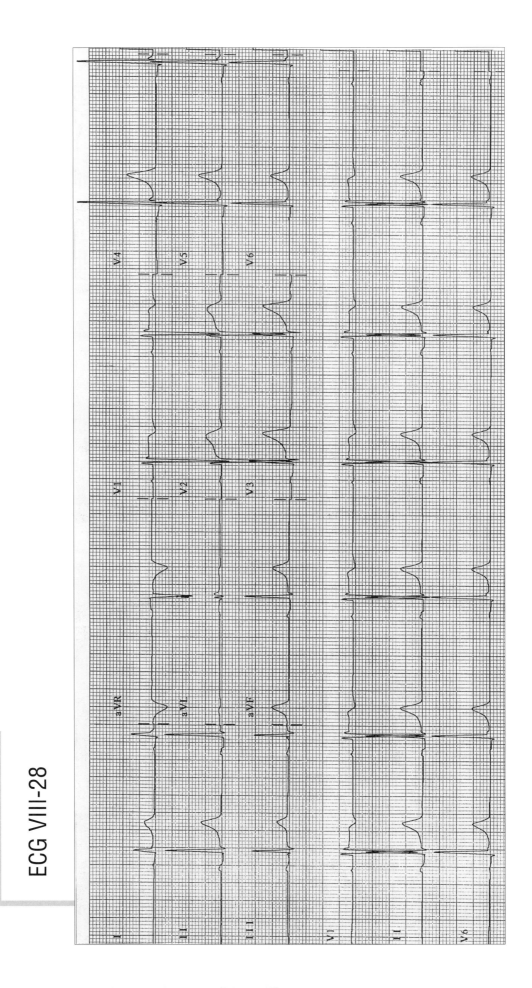

ECG VIII-28

Diagnoses   **ECG VIII-28**

1. Sinus bradycardia (rate = 40/min)

2. Normal variant ("early repolarization")

Clinical Data

29-year-old man; pain in left chest on deep inspiration; afebrile

Comments

The main differential diagnosis includes "early repolarization" (ERP) and pericarditis. It can be impossible to determine the diagnosis from the ECG alone, but the following clues help:

- Clinical picture: ERP occurs almost exclusively in males; absence of tachycardia and fever make pericarditis unlikely.
  - The "fishhook" ST-T pattern (seen here in V4) favors ERP.
  - ST elevation in V6 less than 25% of T height favors ERP.

See also the table of differentiating features at ECG VIII-3.

ECG VIII-29

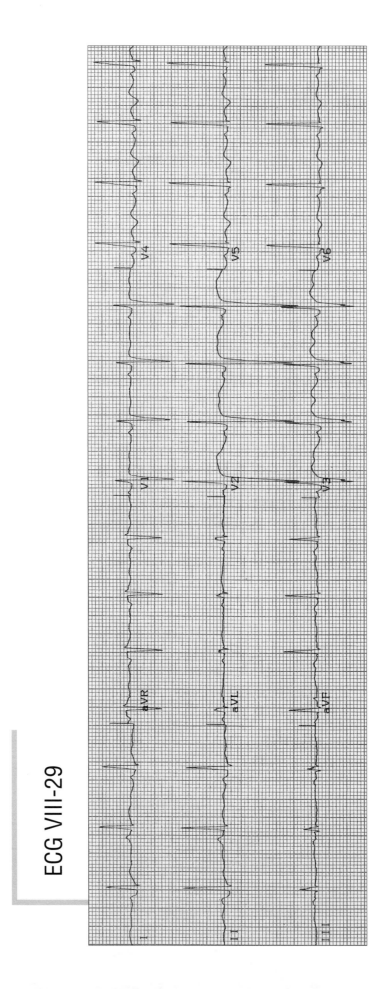

Diagnoses   **ECG VIII-29**

1. Sinus rhythm (rate = 93/min)

2. Hypokalemia (potassium 2.5 meq/L)

Clinical Data

24-year-old man; aspirin overdose

Comment

Note the prominent U waves, especially in the mid-precordial leads, creating the "camel-hump" effect in V3 and V4.

ECG VIII-30

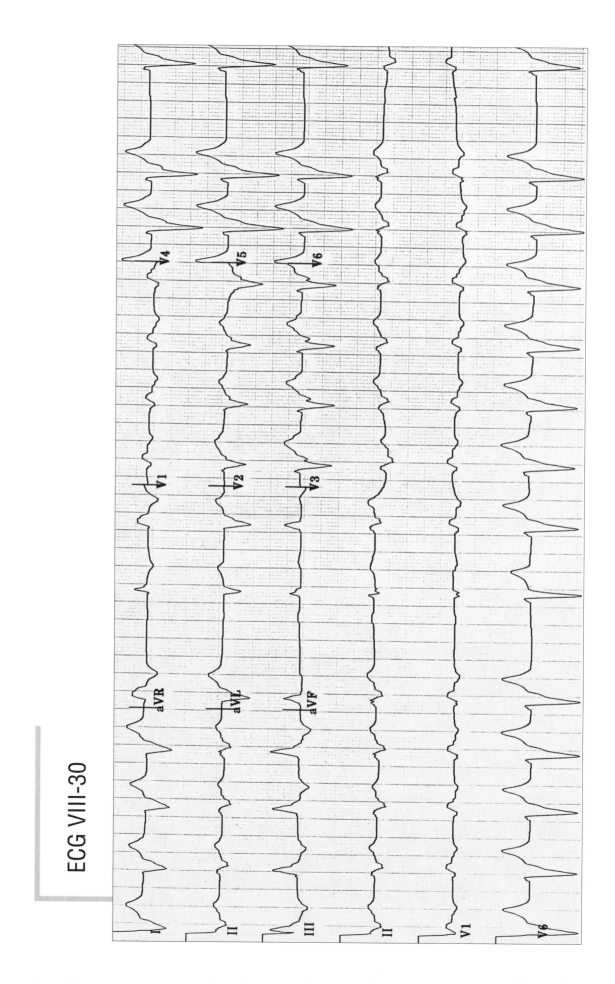

Diagnoses   **ECG VIII-30**

1. Sinus rhythm (rate about 92/min), with . . .

2. . . . type I AV block with long Wenckebach periods (the one period here is 9:8)

3. Hyperkalemia (potassium 9.1 meq/L)

Clinical Data

77-year-old man with chronic renal failure; because of muscular weakness, he decided he needed potassium and took 750 mg t.i.d. for 2 days; he was also on Aldactone and Zestril.

Comments

• Note, in passing, that the hyperkalemia—with its right axis deviation and rS complex in V6—has produced a wide QRS pattern suggestive of ventricular ectopy.

• Note that the QRS after the dropped beat is narrower, presumably because IV conduction is improved after the "breather." It seems that the IV block of potassium intoxication is at least partially rate dependent.

ECG VIII-31

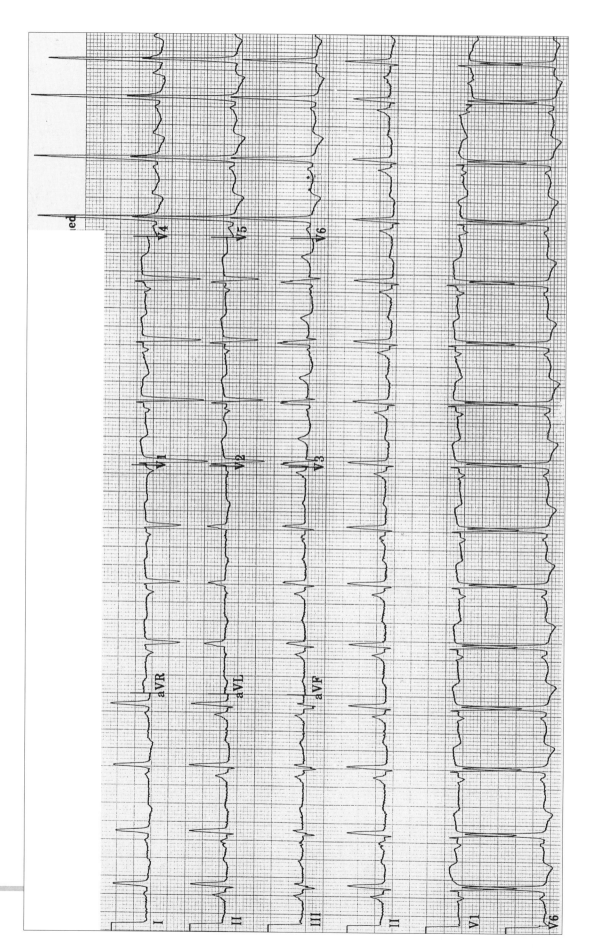

Diagnoses   ECG VIII-31

1. Sinus rhythm (rate = 90/min)

2. Left ventricular hypertrophy with secondary ST-T changes

3. Left atrial enlargement (increased P-terminal force in V1 = 7 mm/sec); P-wave axis +70° ("pseudo-P-pulmonale")

4. Three atrial premature beats with varying coupling

5. Probable old inferior infarction

Clinical Data

59-year-old man

Comments

• The three ABPs (beats 2, 7, and 15) are easily identified by their changed P waves in lead 2 (but not in V1).

• "Pseudo-P-pulmonale" is applied when LVH is present and the P waves simulate P pulmonale, but there is no reason whatever to suspect an underlying cor pulmonale. (See Chou T, Helm RA: The pseudo P pulmonale. Circulation 32:96, 1965.)

ECG VIII-32

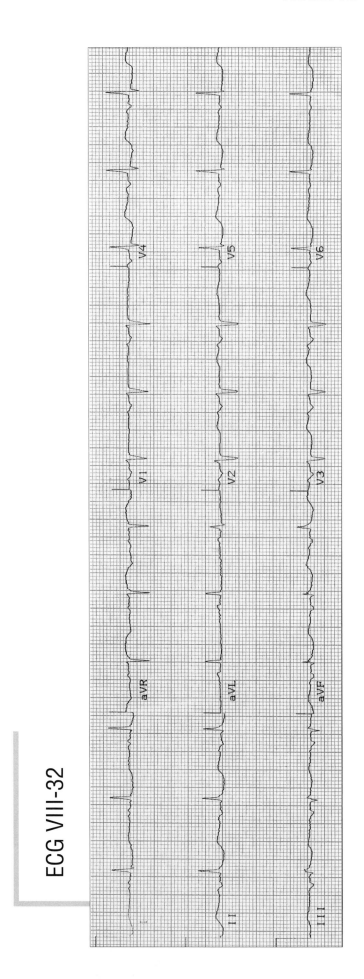

Diagnoses   **ECG VIII-32**

1. Left atrial abnormality/enlargement or ectopic atrial rhythm (rate = 78/min)

2. Hypokalemia

Clinical Data

78-year-old man with carcinoma of colon and intractable diarrhea; potassium 2.7 meq/L

Comments

Signs of left atrial enlargement include:

- P-wave duration of 0.14 s

- Leftward and posterior orientation of the second half of the P wave.

ECG VIII-33

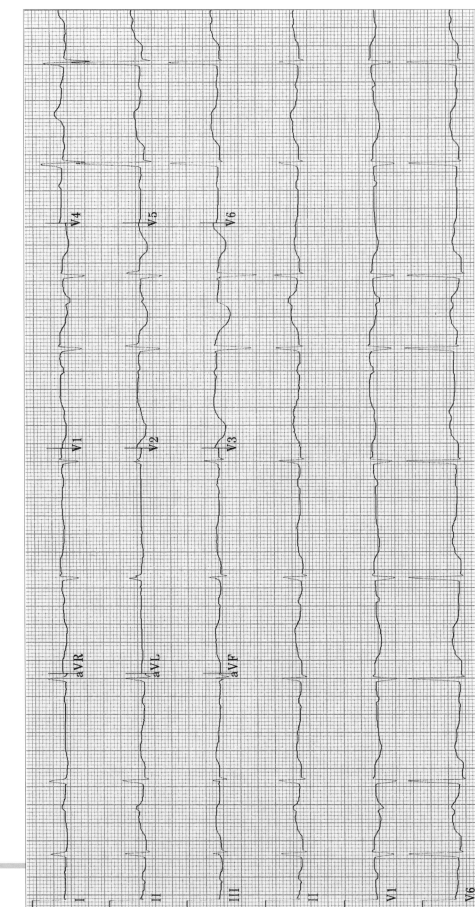

Diagnoses   **ECG VIII-33**

1. Sinus bradycardia with arrhythmia (rate about 50/min)

2. Two atrial premature beats

3. First-degree AV block (PR of sinus beats = 0.26 s, of APBs = 0.31 s)

4. Digitalis and quinidine effects

5. Probable old anteroseptal infarction

Clinical Data

76-year-old woman, recently converted from atrial fibrillation, receiving digoxin and quinidine sulfate

Comments

• With such U waves (see ECG below, *arrows*) that rival, or exceed, the height of the T waves, your first thought should undoubtedly be *severe hypokalemia*—but this patient's potassium was 4.3 meq/L. Your next consideration should be *combined digitalis and quinidine effects*. The third diagnosis to consider is an *intracranial disturbance.*

• The PRs of the APBs are longer than those of the sinus beats because of the associated shorter RP interval—RP/PR reciprocity being the hallmark of AV nodal block (see ECG V-25).

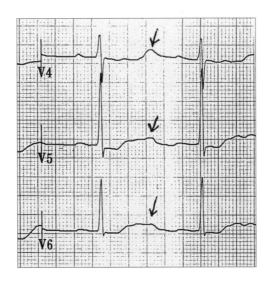

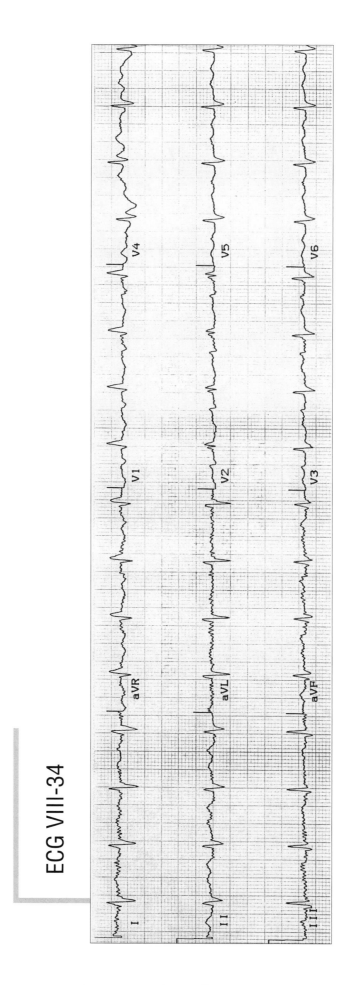

ECG VIII-34

Diagnoses   **ECG VIII-34**

1. Sinus rhythm (rate = 94/min)

2. Left atrial abnormality (increased P terminal force in V1)

3. Right axis deviation/RV hypertrophy

4. Borderline first-degree AV block

5. Low voltage in precordial leads

Clinical Data

30-year-old, 600-pound Pickwickian; at autopsy, heart weighed 830 grams

Comment

PR interval is difficult to measure accurately, but probably slightly prolonged (? 0.22 s).

ECG VIII-35

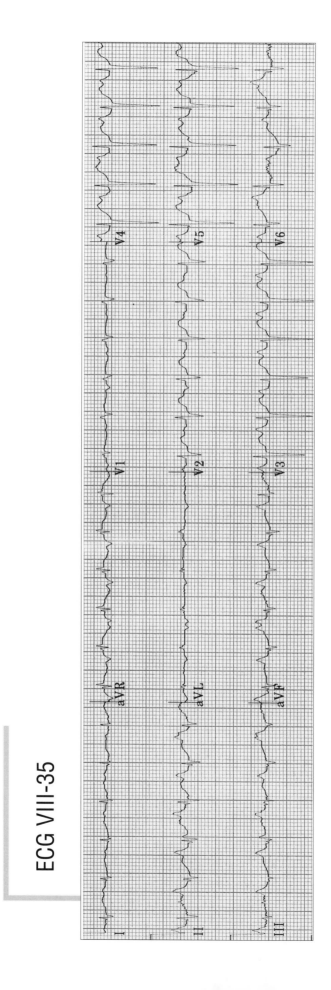

Diagnoses

ECG VIII-35

1. Sinus tachycardia (rate = 144/min)

2. Chronic cor pulmonale

Clinical Data

67-year-old woman with COPD and history of lobectomy for carcinoma of lung

Comments

Features suggesting chronic cor pulmonale include:

- Low voltage in limb leads and in V6
- P-pulmonale with P-wave axis of about $+80°$
- S waves everywhere.

ECG VIII-36

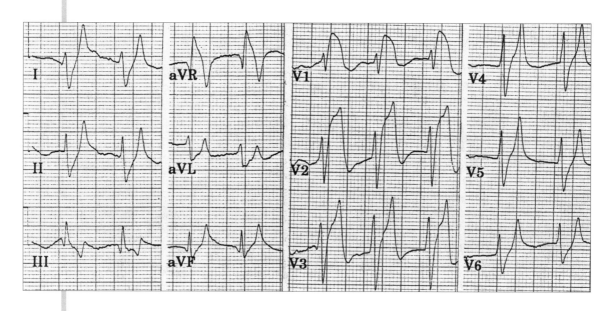

Diagnoses

ECG VIII-36

1. Rhythm uncertain, probably atrial fibrillation (rate = 95/min)

2. Hyperkalemia

Clinical Data

29-year-old diabetic man with sudden onset of vomiting; potassium 8.9 meq/L; thrombolyzed because the ECG suggested an acute anteroseptal infarct, but coronary angiography 3 days later was normal.

Comments

Marked ST elevation is a well documented, but not widely recognized, effect of potassium intoxication. The elevation may be diffuse or localized; and when it is localized—as in this case—it may create the false impression that it represents a discrete anatomical lesion rather than a metabolic disaster.

Index